Your *Clinics* subscription just got better!

You can now access the FULL TEXT of this publication online at no additional cost! Activate your online subscription today and receive...

- Full text of all issues from 2002 to the present
- Photographs, tables, illustrations, and references
- Comprehensive search capabilities
- Links to MEDLINE and Elsevier journals

Activate Your Online Access Today!

Plus, you can also sign up for E-alerts of upcoming issues or articles that interest you, and take advantage of exclusive access to bonus features!

To activate your individual online subscription:

1. Visit our website at **www.TheClinics.com**.

2. Click on "Register" at the top of the page, and follow the instructions.

3. To activate your account, you will need your subscriber account number, which you can find on your mailing label (note: the number of digits in your subscriber account number varies from six to ten digits). See the sample below where the subscriber account nu~~mber~~ ~~is circled~~.

This is your subscriber account number

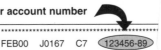

```
************************************************
FEB00   J0167   C7   (123456-89)

J.H. DOE, MD
531 MAIN ST
CENTER CITY, NY  10001-001
```

D1532361

4. That's it! Your online access to the most trusted source for clinical reviews is now available.

theclinics.com

ELSEVIER

theclinics.com

PEDIATRIC CLINICS OF NORTH AMERICA

College Health

GUEST EDITORS
Donald E. Greydanus, MD, FAAP, FSAM
Mary Ellen Rimsza, MD, FAAP
Dilip R. Patel, MD, FAAP, FACCPDM,
FACSM, FSAM

February 2005 • Volume 52 • Number 1

SAUNDERS

An Imprint of Elsevier, Inc.
PHILADELPHIA   LONDON   TORONTO   MONTREAL   SYDNEY   TOKYO

W.B. SAUNDERS COMPANY
A Division of Elsevier Inc.

The Curtis Center • Independence Square West • Philadelphia, Pennsylvania 19106

http://www.theclinics.com

THE PEDIATRIC CLINICS OF NORTH AMERICA   Volume 52, Number 1
February 2005   ISSN 0031-3955
Editor: Carin Davis   ISBN 1-4160-2748-3

The ideas and opinions expressed in *The Pediatric Clinics of North America* do not necessarily reflect those of the Publisher. The Publisher does not assume any responsibility for any injury and/or damage to persons or property arising out of or related to any use of the material contained in this periodical. The reader is advised to check the appropriate medical literature and the product information currently provided by the manufacturer of each drug to be administered to verify the dosage, the method and duration of administration, or contraindications. It is the responsibility of the treating physician or other health care professional, relying on independent experience and knowledge of the patient, to determine drug dosages and the best treatment for the patient. Mention of any product in this issue should not be construed as endorsement by the contributors, editors, or the Publisher of the product or manufacturers' claims.

The Pediatric Clinics of North America (ISSN 0031-3955) is published bi-monthly by W.B. Saunders Company, Corporate and Editorial offices: The Curtis Center, Independence Square West, Philadelphia, PA 19106-3399. Accounting and Circulation offices: 6277 Sea Harbor Drive, Orlando, FL 32887-4800. Periodicals postage paid at Orlando, FL 32862, and additional mailing offices. Subscription prices are $135.00 per year (US individuals), $246.00 per year (US institutions), $177.00 per year (Canadian individuals), $320.00 per year (Canadian institutions), $200.00 per year (international individuals), $320.00 per year (international institutions), $68.00 per year (US students), $100.00 per year (Canadian students), and $100.00 per year (foreign students). To receive student/resident rate, orders must be accompanied by name of affiliated institution, date of term, and the signature of program/residency coordinator on institution letterhead. Orders will be billed at individual rate until proof of status is received. Foreign air speed delivery is included in all Clinics subscription prices. All prices are subject to change without notice. POSTMASTER: Send address changes to *The Pediatric Clinics of North America*, W.B. Saunders Company, Periodicals Fulfillment, Orlando, FL 32887-4800. **Customer Service: 1-800-654-2452 (US). From outside of the US, call 1-407-345-4000.** E-mail: hhspcs@harcourt.com.

The Pediatric Clinics of North America is also published in Spanish by McGraw-Hill Inter-americana Editores S.A., Mexico City, Mexico; in Portuguese by Reichmann and Affonso Editores, Rua Comandante Coelho 1085, CEP 21250, Rio de Janeiro, Brazil; and in Greek by Althayia SA, Athens, Greece.

The Pediatric Clinics of North America is covered in *Index Medicus, Excerpta Medica, Current Contents, Current Contents/Clinical Medicine, Science Citation Index, ASCA, ISI/BIOMED,* and *BIOSIS.*

Printed in the United States of America.

GUEST EDITORS

DONALD E. GREYDANUS, MD, FAAP, FSAM, Professor of Pediatrics and Human Development, Michigan State University College of Human Medicine; Pediatrics Program Director, Kalamazoo Center for Medical Studies; Sindecuse Health Center, Western Michigan University, Kalamazoo, Michigan

MARY ELLEN RIMSZA, MD, FAAP, Director of Health and Research Professor, School of Health Management and Policy, W.P. Carey School of Business, Arizona State University, Tempe; and Professor of Pediatrics, Mayo Clinic College of Medicine, Scottsdale, Arizona

DILIP R. PATEL, MD, FAAP, FACCPDM, FACSM, FSAM, Professor of Pediatrics and Human Development, Michigan State University College of Human Medicine, Kalamazoo Center for Medical Studies, Kalamazoo, Michigan

CONTRIBUTORS

WILLIAM P. ADELMAN, MD, Head, Department of Adolescent Medicine, National Naval Medical Center; Assistant Professor of Pediatrics, Uniformed Services University of the Health Sciences, Bethesda, Maryland

SWATI BHAVE, MD, DCH, FCPS, Professor of Pediatrics and Consulting Pediatrician, Bombay Hospital and Medical Research Center, Mumbai (Bombay), India

HELEN R. DEITCH, MD, Centre Medical and Surgical Associates, State College, Pennsylvania

MARCIA ELLIS, PA-C, MSA, Chief of Staff, Physician Assistant, Sindecuse Health Center, Western Michigan University, Kalamazoo, Michigan

DONALD E. GREYDANUS, MD, FAAP, FSAM, Professor of Pediatrics and Human Development, Michigan State University College of Human Medicine; Pediatrics Program Director, Kalamazoo Center for Medical Studies; Sindecuse Health Center, Western Michigan University, Kalamazoo, Michigan

DANIEL H. HAVLICHEK, MD, Associate Professor, Department of Medicine, College of Human Medicine, Michigan State University, East Lansing, Michigan

PAULA J. ADAMS HILLARD, MD, Professor, Department of Obstetrics and Gynecology, Department of Pediatrics, University of Cincinnati College of Medicine, Cincinnati, Ohio

ALAIN JOFFE, MD, MPH, Director, Student Health and Wellness Center, Johns Hopkins University; Associate Professor of Pediatrics, Johns Hopkins School of Medicine, Baltimore, Maryland

MANMOHAN K. KAMBOJ, MD, Assistant Professor, Pediatrics and Human Development, Michigan State University–College of Human Medicine; Division of Pediatric Endocrinology, Michigan State University–Kalamazoo Center for Medical Studies, Kalamazoo, Michigan

GARY M. KIRK, Division Director of Immunization, Michigan Department of Community Health, Lansing, Michigan

ERICA KROL, PA-C, Clinical Staff, Physician Assistant, Sindecuse Health Center, Western Michigan University, Kalamazoo, Michigan

ASHIR KUMAR, MD, Professor, Department of Pediatrics and Human Development, College of Human Medicine, Michigan State University, East Lansing, Michigan

EUGENE F. LUCKSTEAD, Sr, MD, FACC, FAAP, Professor of Pediatrics and Cardiology, Texas Tech Medical Center, Amarillo, Texas

ASIAH MASON, PhD, Associate Professor, Department of Psychology, Gallaudet University, Washington, DC

MATTHEW MASON, PhD, Clinical Psychologist, Maryland School for the Blind, Columbia, Maryland

LYUBOV MATYTSINA, MD, PhD, Professor of the Postgraduate Chair, Obstetrics, Gynecology, and Perinatology, Donetsk Medical University; Chief, Pediatric and Adolescent Gynecology Department, Donetsk Regional Centre of Maternal and Childhood Care, Donetsk, Ukraine

ANNA-BARBARA MOSCICKI, MD, Department of Pediatrics, Division of Adolescent Medicine, University of California, San Francisco, California

KAREN S. MOSES, MS, RD, CHES, Assistant Director, Health and Wellness Center, Arizona State University, Tempe, Arizona

DENNIS L. MURRAY, MD, Professor, Department of Pediatrics, Medical College of Georgia, Augusta, Georgia

JITENDRA NAGPAL, MD, DNB, Consultant Psychiatrist and Coordinator, Child Development & Adolescent Health Centre, Vidyasagar Institute of Mental Health and Neurosciences, Nehru Nagar, New Delhi, India

DILIP R. PATEL, MD, FAAP, FACCPDM, FACSM, FSAM, Professor of Pediatrics and Human Development, Michigan State University College of Human Medicine, Kalamazoo Center for Medical Studies, Kalamazoo, Michigan

ELAINE L. PHILLIPS, PhD, Professor and Psychologist, University Counseling and Testing Center, Western Michigan University, Kalamazoo, Michigan

HELEN D. PRATT, PhD, Professor, Pediatrics and Human Development, Michigan State University, Kalamazoo Campus, East Lansing, Michigan

MARY ELLEN RIMSZA, MD, FAAP, Director of Health and Research Professor, School of Health Management and Policy, W.P. Carey School of Business, Arizona State University, Tempe; and Professor of Pediatrics, Mayo Clinic College of Medicine, Scottsdale, Arizona

W. BRYAN STAUFER, MD, Sindecuse Health Center, Western Michigan University, Kalamazoo, Michigan

CONTENTS

of student medical care is the campus student health center. The health care providers at student health centers attend to many of the sports-related concerns of student athletes. Preparticipation evaluation provides an opportunity to assess the general health of the student athlete and to identify conditions that might increase the risk of further injury. Sudden cardiac death and sports-associated concussions have generated much interest and are reviewed in this article. Other areas reviewed here include use of drugs and supplements, ankle sprains, acute knee ligament injuries, back pain, and shoulder impingement syndrome.

These problems deserve careful evaluation; they may reflect normal ovulatory menstrual symptoms or be suggestive of significant pathology that can have a major impact on future reproductive and general health. The menstrual cycle is a vital sign whose normalcy suggests overall good health and whose abnormality requires evaluation. Eating disorders and the female athlete triad increase the risk of osteoporosis; polycystic ovary syndrome is associated with future cardiovascular risks. Diagnosis and management of these problems will not only improve a young woman's current health, sense of well-being, and overall quality of life but may also lower her risks for future disease and ill-health. This article addresses normal menstrual function, excessive bleeding, infrequent or absent menses, pain with menses, menstrual-related mood disorders, and recommendations about routine gynecologic examinations and evaluation.

Five percent of all ambulatory visits by men 18 years of age or older include genitourinary symptoms as a reason for the visit. In this article, using typical, unusual, or otherwise instructive cases, the authors review a select group of genitourinary issues in the college-age male. Warts (human papilloma virus), is the most common sexually transmitted infection, and it may mimic other disease. Testicular cancer is one of the most serious diseases to confront health care providers. Varicoceles are the most common scrotal mass. Urethritis is a common presentation of sexually transmitted infection in the young adult male. Acute prostatitis is an unusual condition in the young adult, but it is easily treatable. Sexual dysfunction causes great distress in the young adult, but a systematic approach usually leads to a treatable psychological or environmental cause. With understanding of these medical conditions, the practitioner should feel comfortable addressing the most challenging genitourinary health needs of this population.

Approximately 80% of college-age adolescents are sexually active and at risk for sexually transmitted infections (STIs). Over 4 million STIs occur in teenagers annually and young adults between the ages of 18 and 24, while adolescents 15 to 17 years of age have higher rates of STIs than any other age group in the United States. Thus, the prevention, diagnosis, and treatment of STIs are a critical part of college health care. This article will discuss the epidemiology, diagnosis, and management of some of the most common STIs encountered in the college-age group, with an emphasis on new guidelines for treatment.

FORTHCOMING ISSUES

RECENT ISSUES

PEDIATRIC CLINICS OF NORTH AMERICA FEBRUARY 2005

GOAL STATEMENT

The goal of *Pediatric Clinics of North America* is to keep practicing physicians and residents up to date with current clinical practice in pediatrics by providing timely articles reviewing the state-of-the-art in patient care.

ACCREDITATION

The *Pediatric Clinics of North America* is planned and implemented in accordance with the Essential Areas and Policies of the Accreditation Council for Continuing Medical Education (ACCME) through the joint sponsorship of the University of Virginia School of Medicine and Elsevier Inc. The University of Virginia School of Medicine is accredited by the ACCME to provide continuing medical education for physicians.

The University of Virginia School of Medicine designates this educational activity for a maximum of 90 category 1 credits per year, 15 credits per issue, toward the AMA Physician's Recognition Award. Each physician should claim only those credits that he/she actually spent in the activity.

The American Medical Association has determined that physicians not licensed in the US who participate in this CME activity are eligible for AMA PRA category 1 credit.

Category 1 credit can be earned by reading the text material, taking the CME examination online at http://www.theclinics.com/home/cme, and completing the evaluation. After taking the test, you will be required to review any and all incorrect answers. Following completion of the test and evaluation, your credit will be awarded and you may print your certificate.

FACULTY DISCLOSURE

Disclosure of faculty financial affiliations: As a provider accredited by the Accreditation Council for Continuing Medical Education (ACCME), the Office of Continuing Medical Education of the University of Virginia School of Medicine must ensure balance, independence, objectivity, and scientific rigor in all its individually sponsored or jointly sponsored educational activities. All authors/editors participating in a sponsored activity are expected to disclose to the readers any significant financial interest or other relationship (1) with the manufacturer(s) of any commercial product(s) and/or provider(s) of commercial services discussed in an educational presentation and (2) with any commercial supporters of the activity (significant financial interest or other relationship can include such things as grants or research support, employee, consultant, stock holder, member of speakers bureau, etc.). The intent of this disclosure is not to prevent authors/editors with a significant financial or other relationship from writing an article, but rather to provide readers with information on which they can make their own judgments. It remains for the readers to determine whether the author's/editor's interest or relationships may influence the article with regard to exposition or conclusion.

The authors/editors listed below have identified no professional or financial affiliations related to their presentation: William P. Adelman, MD; Swati Bhave, MD, DCH, FCPS; Carin Davis, Acquisitions Editor; Helen R. Deitch, MD; Marcia Ellis, PA-C, MSA; Donald E. Greydanus, MD; Daniel H. Havlichek, Jr., MD; Alain Joffe, MD, MPH; Manmohan K. Kamboj, MD; Gary M. Kirk, MD.MPH; Erica Krol, PA-C; Ashir Kumar, MB, BS, MD, FAAP; Eugene F. Luckstead, Jr., MD; Asiah Mason, PhD; Matthew Mason, PhD; Lyubov Matytsina, MD, PhD; Anna-Barbara Moscicki, MD; Karen S. Moses, MS, RD, CHES; Jitendra Nagpal, MD, DNB; Dilip R. Patel, MD; Elaine L. Phillips, PhD; Helen D. Pratt, PhD; Mary Ellen Rimsza, MD; and, W. Bryan Staufer, MD.

The authors listed below have identified the following professional or financial affiliation related to their presentations:
Paula Janine Adams Hillard, MD is a consultant & is on the Scientific Advisory Board for Procter & Gamble, Wyeth-Ayerst; has received Post-Grant/Research Support from Berlex, Wyeth-Ayerst; and, is on the speaker's bureau for Wyeth-Ayerst, Berlex, Pharmacia-Upjohn, 3-M Pharmaceuticals, Pfizer, Organon, Ortho-McNeill, Barr Labs, and Tap Pharmaceuticals.
Dennis L. Murray, MD, FAAP will be discussing vaccines and is on the speakers' bureau for Aventis Vaccines; and, is on the Adolescent Vaccine Advisory Board.

Disclosure of Discussion of non-FDA approved uses for pharmaceutical products and/or medical devices: The University of Virginia School of Medicine, as an ACCME provider, requires that all authors identify and disclose any "off label" uses for pharmaceutical and medical device products. The University of Virginia School of Medicine recommends that each physician fully review all the available data on new products or procedures prior to instituting them with patients.

All authors who provided disclosures have indicated that they will not be discussing off-label uses except the following:
Helen R. Deitch, MD will discuss the use of oral contraceptives for treatment of polycystic ovary syndrome.
Donald E. Greydanus, MD will discuss oral contraceptives, ortho evra patch, emergency contraceptives, nuva ring(TM)vaginal ring, vaginal barrier contraceptives, Depo-Provera, Lunelle, Mesigyna, and, Intrauterine devices.
Daniel H. Havlichek, Jr, MD will discuss the use of ciprofloxacin as chemoprophylaxis against Neisseria Meningitis.
Paula Janine Adams Hillard, MD will discuss the use of oral contraceptives and hormonal contraception for medical indications.
W. Bryan Staufer, MD will discuss the use of dextroamphetamine, mixed amphetamine salts, methylphidate, bupropion drugs all commonly used to manage ADHD symptom in adults, drugs 1-3 are approved to manage ADHD in children 6 years and older.

TO ENROLL

To enroll in the *Pediatric Clinics of North America* Continuing Medical Education program, call customer service at **1-800-654-2452** or visit us online at www.theclinics.com/home/cme. The CME program is available to subscribers for an additional fee of $195.00.

PEDIATRIC CLINICS

OF NORTH AMERICA

Pediatr Clin N Am 52 (2005) xv

Dedication

This issue of the *Pediatric Clinics of North America* is dedicated to the clinicians and staff at Sindecuse Health Center of Western Michigan University, Kalamazoo, Michigan. You have taught me the principles of health care for the college student over the past 10 years. I am grateful that you have added the title of college health physician to my other titles of pediatrician and adolescent medicine specialist. I also thank you for allowing me to bring my residents to work with me at Sindecuse to learn about the importance of college health for their future work in medicine. Finally, this issue is specifically dedicated to a wonderful and dedicated college health physician, Dr. Jack Scobey, psychiatrist *par excellence*. You are a beloved member of the Sindecuse family whose time with us was tragically too short—*Requiescat in Pace Cum Deo*.

Donald E. Greydanus, MD, FAAP, FSAM

This issue is also dedicated to the staff of the Arizona State University Student Health and Wellness Center in Tempe, Arizona. It was a great privilege for me to serve as your director for the past 5 years. You have provided the ASU students with excellent health care that is a model for others to follow. I admire your dedication to the students who come to you for care and hope you will continue to do so in the years to come.

Mary Ellen Rimsza, MD, FAAP

doi:10.1016/j.pcl.2004.11.007   *pediatric.theclinics.com*

PEDIATRIC CLINICS

OF NORTH AMERICA

ELSEVIER
SAUNDERS

Pediatr Clin N Am 52 (2005) xvii–xxi

Preface

College Health

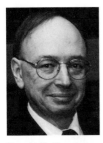
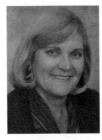
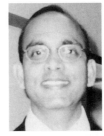

Donald E. Greydanus,
MD, FAAP, FSAM

Mary Ellen Rimsza,
MD, FAAP
Guest Editors

Dilip R. Patel, MD, FAAP,
FACCPDM, FACSM, FSAM

I would there were no age between ten and three and twenty, or that youth would simply sleep out the rest; for there is nothing in between but getting wenches with child, wronging the ancestry, stealing and fighting.

—William Shakespeare (from *A Winter's Tale*)

For millions of individuals and their parents, the transition from childhood to adulthood ends in college. The journey that began for parents with the ecstasy of birth, the delights of childhood, and the oxymoron (a la Shakespeare) of a peacefully troubled adolescence, now enters the final phase of pre-adulthood— the college or university phase of life. The twentieth century added more technology to everyday life in western culture and emphasized the need for a prolonged and more technical education to increase the chances for a successful journey as an adult. Not only is a high school education necessary to make a successful transition to adulthood, but a college and—for many—graduate school education has become necessary to achieve independence and success as an adult. Parents may breathe a sigh of relief as they send their child off to college, but the health care profession must continue its mission to provide optimal health care for these important individuals.

The same problems that this developing person confronted as a child or teen now continue in the college or university life. For example, most children who have a chronic illness now live into adulthood [1]; thus, college students bring with them their asthma, diabetes mellitus, migraine headaches, cardiac disorders, eating disorders, and other medical problems. Various medical problems that have not been identified during a student's childhood or adolescence may become evident during the college years. Roadblocks to efficient learning, such as learning disorders or the controversial condition of attention-deficit/hyperactivity disorder, may be brought to college life, whether or not they have been diagnosed previously. The stress of college life may bring out mental health enigmas such as depression or anxiety disorders; the tragedy of suicide that increased in high school may continue to grow in incidence during the college years—especially in the first year, often the first time away from home. If infectious agents such as the Epstein-Barr virus have not infected an individual as a child or teen, they may invade that individual as a college student, often at a most inopportune time. If the student is not fully immunized, college life provides a new opportunity to get caught up and even make decisions about protection from other microbes (eg, *Neisseria meningitidis*).

The child and adolescent in America lives in an environment that is saturated with media messages that advertise high-risk behavior without consequences. The relentless teaching is to freely enjoy drugs and sex while not worrying about any problems that might result from such potentially precarious behavior. Many high school students succumb to this message because it resonates with their innate biopsychosocial development—and this tendency for high-risk behavior continues into the college years. If they have avoided sex and drugs earlier, in college they may find themselves among peers who accept this behavior, feeling that they are now adults and therefore entitled to the pleasures of sex, drugs, and other conundrums of adult life. Unfortunately, they enter a world with increased risks for unwanted pregnancy, sexually transmitted diseases, sexual assault resulting from the use of date rape drugs, and other hazards. The following lament can be applied to both the teenager and the college student:

> The Youth of today [300 BC] are in character prone to desire and ready to carry any desire they may have into action. Of body desires, it is the sexual to which they are most disposed to give way, and in regard to sexual desire, they exercise no restraint.
>
> —Aristotle [2]

How does the health care profession help our youth as they transit to adulthood while in college? The answer to this important question has been addressed over the course of the twentieth century with the growth of health services for the college student. The first recognized college health physician in the United States was Edward Hitchcock, MD, who was appointed as Professor of Hygiene at Amherst College in Massachusetts in 1860 and ultimately became known as the father of American college health [3–5]. The first comprehensive college health service was developed at the University of California–Berkeley in 1901. The leader in providing guidance to college health programs in the twentieth and now the twenty-first century has been the American College Health Association (ACHA), which was first established in 1920 and acquired its current name in 1948.

By the mid-1950s, many major American campuses had established health centers to care for their students, as reviewed in a landmark article on college health services by Moore and Summerskill [6]. In 1988, Patrick [7] published an important article detailing an overview of university health services that were provided by over 3000 physicians who were part of 27,000 individuals working in college health centers seeking to serve 10 to 12.5 million college students in the United States. In 1990, the Centers for Disease Control and Prevention (US Public Health Service, Division of Adolescent and School Health) identified college health as one of three concepts for study, oversight, and public health intervention [7]. An important treatice on college health was edited by Wallace and colleagues in 1992 outlining concepts of care for the college student [8]. A recent publication edited by Turner and Hurley continued this tradition of providing an *au courant* summary on college health practice [9]. The ACHA has published valuable documents with advice on how to implement the Centers for Disease Control and Prevention's Healthy People 2010 for the college student [10] and health standards for college health services [11].

In 1885, Dr. J.W. Seaver became the Medical Director at the Yale "gymnasium" and provided a careful examination on each college student on an annual basis [9]. Preventive evaluations of young adults, including college students, are still recommended 125 years later, though they are not always accomplished [12–14]. The growth of interest in college health in the twentieth century has also occurred along with an interest in adolescent health in the twentieth century [15]. Today, there are approximately 15 million college students, 58% of whom are between 18 and 24 years of age; nearly half have prolonged times without any health insurance coverage, and about 25% are simply without any type of health insurance throughout their college years. How do we care for them with all their needs and with such limited insurance support?

It is vital that all clinicians in the vicinity of the university contribute to the health care of these important students—the future leaders of America. It is in this spirit that this issue of the *Pediatric Clinics of North America* is written. Important issues in health care of the college student are presented by a variety of experts. Pediatricians who care for their patients before college can prepare them for college life and continue to work with the college health center clinicians in optimizing their health. Other specialists in the college vicinity can also give needed support to these students, providing consultation to their college health clinicians.

I thank the contributors of this issue for their time and expertise. My thanks also to my fellow editors, Mary Ellen Rimsza, MD, and Dilip R. Patel, MD.

Finally, I thank Carin Davis for her encouragement and patience in the development of this inaugural issue on college health for the *Pediatric Clinics of North America*. The flower of youth fades quickly, but if we can help our college students when they need it, the contribution to our society will be priceless and pervasive. Indeed, it is a way of touching immortality.

O youth with song and laughter,

Go not so lightly by.

Have pity and remember,

How soon thy roses die.

—A.W. Peach ("O Youth with Blossoms Laden")

Donald E. Greydanus, MD, FAAP, FSAM
Sindecuse Health Center
Western Michigan University
Michigan State University/Kalamazoo Center for Medical Studies
1000 Oakland Drive
Kalamazoo, MI 49008-1284, USA
E-mail address: greydanus@kcms.msu.edu

Mary Ellen Rimsza, MD, FAAP
Student Health and Wellness Center
Arizona State University
Main Campus, P.O. Box 874506
Tempe, AZ 85287-4506, USA
E-mail address: mrimsza@asu.edu

Dilip R. Patel, MD, FAAP, FACCPDM, FACSM, FSAM
Western Michigan University
Michigan State University/Kalamazoo Center for Medical Studies
1000 Oakland Drive
Kalamazoo, MI 49008-1284, USA
E-mail address: patel@kcms.msu.edu

References

[1] White P. Transition to adulthood: adolescents with disabilities. In: Greydanus DE, Patel DR, Pratt HD, editors. Essentials of adolescent medicine. New York: McGraw-Hill Medical Publishers; 2005, in press.
[2] Welldon JEC. The rhetoric of Aristotle. London: Macmillan Publishing Co.; 1886. p. 1.

[3] Baxter TL. College health. In: Hofmann AD, Greydanus DE, editors. Adolescent medicine. 3rd edition. Stamford (CT): Appleton & Lange; 1997. p. 755–9.

[4] Patrick K. The history and current status of college health. In: Wallace HM, Patrick K, Parcel GS, et al, editors. Principles and practices of student health, Volume 3. Oakland (CA): Third Party Publishing Company; 1992. p. 501–14.

[5] Turner HS, Hurley JL. The history and development of college health. In: Turner HS, Hurley JL, editors. The history and practice of college health. Lexington (KY): University Press of Kentucky; 2002. p. 1–21.

[6] Moore NS, Summerskill J. Health services in American colleges and universities 1953: findings of the American College Health Association Survey. Ithaca (NY): Cornell University Press; 1954.

[7] Patrick K. Student health: medical care within institutions of higher education. JAMA 1988; 260:3301–5.

[8] Wallace HM, Patrick K, Parcel GS, et al, editors. Principles and practice of student health, Volume 3. Oakland (CA): Third Party Publishing Company; 1992. p. 501–851.

[9] Turner HS, Hurley JL, editors. The history and practice of college health. Lexington (KY): University Press of Kentucky; 2002.

[10] American College Health Association. Healthy campus 2010: making it happen. Baltimore (MD): American College Health Association; 2002.

[11] American College Health Association. Standards of practice for health promotion in higher education. Baltimore (MD): American College Health Association; in press.

[12] Erten J, Zaman I. Importance of routine health checkups in young adults. J Adolesc Health 2004;34:2.

[13] Kemper HC, Koppes LL, de Vente W, et al. Effects of health information in youth and young adulthood on risk factors for chronic diseases—20-year study results from the Amsterdam growth and health longitudinal study. Prev Med 2002;35:533–9.

[14] Vinner R, Macfarlane A. Provision of age appropriate health services for young people has been ignored. BMJ 2000;321:1022.

[15] Prescott HM. History of adolescent medicine in the 20th century: from Hall to Elkind. Adolesc Med 2000;11:1–11.

ELSEVIER
SAUNDERS

PEDIATRIC CLINICS
OF NORTH AMERICA

Pediatr Clin N Am 52 (2005) 1–8

A Case Study on the Use of Physician Assistants in College Health

Marcia Ellis, PA-C, MSA*, Erica Krol, PA-C

Sindecuse Health Center, Western Michigan University, 1903 West Michigan Avenue, Kalamazoo, MI 49008-5445, USA

The physician assistant (PA) profession has grown by leaps and bounds since its inception in 1965, when Dr. Eugene Stead formed the very first class at Duke University Medical Center. The American Academy of Physician Assistants (AAPA) estimates there were 50,121 people in clinical practice as PAs at the beginning of 2004 [1]. PAs in general are well accepted and can be found in almost every aspect of medicine. College health is a perfect fit for PAs. They provide high-quality, cost-effective primary care medicine. This article describes the use of PAs at Western Michigan University's Sindecuse Health Center, where the authors have practiced for 21 and 15 years, respectively.

Western Michigan University (WMU) opened its first health center doors in 1927. By 1974, the health center was a 24-hour, full-service facility with food service and an all-male staff of physicians. In 1975, the overnight stays were eliminated and clinic hours reduced to 8 AM to 10 PM. After 10 PM, nurses staffed the clinic for walk-in visits, and clinicians (physicians and PAs) were on-call for emergencies. In 1980, hours were further reduced to 8 AM to 5 PM because of financial constraints and liability concerns. After 5 PM, patients were directed to the local emergency rooms.

During the 1980s, college health across the country was changing. Many clinics were moving away from 24-hour operations, focusing more on health education programs and looking at providing cost-effective, high-quality medicine. HIV was entering the national scene, affecting college health. Other forces behind this change included: "(1) a changing student body with an increasing

---

* Corresponding author.
  E-mail address: ellism@wmich.edu (M. Ellis).

number of older students, particularly women and part-time students; (2) concern about changes in fiscal support for higher education; (3) environmental health and safety requirements from multiple regulatory agencies; and (4) health insurance issues" [2]. These influences made college health a perfect fit for using mid-level practitioners (PAs and nurse practitioners).

Sindecuse Health Center (SHC) has often been at the forefront of national trends. For example, use of PAs began at SHC with the graduation of the first PA class at WMU in 1974 when two male PAs were hired. In 1975, SHC hired its first female provider—a PA.

The presence of PAs at SHC continues today. SHC, accredited by the Accreditation Association for Ambulatory Health Care (AAAHC), is located in the center of the campus of WMU in Kalamazoo, Michigan.

As noted by Dorman and Christmas in *The History and Practice of College Health*:

To respond to student needs and, indeed, to expectations of parents and the college/university administration, 'a well organized and adequately funded college health center should strive to meet the following goals through its medical services activities: 1) accessible medical services; 2) reasonable cost to the student for these services; 3) emphasis on preventive and health education services; 4) integration with (other) student affairs departments (i.e., residential life, counseling center, and international educational services); and 5) confidentiality of medical information preserved.'[3]

These goals are the focus of college health centers, and they help to differentiate the delivery of health services to a campus family from other medical practices in the greater community. PAs and nurse practitioners (mid-level

---

Box 1. Core values of the PA profession*

- PAs promote the public's interests and the patient's needs before any other considerations.
- PAs are ethical health care professionals.
- PAs serve as advocates for patient needs.
- PAs provide patient education and preventative health care services.
- PAs are committed to lifelong learning.
- PAs work with other health care professionals in providing coordinated health care.
- PAs are committed to assuring that health care services are accessible and compassionate.

* From American Academy of Physician Assistants 2003-2004 Membership Information and Resource Handbook, p. 6.

practitioners) are well suited to contribute to these goals (Box 1). The trend in college health is to move toward a managed care practice with a team focus. As dependent practitioners, PAs are exceptionally well suited to function as a member of the team. Because of the cost savings realized when some of the team members are mid-level practitioners, the number of staff members can be increased. Mid-level practitioners are often referred to as "physician extenders" because they help to extend the access to care for the patient.

Box 2. Quotes from SHC medical staff members when asked why they like practicing medicine in college health

"The kids have a ton of potential, and I enjoy helping them maximize that." C. Voytas, MD, Family Practice

"This is an amazing age group. They are young, educated, enthusiastic, goal-oriented, hard-to-please clientele." P. N. Bhatt, MD, Family Practice

"I can see students in addition to employees with on-the-job injuries." S. Cowles, MD, Occupational Medicine

"I love this age group and the opportunity to effect change in their health habits." L. Wiser, PA-C

"I like the collegial atmosphere among providers, the international students, the pure form of medicine, and fewer administrative hassles of regular practice." D. Peirce, MD, Internal Medicine

"They are an educated, motivated population with more insight than patients in my other practice." C. Vyas, MD, Psychiatry

"College students struggle with psychosocial issues, as well as physical illnesses, as they progress through a dramatic maturing process over four years. I enjoy the challenge to help them obtain the confidence they need to grow through this time of their lives." A. Soukup, PA-C

"1. The mutually supportive, non-competitive collegiality among college health clinicians and college health in general.

2. The feeling of being part of the educational mission of the university.

3. The stimulation and anticipation of learning something new/ of having a new experience every day.

4. The tremendous gratification of working with college students and being part of the maturation process during their years of matriculation." B. Staufer, MD, Pediatrics

The majority of mid-level practitioners working in college health has been nurses and nurse practitioners. Over the last 15 years, the number of PAs in college health has been increasing. In the AAPA 2003 census report, there were 111 PAs working in a college health facility. This was 0.6% of the total (18,155) respondents to the survey [4]. A government study looked at the role of PAs and nurse practitioners in hospital outpatient departments and concluded that "Beyond the care they provide in physicians' offices and other non-hospital settings, PAs and NPs make an important contribution to ambulatory health care delivery in hospital outpatient departments" [5].

College students make challenging, but enjoyable patients (Box 2). They are the "cream of the crop," the future leaders and contributing citizens of our country. They are intelligent and inquisitive but often naïve and demanding about their health care. Young adults by nature are risk-takers and tend to believe themselves to be immortal. Their health care providers must provide open, honest communication in a non-judgmental manner while educating them to make healthier lifestyle choices. One of the goals is to help them become discriminating health care consumers.

Clinicians drawn to the college health setting are attracted by interesting and rewarding patient care, reasonable hours, and attractive benefit packages despite notoriously low compensation. It is clearly a lifestyle choice.

Table 1
Clinic visits to the Sindecuse Health Center (SHC)

SHC Activity Profile

		1998–1999	1999–2000	2000–2001	2001–2002	2002–2003
Clinician visits	Appointments	17,095	18,842	20,431	20,651	18,822
	Same-day care	7,903	9,619	10,888	11,108	11,115
	Derm/Psych	1,451	1,360	1,023	1,362	1,288
Nursing visits		7,114	8,869	8,622	8,612	8,612
Health promotion and education contacts	Dietitian appointments	183	264	343	402	*
	Total individual contacts	20,432	20,076	28,929	*	*
	Total program contacts	21,413	21,595	34,413	50,475	*
Sports medicine clinic	Clinician visits	1,221	1,390	1,621	1,735	1,523
	Physical therapy visits	8,228	9,397	10,929	11,642	10,300
Laboratory and radiology	Laboratory procedures	18,387	20,178	20,750	20,312	*
	X-ray procedures	1,994	2,079	2,190	2,117	*
Pharmacy	Total prescriptions	69,783	77,246	84,129	90,784	*

* Data not available.

PAs have been used successfully at SHC to meet the delivery of care demands of the college-aged student. Training in the medical model with focus on primary care gives PAs a strong medical base. This allows them to operate collaboratively with physicians. They have the ability to evaluate and treat patients comprehensively.

From July 2003 through June 2004, the clinicians at SHC saw 31,319 patient visits in appointments and Same Day Care clinic. See Table 1 for a breakdown of clinic visits. The clinicians see a variety of medical complaints, similar to most family practices (Box 1 and 3). They also see the faculty and staff for urgent and preventive needs, along with providing care for all occupational injuries and illness.

The regular staff at the main clinic at SHC includes seven physicians (six Full-Time Equivalents) and four PAs (3.8 FTEs). The physicians are board-certified as follows: one pediatrician, two family practice physicians, two internists, an occupational medicine physician, and a psychiatrist. All the PAs are board-certified in family practice. See Table 2 for information about PA practice. A dermatologist comes one half day every week during the fall and spring semesters and every other week in the summer. The pediatric residency program director

---

Box 3. List of complaints during patient visits

- Preventive care, including periodic examinations, annual gynecologic visits, immunization updates
- Upper and lower respiratory complaints, including asthma, allergy, and ophthalmology problems
- Dermatology, including viral warts, acne, fungal infections, rashes with various causes, including systemic illnesses
- Abdominal pain and complaints with gastrointestinal, urinary, and gynecologic origins
- Musculoskeletal problems, such as back or hip pain, ankle or shoulder injuries, overuse syndromes, problems related to long hours at a computer or studying
- Cardiovascular and endocrine diseases such as hypertension, thyroid disorders, diabetes, and polycystic ovary disease
- Gynecologic issues such as emergency contraception, sexually transmitted infections, and pregnancy testing
- Various constitutional complaints, such as headaches, fatigue, dizziness, etc.
- Mental health and emotional concerns, such as depression, anxiety disorders, obsessive-compulsive disorders, eating disorders, acute stress reactions, post traumatic stress disorders
- Substance abuse, including tobacco and alcohol

Table 2
Physician assistant (PA) practice information

Accredited PA Programs	134 programs are accredited by the Accreditation Review Commission on Education for the Physician Assistant.
Prescribing	Forty-eight states, the District of Columbia, and Guam have enacted laws that authorize PA prescribing. (Indiana, Louisiana, and Ohio do not yet authorize prescribing by PAs.)
State laws	All states plus the District of Columbia and Guam have laws or regulations authorizing PA practice.
Certification and CME	PAs receive their national certification from the National Commission on Certification of Physician Assistants (NCCPA). Only graduates of an accredited PA program are eligible to take the Physician Assistant National Certifying Examination (PANCE). Once a PA is certified, he/she must complete a continuous 6-year cycle to keep her/his certificate current. Every 2 years, a PA must earn and log 100 CME hours and reregister her/his certificate with the NCCPA (second and fourth years), and by the end of the sixth year, recertify by successfully completing either the Physician Assistant National Recertifying Examination (PANRE) or Pathway II. All states require passage of the PANCE for state licensure. Forty-six states have provisions for new graduates to practice prior to passage of PANCE.

From the American Academy of Physician Assistants website. Available at www.aapa.org.

from the Kalamazoo Center for Medical Studies works in the clinic two half days a week during the fall and spring semesters. The Sports Medicine clinic, located on the lower level of the SHC building, is staffed with three physical therapists and an athletic trainer. Two orthopedic surgeons, a podiatrist, and two sports medicine physicians are regular consultants.

The chief of staff (department head of the medical staff) at SHC is a PA with an advanced degree in health care administration. The administrative duties include scheduling clinicians for appointments and Same Day Care, new program or service development, coordinating patient care with other departments (pharmacy, diagnostic services, nursing, health promotion, business office, and sports medicine clinic), educational brochure development, maintaining a policy and procedure manual, conducting staff meetings, and so forth. She spends 20 hours per week in direct patient care.

Providers of health care at SHC (physicians and PAs) refer to themselves as clinicians. With a strong collegial environment, consultations are freely sought among all clinicians. There is no differentiation made in scheduling between providers; PAs and physicians are scheduled in the same manner. The clinicians feel this strengthens their ability to provide quality care and adds to a healthy, supportive work environment. All appointments are 15 or 30 minutes (including physicals, emotional concerns, and minor surgical procedures). The clinicians provide primary care for students in addition to acute and preventive care for faculty, staff, and their dependents over age 11. All clinicians rotate through the Same Day Care clinic in two or three half-day shifts a week and have appointment schedules the remainder of the week. The Health Center is open from 8 AM to 5 PM Monday through Friday, and Saturday mornings during the fall and spring semesters.

At SHC, the PAs precept PA interns and mentor first-year PA students. Most clinicians lecture at the WMU PA program when requested. Interns from the pediatric residency program at Kalamazoo Center for Medical Studies also rotate through SHC.

All of the clinicians meet monthly for a journal club. Discussions center on current topics in college health and adolescent medicine, trends seen in the clinic are discussed and cases presented. Several clinicians have developed special areas of interest. For example, one PA sees patients with eating disorders. Another PA teaches first aid to departments on campus who request this service. A PA and two physicians serve on disaster planning committees at the University and county levels. One physician's focus is on travel medicine, and he serves as a resource to the nursing appointments for travel. Another physician cares for a growing number of students with attention deficit disorders and learning disabilities.

Every clinician is a contributing member of a quality improvement subcommittee, where processes are evaluated for effectiveness and goals are monitored. All clinicians serve on a Medical Executive Committee where peers review medical records for completeness of documentation and aberrant practices. Feedback is given to each clinician monthly. Clinicians develop brochures and other educational materials on health issues for use with patients in the clinic. They have BCLS and code blue refresher training annually to review skills for medical emergencies. All clinicians are certified in cardiopulmonary resuscitation and some clinicians are certified in Advanced Cardiac Life Support. Several "code blue" drills are held throughout the year to practice emergency response skills.

In 1995 S.C. Crane, in his article titled "PAs/NPs: Forging Effective Partnerships in Managed Care Systems," examined three dominant issues in national health policy discussions—how to control health expenditures, how to improve access to care, and how to ensure delivery of high-quality health services [6]. In college health, PAs and nurse practitioners are a credible solution to these issues. In college health, PAs can practice with all of the core values of the PA profession (Box 1).

Many articles have commented on the cost-effectiveness of physician extenders. Physician extenders offer the "advantages of reduced cost and a strong primary care orientation" [7]. The annual budget for SHC is $12,500,000. Of this amount, the medical staff budget is $2,250,000. The average PA salary at SHC is approximately 58% of the average physician salary. Other areas of savings include reduced costs for association memberships, licensing, and recertification fees. The cost of hospital privileges is 50% of physician fees for mid-level practitioners, and malpractice insurance for the PAs is 17% of the cost for physicians. Other benefits such as vacation time, continuing education funds, retirement benefits, and sick leave are equivalent.

Summary

This article describes how SHC uses PAs to maximize high-quality, cost-effective patient care. In addition to serving as staff members of the health care team and in administrative capacities, PAs can serve in a number of functions in college health. Some serve as health educators, consultants, or researchers on their campuses. In some instances, they may be the sole provider for health care to students. For complex cases they maintain referral sources outside their immediate clinic.

Acknowledgments

We would like to thank our colleagues and friends in college health for their contributions to this article.

References

[1] American Academy of Physician Assistants website. Available at: www.aapa.org/glance/html. Accessed May 24, 2004.
[2] Turner HS, Hurley JL. History and development of college health. In: Turner HS, Hurley JL, editors. The history and practice of college health. 1st edition. Lexington, KY: The University Press of Kentucky; 2002. p. 1–21.
[3] Dorman JM, Christmas WA. Primary care issues in college health. In: Turner HS, Hurley JL, editors. The history and practice of college health. 1st edition. Lexington, KY: The University Press of Kentucky; 2002. p. 105.
[4] American Academy of Physician Assistants website. Available at: www.aapa.org/research/03census-content.html#tab17. Accessed May 24, 2004.
[5] McCaig LF, Hooker RS, Sekscenski ES, Woodwell DA. Physician assistants and nurse practitioners in hospital outpatient departments, 1993–1994. Public Health Rep 1998;113(1):75–82.
[6] Crane SC. Forging effective partnerships in managed care systems. Physician Exec 1995;21(10):23–7.
[7] Earle-Richardson GB. Commentary from the front lines; improving the National Health Service Corps' use of nonphysician medical providers. J Rural Health 1998;14(2):91–7.

ELSEVIER
SAUNDERS

PEDIATRIC CLINICS
OF NORTH AMERICA

Pediatr Clin N Am 52 (2005) 9–24

Common Medical Problems of the College Student

Mary Ellen Rimsza, MD, FAAP[a,b,*], Gary M. Kirk, MD, MHPE, MPH[c]

[a]School of Health Services Administration and Policy, Student Health and Wellness Center,
W.P. Carey School of Business, Arizona State University Main Campus, PO Box 872104,
Tempe, AZ 85287-2104, USA
[b]Department of Pediatrics, Mayo Clinic College of Medicine, Scottsdale, AZ, USA
[c]Michigan Department of Community Health, 3423 North Martin Luther King Boulevard,
PO Box 30195, Lansing, MI 48909, USA

The college health physician cares for college students who present with a wide variety of medical disorders. College students can become ill, and it is important that they have health care services designed to deal with their health care issues. This article reviews the management of four common medical problems: *infectious mononucleosis (IM), asthma, migraine headaches,* and *urinary tract infections (UTIs).*

Infectious mononucleosis

IM is one of the most common serious infectious illnesses in the college-age population. IM is caused by Epstein-Barr virus (EBV); however, similar mono-like illnesses can be caused by other infectious agents, including cytomegalovirus, adenovirus, and *Toxoplasma gondii.* The observed rate of heterophil-positive IM has been reported to be 12 per 1000 university students per

* Corresponding author. School of Health Management and Policy, W.P. Carey School of Business, Arizona State University, PO Box 874506, Tempe, AZ 85287-4506.
E-mail address: mrimsza@asu.edu (M.E. Rimsza).

academic year [1]. In a prospective study of entering freshmen at the Chinese University of Hong Kong, 25% of EBV-seronegative students converted to seropositivity during their first academic year [2].

Most adults have acquired EBV infection by age 40. In developing countries, the infection usually is acquired in the first 3 years of life; when the infection is acquired in early childhood, there are usually no symptoms. In more affluent populations, however, approximately one third of EBV infections are first acquired during adolescence and young adulthood, and more than 50% of infected adolescents and young adults are symptomatic. Typical symptoms and signs include fever, sore throat, fatigue, generalized lymphadenopathy, and pharyngitis. The classic syndrome of IM resulting from EBV infection is estimated to occur in 1 of every 1000 young adults per year [3].

EBV is transmitted in oral secretions and can be spread by close oral contact, such as kissing. The virus can be shed for more than 6 months after the initial primary infection, then intermittently throughout life. Approximately 20% to 30% of healthy asymptomatic EBV-infected persons are shedding the virus at any time, and 60% to 90% of immunocompromised EBV-infected persons are shedding the virus at any time. It also is possible to spread the infection by sexual contact because EBV is found in the female genital tract. A study from Edinburgh University suggested that sexual activity and having numerous sexual partners was a highly significant risk factor for EBV seropositivity. Approximately 83% of sexually active students were seropositive compared with 67% of students who had never had intercourse [4].

The incubation period of IM in adolescents is 30 to 50 days. The initial symptoms are often vague and include malaise and fatigue. Other symptoms include fever, sore throat, headache, nausea, abdominal pain, and muscle aches. EBV initially infects the oral epithelial cells, then the entire lymphoreticular system, including the lymph nodes, liver, and spleen. Physical examination findings include generalized lymphadenopathy, pharyngitis, and splenomegaly; more than 90% of patients who have IM have lymphadenopathy. The most commonly affected lymph nodes are the anterior and posterior cervical nodes, but the inguinal, axillary, and epitrochlear nodes also may be enlarged.

Signs of pharyngitis typically include tonsillar enlargement with exudates. Approximately 50% of patients have splenomegaly, usually no more than 2 to 3 cm below the costal margin. The splenic enlargement may be rapid enough to cause right upper quadrant pain, whereas massive splenic enlargement is rare. Approximately 10% of patients also have hepatomegaly, but symptomatic hepatitis and jaundice are uncommon.

The differential diagnosis includes other infections that cause an IM-like illness and other causes of exudative pharyngitis, such as group A beta-hemolytic streptococcal infection. Because approximately 5% of the population may be chronic pharyngeal streptococcal infection carriers, a positive throat culture for group A beta-hemolytic streptococci in a patient who has mono-like symptoms does not exclude the diagnosis of EBV infection. If an adolescent who has symptoms and signs of pharyngitis associated with a positive streptococcal throat culture fails to improve within 3 days of antibiotic therapy, further testing for IM should be considered.

In more than 90% of patients who have IM, the total leukocyte count is 10,000 to 20,000 cells/mm^3 with at least 60% lymphocytes. Approximately 20% to 40% of the lymphocytes are atypical cells, which are larger and have a lower nuclear-to-cytoplasm ratio than normal lymphocytes. Although atypical lymphocytosis can be seen with other infections (including hepatitis A, cytomegalovirus, and rubella), the higher the percent of atypical lymphocytes, the more likely it is that the cause of the infection is EBV. Other abnormal laboratory findings that occur in 50% or more patients include mildly elevated liver transaminases and thrombocytopenia; elevated bilirubin levels and clinical jaundice are rare. Because the platelet count is usually greater than 50,000/mm^3, purpura also is uncommon.

IM is associated with elevated levels of heterophil antibodies. These antibodies agglutinate red blood cells from nonhuman species. The heterophil antibodies in serum from patients who have IM agglutinate sheep and horse red blood cells, but not guinea pig red blood cells. The most widely used heterophil antibody test is a slide test that uses horse red blood cells. Adolescents and young adults who have IM are more likely to have a positive heterophil antibody test than young children. The heterophil test may remain positive for 2 years after the acute infection. The false-positive and false-negative rate of heterophil testing is 5% to 10%. False-negative tests in patients who have clinical symptoms and signs consistent with IM may indicate an infection caused by another infectious agent associated with mono-like illness (eg, cytomegalovirus) instead of EBV.

Antibody testing

EBV-specific antibody testing can be useful in confirming the diagnosis of acute EBV infection (Box 1). During the early, acute phase of IM, the IgM–viral capsid antigen (IgM-VCA), IgG–viral capsid antigen (IgG-VCA), and early antigen (EA) titers usually are elevated. The IgM-VCA can be detected in the first 4 weeks of illness and usually disappears within 3 months. The IgG-VCA titer also can be detected in the first 4 weeks of illness, but persists for life. EA titers peak during convalescence and are detectable for several months after the illness, but may persist at low levels for many years. The IgM antibody to VCA is the most valuable and specific test for the diagnosis of IM resulting from EBV infection and is sufficient to confirm the diagnosis. High levels of antibody to EA

Box 1. Useful antigen tests in infectious mononucleosis

Early antigen (EA)
IgM-viral capsid antigen (IgM-VCA)
IgG-viral capsid antigen (IgG-VCA)
EBV-determined nuclear antigens (EBNA)

may occur in immunocompromised patients who have persistent infection and active EBV replication. High titers of antibodies to the diffuse-staining component of EA occur in patients who have nasopharyngeal carcinoma, and high titers of the cytoplasmic-restricted component of EA occur in patients who have EBV-associated Burkitt's lymphoma. Because EBV-determined nuclear antigen (EBNA) antibodies are the last to develop, absence of these antibodies when other EBV antibodies are present suggests a recent infection, whereas positive EBNA antibody titers suggest that the acute EBV infection occurred more than 3 to 4 months ago.

Management

There is no specific treatment for IM. Decreased physical activity and symptomatic treatment are the mainstays of therapy. Participation in any strenuous athletic activities should be prohibited during the first 2 to 3 weeks of the illness. Activity can be increased gradually as symptoms resolve. Short courses of corticosteroids may be helpful in the treatment of IM complications (Box 2). There are no controlled studies, however, on the efficacy of corticosteroids; because EBV infection is associated with oncogenic complications (eg, nasopharyngeal carcinoma, Burkitt's lymphoma), corticosteroids should not be used in patients who have uncomplicated IM [4].

IM complications are rare. One of the most common complications is airway obstruction secondary to swelling of the tonsils and oropharyngeal lymphoid tissue. Although less than 5% of patients develop this complication, it is the most common reason for hospitalization of patients with IM. Most patients with this complication can be treated successfully with intravenous fluids, humidified air, and corticosteroids. Splenic hemorrhage or rupture occurs in less than 0.5% of adolescent and young adult patients. This dreaded complication happens most commonly during the second week of illness and often is associated with mild abdominal trauma. To avoid this complication, patients who have splenomegaly should be advised to avoid all contact sports until the splenomegaly resolves.

Uncommon complications of IM include a variety of neurologic disorders, such as meningitis, seizures, ataxia, facial nerve palsy, transverse myelitis, and encephalitis. About 50% of patients who have IM complain of headache, but

---

Box 2. Infectious mononucleosis complications that may be improved with corticosteroids

Marked tonsillar hypertrophy
Thrombocytopenia associated with hemorrhage
Autoimmune hemolytic anemia
Seizures
Encephalopathy

serious neurologic complications occur in only 1% to 5% of patients. A perceptual disorder (metamorphopsia or "Alice in Wonderland" syndrome) is a peculiar neurologic manifestation in which spatial relationships and size and shape of objects are distorted. Guillain-Barré syndrome may follow the acute illness.

Approximately 3% of patients develop a Coombs-positive hemolytic anemia. Aplastic anemia, severe neutropenia (<1000 neutrophils/mm^3), and severe thrombocytopenia (platelet count <20,000/mm^3) are rare complications. Aplastic anemia usually presents 3 to 4 weeks after the onset of illness and lasts 4 to 8 days, whereas hemolytic anemia typically appears in the first 2 weeks and lasts 1 month. Other rare complications include myocarditis, pancreatitis, parotitis, and orchitis.

If there are no complications during the acute illness, the prognosis for complete recovery is excellent. Marked fatigue, headache, and pharyngeal symptoms usually resolve in 2 to 4 weeks. Mild fatigue and malaise may persist for a few months, however. Although there are some cases of prolonged fatigue after IM, there is no convincing evidence that EBV infection or recurrence of EBV infection is linked to a chronic fatigue syndrome.

Asthma

Although asthma is the most common chronic disease in children and is becoming increasingly prevalent in children and adults [5], little has been written about asthma in the college-age population. The National Heart, Lung and Blood Institute and World Health Organization, in their 1995 Workshop Report, defined *asthma* as follows [6]:

> [A] chronic inflammatory disorder of the airways in which many cells play a role, in particular mast cells, eosinophils, and T lymphocytes. In susceptible individuals this inflammation causes recurrent episodes of wheezing, breathlessness, chest tightness, and cough particularly at night or in the early morning. These symptoms are usually associated with widespread but variable airflow limitation that is at least partly reversible either spontaneously or with treatment. The inflammation also causes an associated increase in airway responsiveness to a variety of stimuli.

Epidemiology

Asthma is prevalent worldwide in all age groups; its prevalence in children varies greatly in different countries. Some countries have reported prevalence rates among 6- to 7-year-olds of 1.4%, whereas other countries have prevalence rates of 27.1%. This same pattern is seen among 13- to 14-year-old adolescents [7,8]. In the United States, asthma prevalence increased 74% from 1988 to 1994 among children 5 to 14 years old [5]. Measures of morbidity, such as hospitalization rates and emergency department visits, and mortality also have

increased in the United States [9–11]. In addition, children and young adults from
ethnic minority groups and lower socioeconomic groups are known to be at
increased risk for poor outcomes secondary to asthma [12–14]. Asthma occurs in
all races, although rarely in Eskimos [10]. The male and female lifetime
prevalence of asthma diagnosis (in 2001) showed that females are more likely
to be diagnosed with asthma—119 females/1000 population received the diagnosis of asthma versus 107 males/1000 population [15].

General features

The hallmarks of asthma are inflammation and airway responsiveness that
lead to airflow limitations. A patient's history, physical examination, laboratory
evaluation, and response to a trial of therapy all are helpful in making the
diagnosis of asthma. Typically a patient who has asthma complains of chronic
cough, persistent wheezing, or chronic shortness of breath. There is frequently a
history of asthma in other family members and allergies and eczema.

Common triggers that worsen asthma include tobacco smoke, cold air, exercise, and strong scents. Patients with asthma may be able to describe what
happens when their disease worsens, listing not only the most salient consequences (eg, shortness of breath), but also the more subtle results (eg, increased
nocturnal cough). It is important for clinicians to ask about the salient and subtle
manifestations of asthma to improve asthma management.

The physical examination of a patient with asthma may be completely normal
if the patient is well controlled by medications and is not having an exacerbation.
Conversely a patient who has experienced a profound exacerbation may appear
in extremis. In between the two extremes, the pulmonary examination generally
shows diffuse wheezing. The wheezing starts late in the expiratory phase, but
as the disease progresses, it may last throughout expiration and involve the
inspiratory phase as well. With continued progression, the airways may become
so narrow (because of mucus production, airway edema, and smooth muscle
bronchoconstriction) that no wheezing is heard at all. The patient with an asthma
exacerbation often appears anxious and may be using accessory muscles to aid
in breathing. A pulsus paradoxus is found during severe asthma exacerbations.
Other associated findings include hives, eczema, allergic rhinitis, and nasal
polyps (especially in patients with aspirin sensitivity).

The laboratory evaluation of asthma should be specific and straightforward.
Pulmonary function tests are used to confirm the diagnosis of asthma, especially
when used with a fast-acting inhaled β-agonist (eg, albuterol) or a part of a
bronchoprovocation test. Rarely, flexible fiberoptic laryngoscopy is necessary to
rule out vocal cord dysfunction, which may mimic asthma [16,17]. For a patient
in whom the diagnosis has been established, regular, at-home measurements of
the peak expiratory flow rate (PEFR) are helpful for spotting trends that reveal
whether control is adequate; many patients appropriately self-manage their
medications on the basis of their PEFR readings (with prior clinician input).
Spirometry also may be employed to assess asthma severity and help guide the

medication regimen. Other laboratory tests (eg, chest radiographs, allergy testing, blood tests for IgE) should be ordered as indicated.

Management

The approach to asthma management comprises four elements (Box 3), according to the 1997 National Asthma Education and Prevention Program (NAEPP) Expert Panel II [18,19]. *Monitoring* generally refers to PEFR, especially in a patient with moderate-to-severe disease who is seeking a trend as opposed to a determination of airflow limitation [20,21]. Some clinicians use sputum eosinophilia to monitor asthma control and guide therapy, although it is unclear whether sputum eosinophilia independently predicts a patient's response to inhaled or oral corticosteroids [22–25].

Asthma *triggers* are numerous and include allergens, respiratory infections (especially viruses), irritants, chemicals, physical activity, and emotional stress. It is important to identify and avoid or the least limit exposure to the trigger. In cases in which the trigger cannot be avoided and limited exposure is impossible, an additional dose of bronchodilator may be advisable. Influenza vaccination should be administered annually to patients with asthma.

Pharmacologic treatment is an extensive topic, and only a brief outline is offered here. For more extensive information, review the 1997 NAEPP *Guidelines* (updated in 2002) [18]. A patient's asthma typically is categorized into one of four "steps," based on the severity of symptoms (eg, nocturnal awakenings, necessity of bronchodilator use for wheezing or shortness of breath during the day, PEFR [as a percentage of predicted or best] and PEFR variability). *Step 1 disease,* known as *mild intermittent asthma,* is the mildest form and requires no long-term treatment. It has the fewest and least severe symptoms. Therapy for step 1 asthma is a fast-acting inhaled β-agonist as necessary.

Step 2 disease is known as *mild persistent asthma* and is more severe than step 1 disease. Mild persistent asthma requires long-term medication—generally an inhaled corticosteroid—in addition to a fast-acting inhaled β-agonist if control is not maintained. Other types of long-term medications used in step 2 disease (and beyond) include leukotriene-modifying agents, mast cell–stabilizing agents, and long-acting inhaled β-agonists. The last-mentioned are recommended for use only in conjunction with inhaled corticosteroids [26,27].

Box 3. Approach to asthma management

  1. Monitoring
  2. Controlling trigger factors
  3. Pharmacologic treatment
  4. Patient education

Step 3 disease, moderate persistent asthma, is more severe than Step 2 disease and may require high-dose inhaled steroids. The other long-term medications mentioned and theophylline may be a part of the patient's medication regimen. A patient with *step 4 disease, severe persistent asthma,* has symptoms almost continuously and may require regular bursts or daily dosing of oral cortico-steroids, in addition to other long-term medications and fast-acting inhaled β-agonists. In principle, clinicians should get newly diagnosed or poorly con-trolled asthma under control quickly. As the asthma is brought under control, medications, especially corticosteroids, should be weaned to the lowest dose at which there is good control.

Patient education is an essential component of keeping patients with asthma healthy. Patient education consists of teaching patients how to monitor their symptoms, how to identify and avoid their triggers, why and how to use their medications and their devices, and what to do in the event of an emergency or deteriorating control. The last-mentioned is often assisted through the use of an asthma management plan (or asthma action plan). Education is the key to clinician-directed self-management of patients. Motivated, educated patients have reduced hospitalizations because of asthma, improved daily function, and improved patient satisfaction [28].

Challenges of asthma in the college population: potential areas of research

There are a few challenges to the clinician in working with college-age patients with asthma. First, asthma is not well characterized in this population; specifically, data collected on asthma morbidity and mortality do not focus on the college population (eg, the Centers for Disease Control and Prevention and National Center for Health Statistics report 15- to 34-year-old or 18 and older age groups rather than the traditional college age group). Second, college is a time of development from late adolescence to early adulthood. Students may function semi-independently and be educationally "primed," but they also are highly influenced by their peers. In addition, college students may be challenged by sleep deprivation, living in older college buildings with mold and dust mite infes-tation, and the likelihood of increased respiratory infections owing to the close proximity to other students. No studies on the successes or failures of patient education and self-management of the college-age population with asthma exist. These and other areas of interest should provide directions for future research.

Migraine

Migraine is a common neurovascular disorder in the college-age population. It is characterized by severe headache and autonomic nervous system dysfunction and, in some patients, an aura. Although attacks may start at any age, the inci-dence peaks in early to mid adolescence. The 1-year overall prevalence of

---

Box 4. Criteria for migraine without aura

Headaches last 4–72 hours
With ≥ 2 of the following:
   Unilateral location
   Throbbing quality
   Severe enough to inhibit or prohibit daily activities
   Aggravated by routine physical activity (eg. walking stairs)
And during the headache, at least 1 of the following:
   Nausea or vomiting or both
   Photophobia or phonophobia

From International Headache Society Headache Classification Committee. Classification and diagnostic criteria for headache disorders, cranial neuralgias, and facial pain. Cephalgia 1998;8:1–96; with permission.

---

migraine in the United States is 11%; the prevalence is higher in women (15–18%) than in men (6%) [29].

The International Headache Society has developed diagnostic criteria for migraine (Boxes 4 and 5) [30]. The headache begins gradually, often in the morning, and the most common locations are the frontal and temporal regions. The headache episode may last hours to days and is associated with symptoms such as nausea, vomiting, photophobia, and phonophobia. The pain is often uni-

---

Box 5. Criteria for migraine with aura

At least 2 headaches
With at least 3 of the following:
   One or more fully reversible aura symptoms indicating focal
      cerebral cortical dysfunction or brainstem dysfunction
      or both
   At least 1 aura symptom develops gradually over > 4 minutes
      or ≥ 2 symptoms occur in succession
   No single aura symptom lasts > 60 minutes
   Headache follows aura within 60 minutes or before or
      during aura

From International Headache Society Headache Classification Committee. Classification and diagnostic criteria for headache disorders, cranial neuralgias, and facial pain. Cephalgia 1998;8:1–96; with permission.

---

lateral, throbbing, aggravated on movement, and severe [30]. The severity of the pain causes the patient to interrupt activities. The frequency of migraine headaches in affected patients averages 1.5 per month, but 10% have weekly attacks [29].

Migraine without aura is the most common type, but in 15% to 18% of patients, the headache always is preceded or accompanied by an aura; in 13% of patients, the headache is accompanied by an aura sometimes [31]. Prodromal symptoms in patients who have migraine without aura may include mood changes, irritability, increased thirst, fluid retention, or food cravings. Behavioral changes that may result in curtailing activities are the most common prodromal symptoms. Migraine with aura may be associated with visual, sensory, motor, or psychic aura. However, Visual auras are the most common and include transient visual deficits and visual distortions. Sensory auras may consist of numbness or tingling of the extremities, perioral numbness, and dysesthesias. Motor auras include monoparesis and hemiparesis. Psychic auras may be characterized by confusion, dysequilibrium, and amnesia [32].

The differential diagnosis of migraine includes complex partial seizures, intracranial hemorrhage, brain tumor, acute intoxication, and central nervous system infection. Occasionally, migraine presents with dramatic neurologic signs and symptoms, such as hemiparesis, ataxia, blindness, ophthalmoparesis, vertigo, and acute confusional states in addition to severe headache. In these cases, neuroimaging studies often are needed to exclude more ominous neurologic conditions.

Management

The appropriate treatment of a patient who has migraine depends on the frequency, duration, and intensity of the headache and the patient's pain tolerance and disability. A headache calendar in which the patient tracks the frequency and severity of the headaches may be helpful in determining the optimal treatment approach and monitoring its efficacy. In a patient who has migraine, the brain does not seem to tolerate irregular lifestyles well. College students, who often have irregular sleep and eating patterns and increased stress, may benefit particularly from a discussion of the importance of regular sleep, regular meals, adequate exercise, and avoidance of stress as the first step in decreasing the frequency of headaches. Insufficient sleep is associated with increased headache frequency, so counseling the student on the importance of going to bed and getting up at the same time each day may be helpful. The influence of diet on migraine is unclear. About 10% to 30% of migraineurs can identify foods that trigger their migraine episodes. If so, avoiding these foods may be helpful. It is especially important to ask about intake of caffeine because there is a link between caffeine intake and migraine episodes [33]. Alcohol also may precipitate migraine in susceptible individuals.

Drugs used in the treatment of migraine can be divided into two categories: (1) drugs taken at the time of a migraine episode and (2) drugs taken daily to prevent migraine episodes. For an acute migraine episode, drug therapies can be divided further into nonspecific pain relievers and drugs that are used specifically for treatment of migraine. For patients who have infrequent migraine episodes of short duration, an oral analgesic (eg, aspirin, acetaminophen, naproxen, or ibuprofen) may be sufficient. It is important to avoid narcotics because they leave the patient cognitively impaired and can be addictive. The analgesic should be taken at the first sign of a headache and at an appropriate dose (eg, 400–800 mg of ibuprofen; 500–1000 mg of naproxen). Because migraine episodes are associated with decreased gastric motility, which may interfere with absorption of oral analgesics, metaclopromide taken promptly at the onset of the headache along with the analgesic may help increase absorption and control the nausea that often is associated with migraine episodes. If oral analgesics are ineffective or must be taken more often than 2 to 3 days per week, alternative medications should be considered because overuse of analgesics can lead to an increase in headache frequency (analgesic rebound).

If analgesics are ineffective in treating acute episodes, triptans should be considered [34]. Triptans are serotonin 5-HT$_1$ receptor agonists. Their potential mechanism of action includes cranial vasoconstriction, peripheral neuronal inhibition, and inhibition of transmission through second-order neurons of the trigeminocervical complex. The five triptans most commonly used are sumatriptan, naratriptan, rizatriptan, zolmitriptan, and almotriptan. Because absorption of these drugs may be delayed when administered orally during a migraine episode, the use of nonoral formulations, such as nasal sprays, inhalers, injectables, or suppositories, should be considered.

Sumatriptan is available in a formulation for subcutaneous self-injection, an oral formulation, and a nasal spray. The injectable formulation and the nasal spray begin to produce relief in 10 to 15 minutes, whereas the tablet may take 1 to 2 hours to produce relief. Injectable sumatriptan is effective in 70% to 80% of patients who have moderate-to-severe migraine episodes, the nasal spray is effective in 60% of patients within 2 hours, and the oral tablets are effective in 50% to 60% of patients within 2 hours and 70% within 4 hours [34]. A meta-analysis of the triptans revealed that 100 mg of sumatriptan, 2.5 mg of zolmatriptan, 5 mg of rizatriptan, 40 mg of eletriptan, and 12.5 mg of almotriptan were equally effective in providing pain relief within 2 hours of ingestion, whereas higher doses of rizatriptan (10 mg) and eletriptan (80 mg) were more effective than 100 mg of sumatriptan [35].

For patients who have frequent or debilitating headaches, preventive medications should be discussed collaboratively with the patient. Patients who have five or more headaches per month or have acute attacks that are unresponsive to therapy are good candidates for preventive therapy. It is not clear how preventive therapies work, but it is generally thought that they modify the sensitivity of the brain that underlies migraine [35]. A variety of drugs have been used (Box 6), although there are few controlled studies on their efficacy in adolescents. The choice of drug to use for preventive therapy should be made after discussing with the patient the common side effects of each medication. Propranolol is contraindicated in patients who have asthma because it may cause

---

Box 6. Medications used for migraine prevention

β-Adrenergic receptor antagonists
    Propranolol
    Metoprolol
Antidepressants
    Amitriptyline
    Nortriptyline
    Fluoxetine
Anticonvulsants
    Carbamazepine
    Valproate
    Topiramate
    Lamotrigine
    Gabapentin

---

bronchospasm. Other side effects include drowsiness, bradycardia, lightheadedness, and decreased energy. Valproate has teratogenic effects, so it should not be used by women who are at risk for pregnancy owing to unprotected sexual activity. Serious side effects of valproate also include liver and hematologic abnormalities. Amitriptyline side effects include drowsiness, dizziness, postural hypotension, and nausea. The use of methysergide for prophylaxis should be avoided because of the risk of retroperitoneal fibrosis.

Urinary tract infections

UTIs usually are described by their location as urethritis, cystitis, or pyelonephritis. The diagnosis is based on the isolation of a single pathogenic organism in sufficient number from either a clean-catch or catheterized urine specimen. Although UTIs traditionally have been defined by the isolation of greater than 10^5 colony-forming units (CFUs), it has been suggested that for women who have symptoms consistent with a lower UTI (urethritis or cystitis), isolation of at least 10^2 CFUs is sufficient for diagnosis.

Symptoms of an acute UTI include pain or burning on urination (dysuria), frequent voiding of urine (frequency), urge to void urine (urgency), blood in the urine (hematuria), and lower abdominal discomfort. If fever, suprapubic tenderness, or costovertebral tenderness are present, the infection is more likely to involve the upper urinary tract; if these symptoms and signs are absent, the infection is more likely to be limited to the bladder (cystitis) or urethra (urethritis).

Four symptoms significantly increase the probability of UTI: dysuria, frequency, hematuria, and pain [36]. In primary care settings, the probability of cystitis is approximately 90% in women who present with dysuria and frequency without vaginal discharge [36,37]. Physical examination findings are of little value in the diagnosis of UTI; however, the examination may be helpful in the diagnosis of other conditions that are in the differential diagnosis of UTI, including vaginitis, cervicitis, pelvic inflammatory disease, and sexually transmitted infections. Symptoms or signs of vaginal discharge and vaginal irritation significantly decrease the likelihood that a UTI is present [36], but because UTIs are most likely to occur in sexually active women, these diseases frequently overlap. The only physical examination finding that increases the likelihood of UTI is costovertebral angle tenderness, but this finding is characteristic only of upper UTIs.

Although older studies recommended that a urine culture be done in all women with suspected UTI, more recent guidelines suggest that women who have typical symptoms can be diagnosed accurately by urine dipstick and that a urine culture is not necessary [38]. A urine dipstick that is positive for leukocyte esterase or nitrite has a sensitivity of 75% and a specificity of 82% in the diagnosis of UTI [39]. The presence of pyuria on urinalysis has high (95%) sensitivity but relatively low (40–70%) specificity for UTI. The presence of bacteria on microscopic examination of the urine is a more specific (85–95%) but less sensitive test [37].

Cystitis is common in college-age women because the most important risk factor for this infection is sexual activity. Celibate women rarely have cystitis. The risk of acute cystitis during the 48 hours after sexual intercourse increases by a factor of 60. The incidence of cystitis among sexually active young women is approximately 0.5% per year [36]. The risk of UTI and UTI complications is increased in women who have diabetes, immunosuppression, or structural abnormalities of the urinary tract or who are pregnant.

Escherichia coli causes 75% to 90% of acute episodes of cystitis. *Staphylococcus saprophyticus* is the second most common cause and accounts for 5% to 15% of infections. Other organisms include enterococci, *Klebsiella* species, and *Proteus mirabilis*. In the past, a 3-day course of trimethoprim-sulfamethoxazole (TMP-SMX) was effective in eliminating pathogens from the urine in 94% of women who had cystitis [40]. Because of increasing resistance of urinary pathogens to TMP-SMX, however, some authorities now recommend that TMP-SMX be used only if prevalence of resistance in a community is less than 15% to 20% and the patient has not received antibiotics recently.

Ofloxacin is equally or more effective than TMP-SMX, and other fluoroquinolones are likely to be equally efficacious. When TMP-SMX is contraindicated, a 3-day course of ciprofloxacin, levofloxacin, or norfloxacin is a reasonable alternative. These drugs should not be considered first-line therapy, however, because of their higher cost and the concern that using these medications increases the risk of bacterial resistance in the community. Fluoroquinolones are active against *S. saprophyticus* and most typical gram-negative uropathogens, but are effective against only 60% to 70% of enterococci.

Approximately 95% of urinary pathogens are sensitive to nitrofurantoin, but this antibiotic is less active than TMP-SMX against aerobic gram-negative uropathogens other than *E. coli* and is not effective against *Pseudomonas* or

Proteus species. Nitrofurantoin also usually must be taken for 7 days and may cause gastrointestinal upset. The macrocrystalline form must be taken every 6 hours, but the monohydrate macrocrystal is taken just twice daily and causes fewer gastrointestinal symptoms. β-lactams (eg, amoxicillin) should be avoided because bacterial resistance is common.

Women who have acute pyelonephritis should be treated for 14 days with a fluoroquinolone if the organism is susceptible to it. Hospitalization may be necessary for women who are unable to take oral medications, have signs of systemic toxicity, or have underlying structural urinary tract abnormalities or are pregnant. Gram-positive organisms may require treatment with amoxicillin or amoxicillin-clavulanate [40].

Approximately 90% of women have symptomatic relief within 72 hours after initiation of antibiotic therapy. If dysuria is severe, more rapid symptomatic relief can be achieved with the use of phenazopyridine, which is now available without prescription. Routine follow-up is unnecessary after treatment of cystitis unless symptoms persist. Imaging studies and cystoscopy are not indicated.

After an initial UTI, most women have sporadic recurrences, and at least 25% of women have a recurrence within 1 year. Alternative contraceptive methods should be considered by women who have frequent recurrences and use spermicidal-coated condoms or diaphragms because vaginal spermicides increase the risk for UTIs. Continuous or postcoital prophylaxis with low-dose anti-microbial agents may be effective in preventing recurrences. Nitrofurantoin, TMP, TMP-SMX, ciprofloxacin, and norfloxacin all are effective when taken once daily in preventing recurrences. Prophylaxis usually is initiated for 6 months. Postcoital treatment with nitrofurantoin, TMP-SMX, or a fluoroquinolone also is effective in preventing recurrences. Cranberry juice contains proanthocya-nidins, which seem to inhibit attachment of uropathogens to the urinary tract epithelium. Studies have shown that 200 to 750 mL of cranberry juice daily can reduce recurrences by 15% to 20%. Although tablets containing cranberry products are sold commercially, the actual cranberry content of these products is highly variable; the cranberry content of juices marketed as cranberry juice may vary from 5% to 100%.

Although women commonly are advised to void after coitus to prevent UTIs, there is no evidence that this prevents cystitis. There also is no evidence that poor urinary hygiene leads to infection. There is no rationale for advising women who have had a UTI to increase their frequency of urination; change wiping patterns; or avoid pantyhose, douching, or use of hot tubs [37].

References

[1] Chang RS, Char DF, Jones DH, et al. Incidence of infectious mononucleosis at the Universities of California and Hawaii. J Infect Dis 1979;140:479–86.
[2] Dan R, Chang RS. A prospective study of primary Epstein-Barr virus infectins among university students in Hong Kong. Am J Trop Med Hyg 1990;42:380–5.

[3] Jenson HB. Epstein-Barr virus. In: Behrman RE, Kliegman RM, Jenson HB, editors. Nelson textbook of pediatrics. 17th edition. Philadelphia: Saunders-Elsevier; 2004. p. 1062–6.

[4] Crawford DH, Swerdlow AJ. Sexual history and Epstein-Barr virus infection. J Infect Dis 2002;186:731–6.

[5] Mannino DM, Homa DM, et al. Surveillance for asthma—United States, 1960–1995. MMWR Morb Mortal Wkly Rep 1998;1008(47[No. SS-1]):1–28.

[6] National Heart Lung and Blood Institute. Global Initiative for Asthma Management and Prevention. Bethesda (MD): US Department of Health and Human Services, National Institutes of Health; 1995.

[7] Worldwide variation in prevalence of symptoms of asthma, allergic rhinoconjunctivitis, and atopic eczema. ISAAC. Lancet 1998;351:1225.

[8] Worldwide variations in the prevalence of asthma symptoms: the International Study of Asthma and Allergies in Childhood (ISAAC). Eur Respir J 1998;12:315.

[9] Asthma prevalence, health care use and mortality, 2000–2001. Available at: www.cdc.gov/nchs/products/pubs/pubd/hestats/asthma/asthma.htm.

[10] Akinbami L, Schoendorf KC. Trends in childhood asthma: prevalence, health care utilization, and mortality. Pediatrics 2002;110(2 Pt 1):315–22.

[11] CDC. Surveillance for asthma—United States, 1980–1999. MMWR Surveill Summ 2002; 51(SS01):1–13.

[12] Halfon N, Newacheck PW. Childhood asthma and poverty: differential impacts and utilization of health services. Pediatrics 1993;91:56–61.

[13] Evans D, Mellins R. Improving care for minority children with asthma: professional education in public health clinics. Pediatrics 1997;99:157–64.

[14] Yoos HL, McMullen A. An asthma management program for urban minority children. J Pediatr Health Care 1997;11:66–74.

[15] National Center for Health Statistics website. Available at: www.cdc.gov/nchs/products/pubs/pubd/hestats/asthma/asthma.htm.

[16] Christopher KL, Wood RP, et al. Vocal cord dysfunction presenting as asthma. N Engl J Med 1983;308:1566.

[17] Goldman J, Muers M. Vocal cord dysfunction and wheezing. Thorax 1991;46:401.

[18] NAEPP Expert Panel report guidelines for the diagnosis and management of asthma. Bethesda (MD): National Heart Lung and Blood Institute; 2003.

[19] Murphy S, Sheffer AL. National Asthma Education and Prevention Program: highlights of the Expert Panel Report II: guidelines for the diagnosis and management of asthma. Bethesda (MD): National Heart, Lung and Blood Institute; 1997.

[20] Smith HR, Irvin CG. The utility of spirometry in the diagnosis of reversible airways obstruction. Chest 1992;101:1577.

[21] Enright PL, Lebowitz MD. Physiologic measures: pulmonary function test. Am J Respir Crit Care Me 1994;149(S9).

[22] Little SA, Chalmers GW. Non-invasive markers of airway inflammation as predictors of oral steroid responsiveness in asthma. Thorax 2000;55:232.

[23] Green RH, Brightling CE. Asthma exacerbations and sputum eosinophil counts: a randomised controlled trial. Lancet 2002;360:1715.

[24] Meijer RJ, Postma DS, et al. Accuracy of eosinophils and eosinophil cationic protein to predict steroid improvement in asthma. Clin Exp Allergy 2002;32:1096.

[25] Romagnoli M, Vachier I. Eosinophilic inflammation in sputum of poorly controlled asthmatics. Eur Respir J 2002;20:1370.

[26] Simons FE. A comparison of beclomethasone, salmeterol, and placebo in children with asthma. N Engl J Med 1997;337:1659.

[27] Verberne A, Frost C. One year treatment with salmeterol compared with beclomethasone in children with asthma. Am J Respir Crit Care Med 1997;156:688.

[28] Gibson PG, Coughlan J. Self-management education and regular practitioner review for adults with asthma. Cochrane Database Syst Rev 2000.

[29] Stewart WF, Lipton RB. Prevalence of migraine headache in the United States: relation to age, income, race and other sociodemographic factors. JAMA 1992;267:64–9.

[30] International Headache Society Headache Classification Committee. Classification and diagnostic critieria for headache disorders: cranial neuralgias, and facial pain. Cephalgia 1998; 8(Suppl 7):1–96.

[31] Launer LJ, Terwindt GM. The prevalence and characteristics of migraine in a population-based cohort: the GEM study. Neurology 1999;53:537–42.

[32] Lewis DL. Migraine headaches in the adolescent. Adolesc Med 2002;13:413–32.

[33] James JE. Acute and chronic effects of caffeine on performance, mood, headache and sleep. Neuropsychobiology 1998;38:32–41.

[34] New "triptans" and other drugs for migraine. Med Lett 1998;40:97–100.

[35] Goadsey PJ, Lipton RB. Migraines: current understanding and treatment. N Engl J Med 2002;346:257–70.

[36] Bent S, Nallamothu BK. Does this woman have an acute uncomplicated urinary tract infection? JAMA 2002;287:2701–10.

[37] Filn SD. Acute uncomplicated urinary tract infection in women. N Engl J Med 2003;349: 259–66.

[38] Bacheller CD, Bernstein JM. Urinary tract infections. Med Clin North Am 1997;81:452–7.

[39] Hurlbut T, Littenberg G. The diagnostic accurancy of rapid dipstick tests to predict urinary tract infection. Am J Clin Pathol 1991;96:582–8.

[40] Warren JW, Abrutyn E. Guidelines for antimicrobial tretment of uncomplicated acute bacterial cystitis and acute pyelonephritis in women. Clin Infect Dis 1999;29:745–58.

ELSEVIER
SAUNDERS

PEDIATRIC CLINICS
OF NORTH AMERICA

Pediatr Clin N Am 52 (2005) 25–60

The College Athlete

Dilip R. Patel, MD, FAAP, FAACPDM, FACSM, FSAM[a],*,
Donald E. Greydanus, MD, FAAP, FSAM[a],
Eugene F. Luckstead, Sr, MD, FACC, FAAP[b]

[a]*Michigan State University, Kalamazoo Center for Medical Studies, 1000 Oakland Drive, Kalamazoo, MI 49008, USA*
[b]*Texas Tech Medical Center, 1400 S. Coulter Road, Amarillo, TX 79106, USA*

Participation in athletics is an important aspect of life for students during their college years. Student athletes come from different levels of previous experience, physical fitness, and readiness for college sports. The primary source of student medical care is the campus student health center, and college health care providers attend to many of the sports-related medical issues of student athletes [1]. This article reviews preparticipation physical evaluation, use of drugs and supplements by athletes, and selected injuries.

Preparticipation physical evaluation

A preparticipation evaluation by an appropriately qualified health care provider is required of all student athletes before they are allowed to participate in college sports programs. The major goal of such an evaluation is to assess the general health of the student and to identify any conditions that may predispose the athlete to an increased risk of injury or illness from sport participation or increase similar risks to other teammates [1–4]. In most instances, conditions identified in preparticipation physical evaluation (PPE) need further comprehensive assessment before clearing an athlete for sport participation. For many students, a PPE may provide the only opportunity to explore and discuss health risk behaviors such as substance abuse, high-risk sexual behaviors, drinking and

---

* Corresponding author.
E-mail address: patel@kcms.msu.edu (D.R. Patel).

Box 1. Preparticipation physical evaluation history

Past history

    Surgeries (especially chest, abdomen, spine)
    Injuries
    Major medical illness
    Known medical conditions (eg, asthma, diabetes)

Allergies

    Medications, bees, food, other

Dietary History

    Weight loss/gain
    Dietary habits

Cardiovascular History

    Exercise induced presyncope or syncope
    Chest pain, palpitations, undue fatigue, heart
       murmur, hypertension
    Personal or family history of high cholesterol or lipid disorders
    Family history of sudden cardiac death before age 50
    Family history of Marfan syndrome or cardiomyopathy

Neurologic

    Details of any head injury
    Neck injury or burners

Pulmonary

    Exercised related difficulty breathing, wheezing, cough

Health risk behaviors

    Dietary
    Sexual history
    Drug use
    Supplement use

Other

    Hearing or vision problems
    Eye surgery
    Musculoskeletal injuries
    Immunizations
    Menstrual history in female athletes

---

driving, and pathogenic weight control or dietary practices [5–11]. Current guidelines recommend PPE every year, ideally 6 to 8 weeks before the sport season to allow for further assessment or rehabilitation to be completed [10]. For the freshman class planning for fall sports, this may be difficult to accomplish, and some institutions try to collect medical information by way of mail before the students arrive on campus.

Student history remains the cornerstone of PPE; history has identified more than 75% of conditions that may either need further evaluation or limit participation in some sports [2,3]. In addition to history, additional information should also be sought from parents and the student's primary physician. Appropriate consent for release of information should be obtained. Major items to be included in a comprehensive PPE history are listed in Box 1. A complete physical examination should be done during the initial PPE. Subsequent examinations, including orthopedic assessment, may be more focused as indicated by the history [10–12].

Clearance

As specified in the National Collegiate Athletic Association (NCAA) guideline 2a, the final responsibility to determine when to withhold or remove the student athlete from participation rests with the team physician or the team physician's designated representative [13]. If an athlete is medically disqualified from further participation during an NCAA championship, the team physician must notify the athlete, the coach, and the chair of the governing sports committee (or a designated representative). The guideline further stipulates that, in the absence of a team physician, the NCAA tournament physician is responsible for clearance decisions.

Depending on the specific medical problem identified, the athlete either may not participate in any sport or may be allowed limited participation until further evaluation and treatment [10]. Risks of injury to an athlete or teammates or adverse impact on an athlete's health vary, depending on the specific demands of the sport. Sports can be classified based on risk of contact (Box 2) and static or dynamic demands (Table 1) [10]. Such classification of sports forms the basis for allowing limited participation in some sports versus others. Other factors that may influence clearance decisions include: level of competition, position played, athlete's understanding of health risks related to medical condition, inherent risk

Box 2. Examples of sports classified based on likelihood of contact

Contact/collision sports

　Basketball
　Diving
　Field and ice hockey
　Football
　Lacrosse
　Martial arts
　Rugby
　Soccer
　Wrestling

Limited contact sports

　Baseball
　Bicycling
　Cheerleading
　Fencing
　High jump
　Gymnastics
　Pole vault
　Racquetball
　Skating
　Skiing
　Softball
　Volleyball

Noncontact sports

　Archery
　Badminton
　Bowling
　Dancing
　Discus
　Golf
　Running
　Scuba diving
　Swimming
　Tennis
　Weight lifting

Table 1
Examples of sports classified based on peak dynamic and static demands

	A. Low dynamic	B. Moderate dynamic	C. High dynamic
I. Low static	Curling Bowling Golf	Baseball Softball Tennis (doubles) Volleyball	Badminton Cross-country skiing Field hockey Race walking Racquetball Long distance running Soccer Squash Tennis (singles)
II. Moderate static	Archery Diving Equestrian	Fencing Jumping Figure skating Football Rugby Running (sprint) Synchronized swimming	Basketball Ice Hockey Cross-country skiing Lacrosse Middle-distance running Swimming
III. High static	Bobsledding Throwing Gymnastics Karate Luge Water skiing Weight lifting	Body building Downhill skiing Wrestling	Canoeing/kayaking Cycling Decathlon Rowing Speed skating

Modified from Mitchell JH, et al. Classification of sports. Med Sci Sport Exer 1994;26:S244.

of injury from sport participation, availability of alternative activity, and ability to continue to participate with treatment and rehabilitation. The reader is referred to the Preparticipation Physical Evaluation Monograph and other related guidelines for specific conditions [10]. Because of significant interest in literature, sudden cardiac death [14–25] and concussions [26–69] in sports are briefly reviewed here.

Sudden cardiac death

Definition

Sudden cardiac death (SCD) in an athlete is defined as an unexpected death that occurs fewer than 6 hours after exercise in a previously healthy individual [14,15]. The event is not associated with trauma.

Epidemiology

SCD in young athletes (<35 years of age) is uncommon; although the exact incidence in the college-age athlete is not known, the best estimates indicate the

---

Box 3. Causes of sudden cardiac death in young athletes

Hypertrophic cardiomyopathy (most common cause in the
    United States)
Arrhythmogenic right ventricular dysplasia (most common
    cause in Italy)
Brugada syndrome (more prevalent in those of Asian descent)
Wolff-Parkinson-White syndrome
Marfan syndrome
Dilated cardiomyopathy
Anomalous origin of coronary arteries
Aortic dissection
Complete heart block
Aortic stenosis
Congenital long and short QT syndromes
Coronary artery disease
Ebstein anomaly
Myocarditis
Mitral valve prolapse
Drugs of abuse (eg, cocaine, amphetamines, ephedrine, ana-
    bolic steroids)
Commotio cordis (result of blunt chest impact)

---

incidence in young athletes to be 1 to 2 deaths in 200,000 each year [14,22]. In
United States, most sudden cardiac deaths have been reported in male athletes
(male/female ratio of 9:1) in basketball and football, while most sudden deaths in
Europe have been reported in soccer players [22,25].

Studies indicate that the risk for sudden cardiac death increases significantly
with physical exertion in athletes with certain underlying cardiac conditions [18].
Ninety-five percent of sudden deaths in young athletes in United States result
from cardiac conditions. Causes of sudden cardiac death are listed in Box 3
[17,19–25].

Screening of young athletes

Although the incidence of sudden cardiac death in young athletes is low, death
of a young athlete make news headlines. Because of the significant medico-legal
and psychosocial implications associated with SCD, it is imperative to screen all
athletes for risk of SCD based on current guidelines. Again the most important
aspect of the screening is the history. Specific attention to certain aspects of
physical examination is also emphasized. Key points to be included in the
cardiovascular screening of young athletes are listed in Box 4 [14,21–25]. Any

Box 4. Key points in cardiovascular screening of young athletes

Personal history

Exertion-related chest pain
Shortness of breath
Presyncope or syncope
Episodes of dizziness
Palpitations
Undue fatigue with exercise
Known history of congenital heart disease or surgery
Known history of heart murmur
History of high cholesterol
History of high blood pressure
Recent febrile illness

Family history

Premature cardiac death before age 50
Marfan syndrome
Cardiomyopathy
Hypertension
Lipid disorders
Rheumatic fever
Congenital heart disease

Medications, dietary supplement, drugs of abuse

Some have cardiovascular effects such as beta-blockers, albuterol and other beta-agonists, some of the ingredients in common cough and cold preparations (eg, ephedrine, excess caffeine)
Drug of abuse (eg, cocaine, amphetamines, anabolic steroids)

Cardiovascular examination

Heart rate and rhythm
Blood pressure measurement
Signs of Marfan syndrome
Femoral pulses palpated simultaneously with radial or brachial pulse (delay or diminished in coarctaion of aorta)

Murmurs
  Systolic ejection murmur that intensifies with standing or
      Valsalva maneuver and decrease with squatting suggest
      hypertorphic cardiomyopathy.
  Aortic (decrescendo diastolic) or mitral insufficiency (holosys-
      tolic) murmurs may be noted in Marfan's syndrome
  Systolic ejection or midsystolic clicks

significant finding in the history or physical examination is an indication for withholding the athlete from sport participation pending more definitive evaluation by a cardiologist, and recommendation for sport participation will be based on findings of such evaluation. Additional cardiac tests such as electrocardiography, echocardiography, and exercise stress testing are indicated based on history and examination findings on an individual basis. Studies do not support the inclusion of such tests for mass screening of all athletes [19–21].

In athletes who have been diagnosed with a specific cardiovascular condition, the decision to allow participation in a given sport and the level of physical activity is guided largely by several student athlete participation reference sources [14,15,17,18,21,23] and the 26th Bethesda Guidelines [24]. Although a careful cardiovascular screening is recommended and is routinely performed as part of the PPE, it must be recognized that such screening has significant limitations in predicting the likelihood of sudden cardiac death in an individual athlete, even with all normal findings [21,22]. A recent study concluded that preparticipation screening in many colleges and universities in the United States was inadequate to identify cardiovascular conditions with potential risk for sudden cardiac death in competitive student athletes [16].

Sports-associated concussions

Definition

There is no generally accepted definition of concussion. The American Academy of Neurology has defined concussion as a transient alteration in mental status not necessarily associated with loss of consciousness [26]. Confusion and amnesia are considered to be the hallmarks of concussion. Concussion is a result of diffuse injury to the brain and although typically result from direct impact to head, it can also occur in the absence of such direct impact, from sudden deceleration, acceleration or shearing stress to the brain [26–30]. There is no evidence of gross structural alteration of brain structure and neuroimaging studies are normal.

Epidemiology

In the United States more than 300,000 sports-related concussions are reported each year [29,31]. This likely represents an underestimate, as many athletes fail to understand the significance of head injury and do not report such instances. Overall, concussions account for 90% of head injuries in sports. Most concussions have been reported in American football. Other sports with high incidence of concussions include soccer, ice hockey, martial arts, wrestling, and lacrosse [32,34].

Grading systems

Numerous concussion grading criteria and management guidelines (23 by some account) have been published to assess the severity of concussion and develop return to play criteria based on severity [35–41]. None of the grading systems or return to play guidelines has been validated by research [27,35]. Most are based on consensus and expert opinion. Two of the commonly used grading systems are shown in Table 2 [26,38].

Assessment and management guidelines

Initial assessment is based on a meticulous history and neurologic examination. Symptoms and signs of acute cerebral concussion based on Concussion in Sport Group (CISG) guidelines are listed in Box 5 [27]. In athletes with a history of head impact and normal findings on initial assessment, it is critical to watch for evolving symptoms or signs over the next several minutes to hours following the impact [26,27]. The athlete should not be left alone unobserved on the sideline or in the locker room or training room. The athlete may also present in the office setting, with late-onset nonspecific symptoms and

Table 2
Concussion grading systems

Grade	Cantu	American Academy of Neurology
1	No LOC; PTA <30 minutes	No LOC; transient confusion; concussion symptoms or mental status abnormality resolve in <15 minutes
2	LOC <5 minutes; PTA >30 minutes and <24 hours	No LOC; transient confusion; concussion symptoms or mental status abnormality last >15 minutes
3	LOC >5 minutes or PTA >24 hours	Any LOC, either brief or prolonged

Abbreviations: LOC, loss of consciousness; PTA, posttraumatic amnesia.

Box 5. Symptoms and signs of acute cerebral concussion

Cognitive features

　　Unaware of period, opposition, score of game
　　Confusion
　　Amnesia
　　Loss of consciousness
　　Unaware of time, date, place

Typical symptoms

　　Headache
　　Dizziness
　　Nausea
　　Unsteadiness/loss of balance
　　Feeling stunned, "dinged," or "dazed"
　　"Having my bell rung"
　　Seeing stars or flashing lights
　　Ringing in the ears
　　Double vision

Physical signs

　　Loss of consciousness/impaired conscious state
　　Poor coordination or balance
　　Concussive convulsion/impact seizure
　　Gait unsteadiness/loss of balance
　　Slow to answer questions or follow directions
　　Easily distracted, poor concentration
　　Displaying unusual or inappropriate emotions, such as laughing
　　　　or crying
　　Nausea/vomiting
　　Vacant stare/glassy eyes
　　Slurred speech
　　Personality changes
　　Inappropriate playing behavior (eg, running in the wrong direction)
　　Appreciably decreased playing ability

Adapted from Aubry M, Cantu R, Dvorak J, et al. Summary and agreement statement of the First International Conference on Concussion in Sport, Vienna 2001. Phys Sportsmed 2002;30: 57–63; with permission.

signs such as academic difficulties, deteriorating grades, difficulties in attention and concentration, mood disturbances, easy fatigueability, irritability, and sleep disturbances [26,28,33].

An athlete with any symptoms or signs should be removed from sport participation and evaluated further. The Sport in Concussion Group recommends a gradual return to sport, following a stepwise approach starting with complete rest and progressing from light activity, sport-specific activity, noncontact training, and contact sport to full participation [27]. It is recognized that each athlete may progress at his or her individual rate through recovery phase; hence no specific timeline is proposed in terms of return to play. The athlete must be asymptomatic both at rest and on exertion before starting any training [26,27,36,38].

The NCAA does not endorse any of the current grading systems or return to play guidelines because of lack of scientific validity or consensus among experts [13]. Although one or more of the current guidelines may provide a framework for initial assessment and return to play decisions (Tables 3 and 4), the final decision is based on the clinical judgment of the physician, which is based on his or her assessment of the individual athlete [26,27,36,38].

Increasingly, in recent years neuropsychologic testing is being recognized as a valuable tool to objectively assess and monitor recovery after concussion [42–53]. A baseline neuropsychologic profile of an athlete is obtained before that athlete begins sport participation. Neuropsychologic testing is performed soon after concussion and periodically thereafter over the next several months. A return-to-baseline profile suggests recovery and guidance regarding return-to-play decisions. Cost, accessibility, and lack of baseline data for most collegiate

Table 3
Return-to-play criteria following first concussion

	Grade and criteria		
	1	2	3
Cantu guideline	RTP if asymptomatic for 1 week. Terminate season if CT/MRI scan is abnormal	RTP if asymptomatic for 2 weeks; terminate season if CT/MRI scan is abnormal	May not RTP for at least 1 month. After 1 month, RTP if asymptomatic for 1 week
American Academy of Neurology guideline	RTP if asymptomatic for 15 minutes	RTP if asymptomatic for 1 week	Transport to a hospital emergency department. With brief LOC (seconds), may RTP when asymptomatic for 1 week; with prolonged LOC (minutes), may RTP when asymptomatic for 2 weeks

Athlete must be asymptomatic both at rest and on provocative exertion.
Abbreviations: LOC, loss of consciousness; RTP, return to play.

Table 4
Return-to-play criteria: multiple concussions in the same season

Guideline	Frequency	Return to play criteria		
		Grade 1	Grade 2	Grade 3
Cantu	Second concussion	RTP in 2 weeks if asymptomatic for 1 week	May not RTP for at least 1 month; may then RTP if asymptomatic for 1 week; consider terminating season	Terminate season; may RTP next season if asymptomatic
	Third concussion	Terminate season; may RTP next season if asymptomatic	Terminate season; may RTP next season if asymptomatic	Consider no further contact sports
American Academy of Neurology	Second	RTP if asymptomatic for 1 week	Athlete may RTP if asymptomatic for 2 weeks; terminate season if CT/MRI scan is abnormal	May RTP if asymptomatic for 1 month or longer; terminate season if CT/MRI scan is abnormal
	Third concussion	No recommendation	No recommendation	No recommendation

Athlete must be asymptomatic both at rest and on provocative exertion.
Abbreviations: LOC, loss of consciousness; RTP, return to play.

athletes are at present potential barriers to widespread application of neuro-psychologic testing in the management of concussion.

Current guidelines do not recommend routine use of neuroimaging in the evaluation of concussions [26,27,41,54–56]. Neuroimaging is indicated in athletes with loss of consciousness, persistent symptoms and signs, and focal neurologic findings [26,38,54,55].

Complications

Case reports of a potential acute complication called *second impact syndrome* following concussion have been reported in athletes who sustain a second blow to the head while they are still symptomatic from the first concussion [34,38,56,57,58]. It is hypothesized that following a second blow to the head, a cascade of pathophysiologic events leads to increased intracranial pressure, cerebral edema, and herniation with high mortality, more than 50% of which are reported to occur within minutes [34,38]. All such cases have been reported in young male athletes. Some studies have identified a potential genetic pre-disposition for adverse outcome following head injury in some individuals [57,62–69]. Awareness and education about this potential complication is important, and the athlete should not be allowed to resume sport participation before he or she is fully asymptomatic and has had a normal examination.

Many studies have reported that recurrent concussions impart cumulative effects on brain resulting in long-term deterioration in neurocognitive functioning [40,57,58,60,63,66–69]. The importance of subtle long-term adverse effects of concussions must be discussed with all athletes who sustain or are at risk for head injury. Depending on the severity of initial neurocognitive deficits, the recovery may take from weeks to months, with significant impact on college athlete's academic and social functioning.

Use of drugs and dietary supplements

Use of drugs and dietary supplements by athletes at all levels of participation remains a persistent problem, and the trend in drug and supplement use changes over time [70–76]. The enormous temptation for using performance-enhancing substances is supported by a highly sophisticated underground network for manufacturing and distribution of such agents as exemplified by the recent discovery of the designer steroid tetrahydrogestrinone [77]. The NCAA conducts drug-use surveys of student athletes in all sports every 4 years [13]. Drug use spans the spectrum of substances used for sport performance enhancement (such as anabolic steroids) to recreational agents (such as alcohol and marijuana). Alcohol and marijuana remain the most commonly used drugs on college campuses; 80% of students report use of alcohol, and 28% report use of marijuana [13].

The NCAA maintains a list of substances banned in sports and conducts drug testing at championship events as well as year-round random testing. The NCAA guideline 2i recommends that drug education and testing programs be established and implemented by all member institutions [13].

Some of the drugs known to be relatively more commonly used by athletes are listed in Box 6 [70,73,74,78–82]. NCAA guideline 2k and 2l addresses the use of local anesthetics and injectable corticosteroids in student athletes [13]. The use of these agents locally is left to the discretion of the treating physician with the full understanding of risks and benefits of such use in the context of sport injuries.

The use of dietary supplements is widespread in the general United States population, ranging from 40% to 60% [72,75,83]. The exact prevalence of various dietary supplements used by college athletes is not known. Dietary supplements are easily and legally available and are not regulated by the US Food and Drug Administration, and research-based data on their safety and effectiveness are limited [83]. Although some dietary supplements constitute part of a normal diet (eg, proteins, carbohydrates, vitamins, and some minerals) and as such are known to be essential and safe, others (eg, creatine, androsteinedione, and numerous others) are not. Some of the currently popular supplements are listed in Box 7 [72,74,84–110].

In general, no drugs or nutritional supplements are recommended to enhance athletic performance. The long-term effects of many of the performance-

Box 6. Drugs abused in sports

Alcohol

Moderate amounts theorized to decrease anxiety, improve hand steadiness. Adverse impact on coordination, balance, reaction time, endurance. Predispose to dehydration and hypoglycemia, impaired mental judgment. Formally prohibited only in pentathlon. Sanctions likely in archery and shooting events.

Amphetamines

Potent central nervous system stimulants. Improve alertness, arousal, concentration, self-confidence. Improve muscle contractility; decrease or postpone fatigue. Appetite suppressant. Adverse effects include hypertension, sudden cardiac death, stroke, psychotic reactions, heat illness, and heat stroke. Available as a tablet and a powder. Swallowed, inhaled, or injected.

Anabolic–androgenic steroids

Increase muscle mass, strength, and power when used in conjunction with regular resistance training and appropriate diet. Continued use remains a major problem at all levels of sports. Dangerous adverse effects include hepatotoxicity, atherosclerosis, hypertension, myocardial ischemia, sudden cardiac death, psychotic reactions.

Testosterone

Oral, injectable, patch. Used for its anabolic, androgenic effects. Increases bone density, decreases fat mass, increases lean muscle mass. Effective when used in conjunction with regular resistance training and appropriate diet. Dangerous side effects similar to those of anabolic–androgenic steroids.

Blood-doping and erythropoietin

Blood needs storage and infusion. Erythropietin needs to be injected. Very expensive. Use is a continued problem in endurance sports. Increases oxygen-carrying capacity of blood. Improves endurance and aerobic capacity. Difficult to detect with current urine tests. Associated with sudden death, blood-borne infections, hypertension, thromboembolic events, myocardial infarction, stroke.

Human growth hormone

Used for its anabolic effects. Injectable form. Expensive. Increases lean muscle mass, decreases fat mass, enhances strength and power. Ergogenic effects not susbstantiated. Side effects are well documented and include pseudotumor cerebri, carpal tunnel syndrome, arthralgias, myopathy, worsening scoliosis/kyphosis, hyperglycemia, insulin resistance, hypothyroidism, adrenal insufficiency, acute pancreatitis, hepatotoxicity, increased risk for certain malignancies.

---

enhancing substances are not fully elucidated, and their use by young athletes is strongly discouraged by all major sport-governing bodies and scientific societies.

NCAA injury surveillance system

The NCAA Injury Surveillance System collects injury data from a representative sample of member institutions every year [13]. Data is analyzed to identify incidence and trends of various injuries in different sports. For the purpose of the Injury Surveillance System, a reportable injury is one that "occurs as a result of participation in an organized intercollegiate practice or game; requires medical attention by a team athletic trainer or physician; and results in restriction of the student-athlete's participation or performance for one or more days beyond the day of injury" [13]. Injury rates for 2002–2004 are shown in Figs. 1 and 2 [13]. Practice injuries resulting in 7 or more days of time loss were highest in spring football (4.4%), followed by wrestling (2.2%), women's gymnastics (2.0%), football (1.6%), and women's soccer (1.4%). Game injuries resulting in 7 or more days of time loss were highest in football (14%), followed by wrestling (11.6%), men's ice hockey (5.4%), men's soccer (4.8%), and women's soccer (4.8%). Injuries resulting in surgery were most frequent in football, both during practice (1.0%) and during a game (3.3%) [13].

Ankle sprains

Ankle sprains are the most common acute sport injury and account for 10% to 30% of all musculoskeletal injuries reported in sports [111,112]. Sprains account for most ankle injuries in sports; 85% are inversion or lateral sprains, while 15% are eversion or medial sprains. Ankle sprains are seen most frequently in soccer, dance, volleyball, running, football, basketball, hockey, baseball, and gymnastics [111,112].

Box 7. Summary of common supplements

Arginine

Promoted to increase growth hormone secretion. Oral arginine not effective. No evidence of increased muscle mass or improved sports performance.

Androsteinedione and dehydroepiandrosterone

Androsteinedione and dehydrepioandrosterone are precursors of testosterone. No evidence of increased testosterone levels. Serious side effects similar to those associated with anabolic–androgenic steroid use. US Food and Drug Administration recently issued a warning concerning serious side effects of androsteinedione.

Conjugated linoleic acid

No increase in lean body mass or strength. No effects on improving immunity. Inconclusive evidence on effectiveness to reduce body fat.

Creatine

Effective in increasing weight. Effective in improving performance in short-term high-intensity, intermittent activities. Improves recovery time. Effective only if used with regular resistance training. Some evidence shows improved lean mass and strength. No serious side effects with short-term use in persons with no renal disease. Effects of long-term use not known. Associated with cases of dehydration, heat illness, hypertension, muscle cramps. No effects on long-term aerobic activities.

Ephedrine and ephedra

Increases endurance and postpones fatigue. Increases sense of energy. Effective weight loss shown in studies of at least 6 months' duration. Enhances weight loss when used with caffeine. Increases risk for pychosis, anxiety, insomnia, headaches. Rare but serious risks include death, myocardial infarction, cardiac arrythmias, stroke, hypertension, and seizures. Banned by the US Food and Drug Adminisration from over-the-counter products.

Garcinia cambogia

Herbal compound found in many weight loss products. Active ingredient is hydroxycitric acid. No conclusive evidence of effectiveness.

Glutamine

Promoted to increase muscle mass and strength and to improve immune function. Some studies suggest improved high-intensity resistance training effects. No evidence of improved immunity.

Protein

Increased need for both resistance training and endurance training. Effective in increasing muscle mass and strength. For strength/resistance training, should be consumed immediately before and following exercise; for aerobic activities, should be taken after exercise. No serious side effects in persons with no renal disease. Daily intake exceeding 1.8 g/kg/body weight is not recommended.

Tribulus terrestris

Herb containing glycosides/saponins. No evidence of improved strength or exercise performance. Potential hepatic and neuro-toxicity based on animal studies.

Typical inversion sprain occurs when the foot is suddenly turned in when landing from a jump, stepping or landing on one foot, suddenly changing direction, suddenly decelerating, or losing balance [113–116]. A history of previous ankle sprain and inadequate rehabilitation increases the risk for subsequent sprain.

The athlete typically gives a history of sudden inversion of the foot associated with pain. There may or may not be a history of feeling or hearing a "pop." The athlete may not be able to continue to play depending on the severity of the injury. There is typically a diffuse swelling around the ankle that may be less apparent if ice was applied immediately. The athlete may have pain on weight bearing. Pain is elicited on active and passive movements of the ankle. Apparent deformity or joint effusion is indicative of a more severe underlying injury. In a typical inversion sprain, tenderness can be localized over the anterior talofibular ligament. Tenderness over the talus, 5th metatarsal, or malleolus indicates a need for radiographic examination to rule out a fracture. In an inversion sprain the

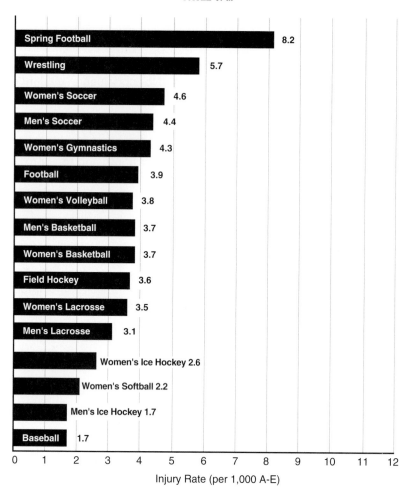

Fig. 1. Average practice injury rate (expressed as injuries per 1000 athlete exposures) for all sports analyzed in the Injury Surveillance System in the 2002–2003 season. A-E, athletic exposure (one athlete participating in one practice or contest in which said athlete is exposed to the possibility of athletic injury). (*From* National Collegiate Athletic Association. NCAA sports medicine handbook 2003–2004. Indianapolis (IN): National Collegiate Athletic Association; 2004; with permission.)

anterior talofibular ligament (ATFL) is the most commonly injured ligament, followed by the calcaneofibular and posterior talofibular, in that order (Fig. 3) [117–119]. An anterior drawer test (Fig. 4) assesses the integrity of the ATFL. A soft end point with increased anterior movement on anterior drawer test is noted in severe ATFL sprains [111,113]. Inability to bear weight, apparent deformity, eversion sprain, and bony tenderness are indications for radiographic examination; antero-posterior, lateral, and mortise views should be obtained [111,112,119].

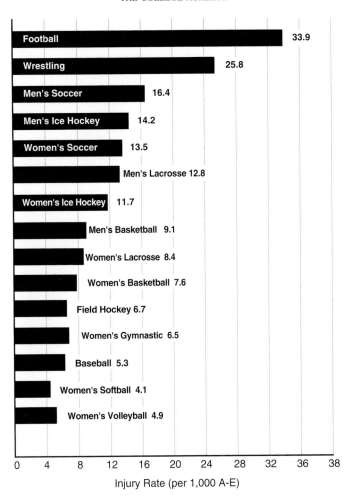

Fig. 2. Average game injury rate (expressed as injuries per 1000 athlete exposures) for all sports analyzed in the Injury Surveillance System in the 2002–2003 season. (*From* National Collegiate Athletic Association. NCAA sports medicine handbook 2003–2004. Indianapolis (IN): National Collegiate Athletic Association; 2004; with permission.)

Immediate treatment consists of local application of ice, compression, elevation, and protective bracing with a lace-up or stir-up brace. The athlete may need crutches depending on pain and severity of the injury. The athlete should be referred for full ankle rehabilitation. Typical recovery can take between 3 and 8 weeks before full return to sports. Failure to recover as expected and persistent disability or pain should prompt reassessment and consideration of associated injuries or complications such as anterior talar impingement, impingement spurs, peroneal tendonitis or subluxation, osteochonral fracture of the talus, tibio-fibular syndesmosis sprain, and functional or mechanical ankle

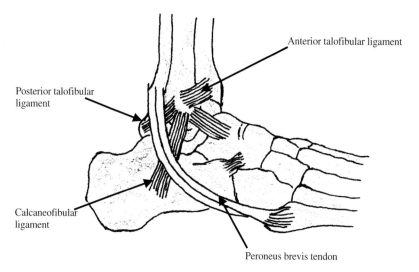

Anterior talofibular ligament

Posterior talofibular
ligament

Calcaneofibular
ligament

Peroneus brevis tendon

Fig. 3. Lateral view of ankle.

instability [111,112,114,116,118]. Various approaches for prevention of ankle sprains, such as high ankle shoes, taping, braces, and correcting foot bio-mechanics have been investigated, and data provide equivocal evidence in support of efficacy of any one or more of these preventive measures [120–125]. Sports-specific training and adequate rehabilitation of ankle sprain have been shown in some studies to be effective strategies in reducing incidence of ankle sprains.

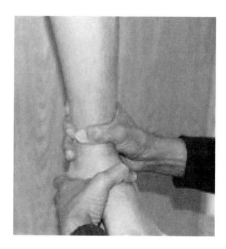

Fig. 4. Anterior drawer test for ankle.

Acute knee injuries

Acute injuries of the knee are common in both contact as well as noncontact sports and are relatively frequent in soccer, rugby, hockey, and football [111,112,126,127]. Acute injuries may involve any of the ligaments, menisci, or bony structures in and around the knee joint (Fig. 5). Anterior cruciate ligament, medial collateral ligament, and medial meniscal injuries are common and are briefly reviewed here.

Anterior cruciate ligament (ACL) sprains are common in sports, and most are noncontact injuries [111,112,127]. The typical mechanism is a sudden deceleration and pivoting movement. The athlete feels sudden pain and the knee gives out. The athlete is not able to continue to play because of knee instability and pain. Within a few minutes to hours, the knee swelling is noted due to acute hemarthrosis. Other causes of acute hemarthrosis include a fracture, patellar dislocation, and peripheral tear of a meniscus. The athlete may or may not be able to bear weight. The athlete may not be able to fully extend or flex the knee

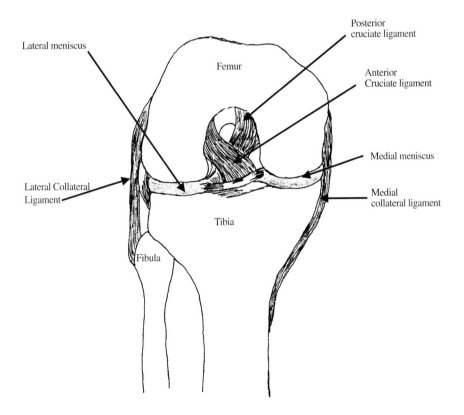

Fig. 5. Anterior view of open knee.

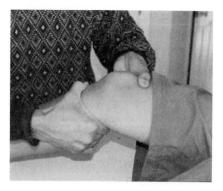

Fig. 6. Lachman test for the ACL. With the patient supine, knee flexed at approximately 20°, stabilize femur with one hand and move tibia forward with the other. Increased forward movement and loss of end point indicate an ACL tear.

because of knee effusion and hamstring spasm. In an isolated ACL sprain, there usually is no peripatellar or joint line tenderness. The Lachman test (Fig. 6) is highly specific and sensitive for assessing a complete tear of the ACL [111–113]; it is performed with the knee in 15° to 30° flexion while the athlete is supine on a table with one hand stabilizing the femur and the other attempting anterior translation of the tibia over the femur. There is loss of end point and increased anterior translation of the tibia over the femur in a complete tear of the ACL. MRI is diagnostic and also helps delineate the extent of associated injuries. The knee may be placed in an immobilizer and the athlete may need crutches. All suspected or diagnosed ACL sprains should be referred to an orthopedic surgeon for definitive treatment, which in most young athletes is reconstruction of the ACL followed by appropriate rehabilitation [112].

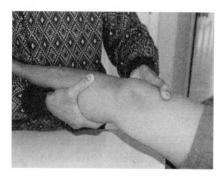

Fig. 7. Valgus stress for the medial collateral ligament. With the patient supine, knee extended, stabilize femur with one hand and apply valgus stress with other hand distal to knee.

A medial collateral ligament sprain typically occurs when the athlete sustains a sudden forceful impact on the lateral aspect of the knee, usually from a collision with another athlete. The athlete presents with pain and localized tenderness over the medial aspect of the knee over the ligament. There is no instability or swelling of the knee. The athlete is generally able to walk with full weight bearing. Full range of motion is maintained. The pain is elicited through valgus stress applied to the knee (Fig. 7). In a complete tear, gaping or increased laxity is noted on valgus stress. A hinged brace may allow for early range of motion, strengthening, and endurance exercises. Healing occurs within a few days, and the athlete is allowed to return to sports when pain-free and examination is normal.

A medial meniscus injury may occur as an isolated injury or may be associated with other injuries, most commonly with a sprained ACL. A sudden deceleration, stop, and twisting of the knee is the typical mechanism of injury [111,112]. The athlete presents with minimal or no swelling, medial knee pain, and locking of knee. Medial joint line tenderness is noted and McMurray test is positive

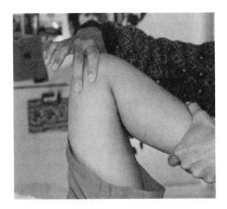

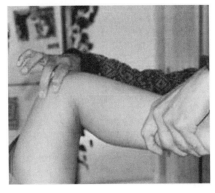

Fig. 8. McMurray test. With the patient supine, the knee and hip are flexed, with one hand over the knee with fingers over the medial joint line and thumb over the lateral, and the knee is extended and externally rotated. The patient may feel pain medially or the examiner may feel the torn posterior horn of medial meniscus. To assess lateral meniscus, knee is internally rotated.

[113]. With the athlete supine on a table, hip and knee flexed as a starting position, gently extend and externally rotate the knee, with fingers on the medical joint line (Fig. 8). The athlete will have acute pain medially and the examiner may feel the torn posterior horn of the medical meniscus. MRI is usually diagnostic, although arthroscopy may be needed in some cases. An orthopedic consultation is generally indicated, because most meniscal tears have poor potential for healing and need definitive repair in young active athletes. Indications for orthopedic consultation for knee injuries include: complete tear of anterior cruciate or collateral ligaments, torn meniscus, patellar dislocation,

---

Box 8. Causes of low back pain in young athletes

Muscle/soft tissue
  Muscle strains/ligamentous sprains (most common cause)
Psychosomatic
Disk conditions
  Disk rupture/herniation
  Diskitis
  Disk degeneration
  Hypermobility syndrome
  Postural kyphosis
Vertebral and spinal cord
  Spondylolysis and spondylolisthesis
  Idiopathic juvenile osteoporosis
  Lumbarization or sacralization
  Spina bifida occulta
  Vertebral osteomyelitis
  Sacroiliac joint disorders/sacral stress fractures
  Facet syndrome/stress fracture
  Spine fracture
  Benign and malignant tumors of the spine or cord
Inflammatory conditions
  Spondyloarthropathy
  Ankylosing spondylitis
  Rheumatoid arthritis
  Osteoarthritis of spine
Intra-abdominal conditions
  Inflammatory bowel disease
  Renal disease
  Urinary tract infection
  Gynecologic conditions
  Intra-abdominal neoplasms

Box 9. Specific examination of the young athlete with lower back pain

Standing

- Gait: observe for limping or other gait abnormalities; degree of pain or discomfort during ambulation or during examination should be noted
- Posture
- Spine curvature (scoliosis, kyphosis, lordosis)
- Alignment of iliac crests
- Active range of movements of lumbo-sacral spine (flexion, extension, lateral flexion, rotation)
- One-legged hyperextension test, which may elicit localized lumbar pain in many athletes with spondyloysis of lumbar spine
- Trendelenburg test; side with weak gluteus medius (S 1) will sag.
- Test strength of calf muscles by repeated unilateral heel raises (S1)
- Test strength of anterior tibialis by heel walking (L5)
- Palpate and localize soft tissue or bony tenderness

Supine

- Note level of anterior superior iliac spines
- Measure leg length (from anterior superior iliac spine to lateral malleolus)
- Note thigh or leg atrophy (measure girth)
- Note hamstring flexibility
- Test strength of following muscles:
  Abdominals (T6-L1)
  Hip flexors (L2)
  Quadriceps (knee extension, L3)
  Anterior tibialis (foot/ankle dorsiflexion, L4)
  Extensor hallucis longus (toe extension, L5)
  Hamstrings (knee flexion, S2)
- Test sensation to touch:
  Medial mid-thigh (L2)
  Superior aspect of medial knee (L3)
  Dorsum of foot (L4)
  Lateral border/outer plantar aspect of foot (S1)
  Popliteal fossa (S2)

- Test reflexes:
  Deep tendon reflexes (patellar [L4], Achilles [S1])
  Superficial reflexes (abdominal, cremasteric)
  Pathologic (plantar)
- Straight leg raise (increased tension on sciatic nerve roots cause pain radiating in the nerve root distribution in lower extremity)
- Sacroiliac tests:
  Patrick or FABER test (Fig. 9)
  Gaenslin test (Fig. 10)

Prone

- Hyperextension of the back to differentiate between postural round back (deformity disappears on hyperextension) and kyphosis (deformity persists on hyperextension)

fractures in and around the knee, ruptured or avulsed quadriceps or patellar tendon, intra-articular loose body, osteochondritis dessicans, osteomyelitis, and septic arthtitis [111,112,126,127].

Back pain in athletes

The prevalence of lower back pain is higher in athletes than in the general population. The reported range of prevalence of back pain in athletes ranges from

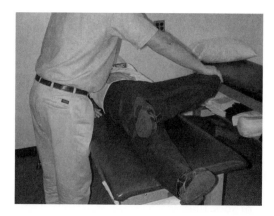

Fig. 9. Patrick or FABER test for sacroiliac joint. Pain in sacroiliac or hip may be elicited with patient supine, knee partially flexed, and hip flexed, abducted and externally rotated with gentle posteriorly directed pressure.

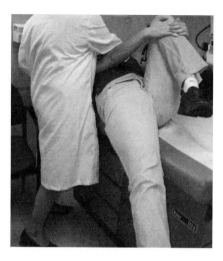

Fig. 10. Gaenslin test. With the patient supine and one leg flexed at the knee and hip, the other leg extended at the hip is lowered from the edge of the examination table. Pain is elicited in the sacroiliac area on the side where the leg is lowered.

1% to more than 30% depending on sport, sex, level of training, and specific techniques involved [128,129]. Lower back pain is relatively more common in gymnastics, wrestling, tennis, soccer, golf, rowing, weight lifting, and football. The recurrence rate is also higher in those athletes who have a past history of back pain [111,113,128,129].

The most common cause of lower back pain in college-age athletes is acute or chronic strain or sprain [128]. In the absence of other injuries these athletes recover rapidly following a brief period of relative rest followed by back flexibility and strengthening exercises. Prevention strategies should address regular training and conditioning, posture, and correct sport techniques [130]. The athlete should work with a physical therapist or athletic trainer to develop an individualized rehabilitation and conditioning program. The differential diagnosis of chronic or recurrent lower back pain in the athlete should include careful consideration of the conditions listed in Box 8 [111,112,128,129,131]. The mainstay of evaluation is history and physical examination.

History

History should ascertain the nature of the pain, location, onset, duration, course, and aggravating and relieving factors. Radiation of pain in the lower extremities, paresthesias, and weakness may suggest neurologic involvement. The mechanism of injury will further help delineate the nature of the underlying injury. A sudden increase in the volume and intensity of activity or a change in the nature of activity may contribute to back pain. One should ascertain limitations of daily activities or sport participation as an indicator of severity of the injury or pain. Also inquire about previous history of treatment and response: medications, brace, physical therapy. Ask the athlete about any abdominal, genitourinary, or constitutional symptoms.

Physical examination

In addition to general physical examination as indicated by history (abdomen, genitourinary), specific examination of the young athlete who presents with lower back pain should include the items listed in Box 9 [111–113].

Shoulder impingement syndrome

Shoulder pain is a common complaint in collegiate athlete resulting from a number of underlying causes (Box 10) [111,112,132–135]. A relatively common cause of shoulder pain in athletes is shoulder or rotator cuff impingement

---

Box 10. Causes of chronic/recurrent shoulder pain

Intrinsic causes

    Glenohumeral joint instability
    Long head of biceps tendonitis
    Rotator cuff impingement, tendonitis, tear
    Scapular dyskinesis
    Subacromial bursitis
    Arthritis of glenohumeral joint, acromioclavicular joint
    Acromioclavicular joint sprain
    Atraumatic osteolysis of distal clavicle
    Stress fracture of scapula, proximal humerus

Referred pain

    Conditions affecting cervical cord; spinal cord or nerve root impingement; spinal cord tumor; syringomyelia
    Cervical disk herniation
    Cardiac disease
    Lung disease
    Thoracic outlet syndrome
    Cervical rib
    Vascular pain (eg, effort thrombosis)
    Brachial plexus injuries
    Suprascapular neuropathy

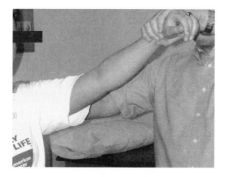

Fig. 11. Neer impingement sign. Forced forward flexion of shoulder will elicit shoulder pain.

syndrome. The muscles of rotator cuff are supraspinatus, infraspinatus, subscapu-laris, and teres minor, which along with the long head of biceps tendon act as dynamic stabilizers during glenohumeral joint movements [111,112,132,133].

Lesions of rotator cuff, especially the supraspinatus tendon underneath the coracoacromial arch, can occur as a result of overuse and glenohumeral joint instability. Shoulder impingement is relatively more common in sports involving repeated overhead activity, such as baseball pitching, swimming, and tennis. The athlete typically presents with pain associated with overhead activity that may be severe enough to limit continued sport participation. There may be pain extending into the arm, night pain, and feeling of shoulder stiffness. The athlete notices deterioration in sport performance. On examination pain is elicited on abduction and external rotation of the shoulder, and the Neer (Fig. 11) and Hawkins (Fig. 12) impingement signs are positive [111–113]. Test of supra-spinatus (Fig. 13) may result in pain or detect weakness. In patients with anterior glenohumeral instability, pain may be elicited with patient supine and abduction and external rotation of the arm, which may be relieved with moving the humeral

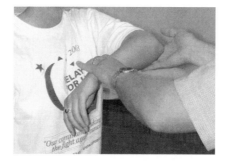

Fig. 12. Hawkins impingement sign. Shoulder pain is elicited upon forcible internal rotation of the arm flexed forward 90°.

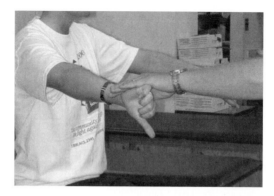

Fig. 13. Supraspinatus test. With the elbow extended and the arm at 90° abduction, forward flexed, and internally rotated (empty can sign), manual resistance is applied. In a supraspinatus lesion pain is felt in the shoulder or weakness in abduction is detected.

head back into glenoid by a posteriorly directed force (Fig. 14). Typically, there is no swelling of the shoulder joint. Injection of xylocaine in the subacromial bursa may relieve the pain temporarily. Shoulder radiographs may be normal in most young athletes with acute impingement. MRI scans may show evidence of tendonitis, subacromial bursitis, or rotator cuff or labral tears if present in severe acute injuries, and may help in the differential diagnosis.

Treatment requires a period of relative rest which may include no sports participation and short-term use of nonsteroidal anti-inflammatory drugs. Rotator cuff rehabilitation exercises are started with a physical therapist as soon as the patient can tolerate them. Most young athletes respond well to a short period of physical therapy [136,137].

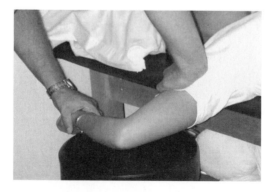

Fig. 14. Jobe's relocation test (Fowler's sign). With the patient supine, the arm is abducted and externally rotated until the patient feels pain or apprehension. Pain is relieved with the arm supported in the posterior direction.

Acknowledgments

The authors thank Cori Edgecomb for administrative assistance in the preparation of the manuscript.

References

[1] Jenkins M. Special issues in athletic medicine. In: Turner HS, Hurley JL, editors. The history and practice of college health. Lexington (KY): The University Press of Kentucky; 2002. p. 263–301.

[2] Joy EA, Paisley TS, Price R, et al. Optimizing the collegiate preparticipation physical evaluation. Clin J Sport Med 2004;14:183–7.

[3] Greydanus DE, Patel DR, Luckstead EF, et al. Value of sports pre-participation examination in health care for adolescents. Med Sci Monit 2004;10:1–11.

[4] Lively MW. Preparticipation physical examinations: a collegiate experience. Clin J Sport Med 1999;9:3–8.

[5] American Academy of Family Physicians, American Academy of Orthopedic Surgeons, American College of Sports Medicine, American Medical Society for Sports Medicine, American Orthopedic Society for Sports Medicine, American Osteopathic Academy of Sports Medicine. Female athlete issues for the team physician: a consensus statement. Med Sci Sports Exerc 2003;35:1785–93 [erratum: Med Sci Sports Exerc 2003;35:2122].

[6] Greydanus DE, Patel DR. The female athlete. Before and beyond puberty. Pediatr Clin North Am 2002;49:553–80.

[7] Nattive A, Puffer J, Green G. Lifestyle and health risks of collegiate athletes: a multi-center study. Clin J Sport Med 1997;7:262–72.

[8] Kokotailo P, Henry B, Koscik R, et al. Substance abuse and other risk behaviors in collegiate athletes. Clin J Sport Med 1996;6:183–9.

[9] Patel DR, Luckstead EF. Sports participation, risk taking, and health risk behaviors. Adol Med 2000;11:141–55.

[10] American Academy of Pediatrics, American Academy of Family Physicians, American Medical Society for Sports Medicine, American Orthopedic Society for Sports Medicine, American Osteopathic Association for Sports Medicine. Preparticipation physical evaluation monograph. 3rd edition. Minneapolis (MN): McGraw-Hill Medical Publishing; 2004.

[11] Wingfield K, Matheson GO, Meeuwisse WH. Preparticipation evaluation. Clin J Sport Med 2004;14:109–22.

[12] Garrick JG. Preparticipation orthopedic screening evaluation. Clin J Sport Med 2004;14:123–6.

[13] National Collegiate Athletic Association. Sports medicine handbook. 16th edition. Indianapolis (IN): National Collegiate Athletic Association; 2004.

[14] Luckstead EF. Cardiac risk factors and participation guidelines for youth sports. Pediatr Clin North Am 2002;49:681–708.

[15] Pfister GC, Puffer JC, Maron BJ. Preparticipation cardiovascular screening for US collegiate student-athletes. JAMA 2000;283:1597–9.

[16] Coris EE, Sahebzamani F, Walz S, et al. Automated external defibrillators in National Collegiate Athletic Association division I athletics. Am J Sports Med 2004;32:744–54.

[17] Hipp AA, Heitkamp HC, Rocker K, et al. Hypertrophic cardiomyopathy–sports-related aspects of diagnosis, therapy, and sports eligibility. Int J Sports Med 2004;25:20–6.

[18] Corrado D, Basso C, Rizzoli G, et al. Does sports activity enhance the risk of sudden death in adolescents and young adults? J Am Coll Cardiol 2003;42:1959–63.

[19] Hosey RG, Armsey TD. Sudden cardiac death. Clin Sports Med 2003;22:51–66.

[20] Seto CK. Preparticipation cardiovascular screening. Clin Sports Med 2003;22:23–35.

[21] Beckerman J, Wang P, Hlatky M. Cardiovascular screening of athletes. Clin J Sport Med 2004;14:127–33.

[22] Maron BJ. Sudden death in young athletes. N Engl J Med 2003;349:1064–75.

[23] Maron BJ, Thompson PD, Puffer JC, et al. Cardiovascular preparticipation screening of competitive athletes: a statement for health professionals from the Sudden Death Committee (Clinical Cardiology) and Congenital Cardiac Defects Committee (Cardiovascular Diseases in the Young). American Heart Association. AHA Medical/Scientific Statement. Circulation 1996; 94:850–6.

[24] American Heart Association. 26th Bethesda Conference. Recommendations for determining eligibility for competition in athletes with cardiovascular abnormalities. J Am Coll Cardiol 1994;24:845–99.

[25] Maron BJ, Shirani J, Poliac LC, et al. Sudden death in young competitive athletes: clinical, demographic and pathological profiles. JAMA 1996;276:199–204.

[26] Quality Standards Subcommittee of the American Academy of Neurology. The management of concussion in sports. Neurology 1997;48:581–5.

[27] Aubry M, Cantu R, Dvorak J, et al. Summary and agreement statement of the first International Conference on Concussion in Sport, Vienna 2001. Phys Sportsmed 2002;30:57–63.

[28] Wojtys EM, Hovda D, Landry G, et al. Concussion in sports. Am J Sports Med 1999;27: 676–87.

[29] Kelly JP. Traumatic brain injury and concussion in sports. JAMA 1999;282:989–91.

[30] Grindel SH. Epidemiology and pathophysiology of minor traumatic brain injury. Curr Sports Med Rep 2003;2:18–23.

[31] Koh JO, Cassidy JD, Watkinson EJ. Incidence of concussion in contact sports: a systematic review of the evidence. Brain Inj 2003;17:901–17.

[32] McCrory P, Johnston K, Meeuwisse W, et al. Evidence based review of sport related concussion: basic science. Clin J Sport Med 2001;11:160–6.

[33] Johnston K, McCrory P, Mohtadi N, et al. Evidence based review of sport related concussion: clinical science. Clin J Sport Med 2001;11:150–60.

[34] Bailes JE, Cantu RC. Head injury in athletes. Neurosurgery 2001;48:26–46.

[35] Leclerc S, Lassonde M, Delaney JS, et al. Recommendations for grading of concussion in athletes. Sports Med 2001;31:629–36.

[36] Collins MW, Hawn KL. The clinical management of sports concussion. Curr Sports Med Rep 2002;1:12–22.

[37] Johnston KM, Lassonde M, Ptito A. A contemporary neurosurgical approach to sport related head injury: the McGill concussion protocol. J Am Coll Surg 2001;192:515–24.

[38] Cantu RC. Guidelines for return to contact sports after a cerebral concussion. Phys Sportsmed 1986;14:75–83.

[39] Colorado Medical Society. Guidelines for the management of concussion in sports. Denver (CO): Colorado Medical Society; 1991.

[40] Gebke KB. Mild traumatic brain injury. Curr Sport Med Rep 2002;1:23–7.

[41] Canadian Academy of Sports Medicine Committee. Canadian Academy of Sports Medicine Guidelines for assessment and management of sport-related concussion. Clin J Sport Med 2000; 10:209–11.

[42] Maroon JC, Lovell MR, Norwig J, et al. Cerebral concussion in athletes: evaluation and neuropsychological testing. Neurosurgery 2000;47:659–72.

[43] Grindel SH, Lovell MR, Collins MW. The assessment of sport-related concussion: the evidence behind neuropsychological testing and management. Clin J Sport Med 2001;11:134–43.

[44] Collie A, Darby D, Maruff P. Computerised cognitive assessment of athletes with sports related head injury. Br J Sports Med 2001;35:297–302.

[45] Capruso DX, Levin HS. Cognitive impairment following closed head injury. Neurologic Clinic 1992;10:879–91.

[46] Hinton-Bayre AD, Geffen G. Severity of sports-related concussion and neuropsychological test performance. Neurology 2002;59:1068–70.

[47] Schatz P, Zillmer EA. Computer-based assessment of sports-related concussion. Appl Neuropsychol 2003;10:42–7.

[48] Field M, Collins MW, Lovell MR, Maroon J. Does age play a role in recovery from sports-

related concussion? A comparison of high school and collegiate athletes. J Pediatr 2003;142: 546–53.

[49] Daniel JC, Olesniewicz MH, Reeves DL, et al. Repeated measures of cognitive processing efficiency in adolescent athletes: implications for monitoring recovery from concussion. Neuropsychiatry Neuropsychol Behav Neurol 1999;12:167–9.

[50] Ryan JP, Atkinson TM, Dunham KT. Sports-related and gender differences on neuro-psychological measures of frontal lobe functioning. Clin J Sport Med 2004;14:18–24.

[51] Echemendia RJ, Putukian M, Mackin RC, et al. Neuropsychological test performance prior to and following sports-related mild traumatic brain injury. Clin J Sport Med 2001;11:23–31.

[52] Downs DS, Abwender D. Neuropsychological impairment in soccer athletes. J Sport Med Phys Fitness 2002;42:103–7.

[53] Aster EJT, Kessels AG, Lezak MD, et al. Neuropsychological impairment in amateur soccer players. JAMA 1999;282:971–3.

[54] Haydel MJ, Preston CA, Mills TJ, et al. Indications for computed tomography in patients with minor head injury. N Engl J Med 2000;343:100–5.

[55] Chen SHA, Kareken DA, Fastenau PS, et al. A study of persistent post-concussion symptoms in mild head trauma using positron emission tomography. J Neurol Neurosur Psychiatry 2003;74: 326–32.

[56] McCrory P. Treatment of recurrent concussion. Curr Sport Med Rep 2002;1:28–32.

[57] McCrory P. What advice should we give to athletes postconcussion? Br J Sports Med 2002; 36:316–8.

[58] Kelly JP, Rosenberg JH. The diagnosis and management of concussion in sports. Neurology 1997;48:575–80.

[59] Bruno LA, Gennarelli TA, Torg JS. Management guidelines for head injuries in athletics. Clin Sports Med 1987;6:17–29.

[60] Landry GL. Central nervous system trauma: management of concussions in athletes. Pediatr Clin North Am 2002;49:723–41.

[61] Kelly JP, Nichols JS, Filley CM, et al. Concussion in sports: guidelines for the prevention of catastrophic outcome. JAMA 1991;266:2867–9.

[62] Webbe FM, Ochs SR. Recency and frequency of soccer heading interact to decrease neurocognitive performance. Appl Neuropsychol 2003;10:31–41.

[63] Webbe FM, Barth JT. Short-term and long-term outcome of athletic closed head injuries. Clin Sports Med 2003;22:577–92.

[64] McCrory PR, Berkovic SF. Second impact syndrome. Neurology 1998;50:677–83.

[65] Ferguson RJ, Mittenberg W, Barone DF. Postconcussion syndrome following sports related head injury: expectation as etiology. Neuropsychology 1999;13:582–9.

[66] Macciocchi SN, Barth JT, Littlefield LM. Outcome after mild head injury. Clin Sports Med 1998;17:27–36.

[67] Robadi MH, Jordan BD. The cumulative effect of repetitive concussion in sports. Clin J Sport Med 2001;11:194–8.

[68] Guskiewicz KM, McCrea M, Marshall SW, et al. Cumulative effects associated with recurrent concussion in collegiate football players: The NCAA Concussion Study. JAMA 2003;290: 2549–55.

[69] Master JT, Kessels AGH, Jordan BD, et al. Chronic traumatic brain injury in professional soccer players. Neurology 1998;51:791–6.

[70] Tokish JM, Kocher MS, Hawkins RJ. Ergogenic aids: a review of basic science, performance, side effects, and status in sports. Am J Sports Med 2004;32:1543–53.

[71] Froiland K, Koszewski W, Hingst J, et al. Nutritional supplement use among college athletes and their sources of information. Int J Sport Nutr Exerc Metab 2004;14:104–20.

[72] Patel DR, Greydanus DE. Nutritional supplement use young athletes: an update. Int Pediatr 2005;20(1).

[73] Williams MH. The ergogenics edge: pushing the limits of sport performance. Champaign (IL): Human Kinetics; 1998.

[74] Congeni J, Miller S. Supplements and drugs used to enhance athletic performance. Pediatr Clin North Am 2002;49:435–61.

[75] Greydanus DE, Patel DR. Sport doping in the adolescent athlete: the hope, hype and hyperbole. Pediatr Clin North Am 2002;49:829–56.

[76] Miller BE, Miller MN, Verhegge R, et al. Alcohol misuse among college athletes: self-medication for psychiatric symptoms? J Drug Educ 2002;32:41–52.

[77] Handelsman DJ. Designer androgens in sport: when too much is never enough. Sci STKE 2004;27:pe41.

[78] Pascual JA, Belalcazar V, de Bolos C, et al. Recombinant erythropoietin and analogues: a challenge for doping control. Ther Drug Monit 2004;26:175–9.

[79] Minuto F, Barreca A, Melioli G. Indirect evidence of hormone abuse. Proof of doping? J Endocrinol Invest 2003;26:919–23.

[80] Jelkmann W. Erythropoietin. J Endocrinol Invest 2003;26:832–7.

[81] Corrigan B, Beyond EPO. Clin J Sport Med 2002;12:242–4.

[82] Kazlauskas R, Howe C, Trout G. Strategies for rhEPO detection in sport. Clin J Sport Med 2002;12:229–35.

[83] National Institutes of Health. Office of Dietary Supplements. 2004. Available at: http://odp.od.nih.gov.

[84] Lemon P, Berardi JM, Noreen EE. The role of protein and amino acid supplements in the athlete's diet: does type of timing of ingestion matter? Curr Sports Med Rep 2002;4:214–21.

[85] Wagenmakers AJ. Amino acid supplements to improve athletic performance. Curr Opin Clin Nutr Metab Care 1999;2:539–44.

[86] Chromiak JA, Antonio J. Use of amino acids as growth hormone-releasing agents by athletes. Nutrition 2002;18:657–61.

[87] Candow DG, Chilibeck PD, Burke DG, et al. Effect of glutamine supplementation combined with resistance training in young adults. Eur J Appl Physiol 2001;86:142–9.

[88] Corrigan B. DHEA and sport. Clin J Sport Med 2002;12:236–41.

[89] Bhasin S, Woodhouse L, Storer TW. Proof of the effect of testosterone on skeletal muscle. J Endocrinol 2000;170:27–38.

[90] Brown GA, Vukovich MD, Reifenrath TA, et al. Effects of anabolic precursors on serum testosterone concentrations and adaptations to esistance training in young men. Int J Sport Nutr Exerc Metab 2000;10:340–59.

[91] Storer TW, Magliano L, Woodhouse L, et al. Testosterone dose-dependently increases maximal voluntary strength and leg power, but does not affect fatigability or specific tension. J Clin Endocrinol Metab 2003;88:1478–85.

[92] Leder BZ, Longcope C, Catlin DH, et al. Oral androstenedione administration and serum testosterone concentration in young men. JAMA 2000;283:779–82.

[93] Kelly GS. Conjugated linoleic acid: a review. Altern Med Rev 2001;6:367–82.

[94] Kreider RB, Ferreira MP, Greenwood M, et al. Effects of conjugated linoleic acid supplementation during resistance training on body composition, bone density, strength, and selected hematological markers. J Strength Cond Res 2002;16:325–34.

[95] Smedman A, Vessby B. Conjugated linoleic acid supplementation in humansmetabolic effects. Lipids 2001;36:773–81.

[96] Thom E, Wadstein J, Gudmundsen O. Conjugated linoleic acid reduces body fat in healthy exercising humans. J Int Med Res 2001;29:392–6.

[97] Terpestra AH. Effects of conjugated linoleic acid on body composition and plasma lipids in humans: an overview of the literature. Am J Clin Nutr 2004;79:352–61.

[98] Burke DG, Chilibeck PD, Davidson KS, et al. The effect of whey protein supplementation with and without creatine monohydrate combined with resistance training on lean tissue mass and muscle strength. Int J Sport Nutr Exerc Metab 2001;11:349–64.

[99] Dempsey RL, Mazzone MF, Meurer LN. Does oral creatine supplementation improve strength? A metaanalysis. J Fam Pract 2002;51:945–51.

[100] Poortmans JR, Francaux M. Adverse effects of creatine supplementation: fact or fiction? Sports Med 2000;30:155–70.

[101] American College of Sports Medicine Roundtable. The physiological and health effects of oral creatine supplementation. Med Sci Sport Exer 2000;32:706–17.

[102] Lenz TL, Hamilton WR. Supplemental products used for weight loss. J Am Pharm Assoc 2004;44:59–67.

[103] Jacobs I, Pasternak H, Bell DG. Effects of ephedrine, caffeine, and their combination on muscular endurance. Med Sci Sports Exerc 2003;35:987–94.

[104] Shekelle PG, Hardy ML, Morton SC, et al. Efficacy and safety of ephedra and ephedrine for weight loss and athletic performance: a meta-analysis. JAMA 2003;289:1537–45.

[105] Cupp MJ. Herbal remedies: adverse effects and drug interactions. Am Fam Physician 1999;59:1239–45.

[106] Heymsfield SB, Allison DB, Vasselli JR, et al. *Garcinia cambogia* (hydroxycitric acid) as a potential antiobesity agent: a randomized controlled trial. JAMA 1998;280:1596–600.

[107] Bucci LR. Selected herbals and human exercise performance. Am J Clin Nutr 2000;72:624S–36S.

[108] Wolfe RR. Protein supplements and exercise. Am J Clin Nutr 2000;72:551S–7S.

[109] Antonio J, Uelmen J, Rodriguez R, et al. The effects of *Tribulus terrestris* on body composition and exercise performance in resistance-trained males. Int J Sport Nutr Exerc Metab 2000;10:208–15.

[110] Antonio J, Uelmen J, Rodriguez R, et al. The effects of Tribulus terrestris on body composition and exercise performance in resistance trained males. Int J Sport Nutr Exer Metab 2000;10:208–15.

[111] Reid DC. Sport injury assessment and rehabilitation. New York: Churchill Livingstone; 1992.

[112] DeLee JC, Drez Jr D, Miller MD, editors. DeLee and Drez's orthopedic sports medicine: principles and practice. 2nd edition. Philadelphia: WB Saunders-Elsevier Science; 2004.

[113] Mcgee DJ. Orthopedic physical assessment. 4th edition. Philadelphia: WB Saunders; 2000.

[114] Mizel MS, Hecht PJ, Marymont JV, et al. Evaluation and treatment of chronic ankle pain. Instr Course Lect 2004;53:311–21.

[115] Safran MR, Benedetti RS, Bartolozzi 3rd AR, et al. Lateral ankle sprains: a comprehensive review: part 1: etiology, pathoanatomy, histopathogenesis, and diagnosis. Med Sci Sports Exerc 1999;31(7 Suppl):S429–37.

[116] Safran MR, Zachazewski JE, Benedetti RS, et al. Lateral ankle sprains. Part 2. MSSE 1999;31:S438–47.

[117] Frey C. Ankle sprains. Instr Course Lect 2001;50:515–20.

[118] Baker JM, Ouzounian TJ. Complex ankle instability. Foot Ankle Clin 2000;5:887–96.

[119] Wolfe MW, Uhl TL, Mattacola CG, et al. Management of ankle sprains. Am Fam Physician 2001;63:93–104 [erratum: Am Fam Physician 2001;64:386].

[120] Thacker SB, Stroup DF, Branche CM, et al. The prevention of ankle sprains in sports. A systematic review of the literature. Am J Sports Med 1999;27:753–60.

[121] Kerkhoffs GM, Handoll HH, de Bie R, et al. Surgical versus conservative treatment for acute injuries of the lateral ligament complex of the ankle in adults. Cochrane Database Syst Rev 2002;(3):CD000380.

[122] Kerkhoffs GM, Struijs PA, Marti RK, et al. Different functional treatment strategies for acute lateral ankle ligament injuries in adults. Cochrane Database Syst Rev 2002;(3):CD002938.

[123] Kerkhoffs GM, Rowe BH, Assendelft WJ, et al. Immobilisation and functional treatment for acute lateral ankle ligament injuries in adults. Cochrane Database Syst Rev 2002;(3):CD003762.

[124] Ubell ML, Boylan JP, Ashton-Miller JA, et al. The effect of ankle braces on the prevention of dynamic forced ankle inversion. Am J Sports Med 2003;31:935–40.

[125] Gross MT, Liu HY. The role of ankle bracing for prevention of ankle sprain injuries. J Orthop Sports Phys Ther 2003;33:572–7.

[126] Jackson JL, O'Malley PG, Kroenke K. Evaluation of acute knee pain in primary care. Ann Intern Med 2003;139:575–88.

[127] Griffin LY, Agel J, Albohm MJ, et al. Noncontact ACL injuries: risk factors and prevention strategies. J Am Acad Orthop Surg 2000;8:141–50.

[128] Bono CM. Low-back pain in athletes. Journal of Bone and Joint Surgery 2004;86A:382–96.
[129] Trainor TJ, Trainor MA. Etiology of low back pain in athletes. Curr Sports Med Rep 2004;3:41–6.
[130] Standaert CJ, Herring SA, Pratt TW. Rehabilitation of the athlete with low back pain. Curr Sports Med Rep 2004;3:35–40.
[131] Brolinson PG, Kozar AJ, Cibor G. Sacroiliac joint dysfunction in athletes. Curr Sports Med Rep 2003;2:47–56.
[132] Chang WK. Shoulder impingement syndrome. Phys Med Rehabil Clin N Am 2004;15:493–510.
[133] Almekinders LC. Impingement syndrome. Clin Sports Med 2001;20:491–504.
[134] Ruotolo C, Penna J, Namkoong S, et al. Shoulder pain and the overhand athlete. Am J Orthop 2003;32:248–58.
[135] Jazrawi LM, McCluskey 3rd GM, Andrews JR. Superior labral anterior and posterior lesions and internal impingement in the overhead athlete. Instr Course Lect 2003;52:43–63.
[136] Desmeules F, Cote CH, Fremont P. Therapeutic exercise and orthopedic manual therapy for impingement syndrome: a systematic review. Clin J Sport Med 2003;13:176–82.
[137] Wilk KE, Meister K, Andrews JR. Current concepts in the rehabilitation of the overhead throwing athlete. Am J Sports Med 2002;30:136–51.

ELSEVIER
SAUNDERS

Pediatr Clin N Am 52 (2005) 61–70

PEDIATRIC CLINICS

OF NORTH AMERICA

Understanding College Students with Learning Disabilities

Asiah Mason, PhD[a],*, Matthew Mason, PhD[b]

[a]Department of Psychology, Gallaudet University, 800 Florida Avenue NE,
Washington, DC 20002, USA
[b]Maryland School for the Blind, 12007 Yellow Bell Lane, Columbia, MD 21044, USA

Following is an excerpt from a textbook on behavior and learning disorders [1], describing a how a college student's academic efforts were affected by his learning disabilities:

> ... Imagine the inability to memorize times tables, not being able to "tell time" until the ninth grade, and taking several days to read a simple chapter from a school textbook. I was terrified of math ... I dreaded the class time itself for inevitably the teacher would call on me for an answer to a simple problem. When I was a sophomore ... I learned that I think, perceive, and process information differently. I have problems with processing speed, short-term memory and fluid reasoning. ... I take untimed tests ... use a calculator ... tape record lectures ... and use transparent blue-green plastic sheets when I read. (p. 215)

To many persons with learning disabilities, this excerpt relates a familiar story. Often a learning disability remains undiagnosed for many years, and the individual feels the brunt of the impact of the disability during the lengthy time in which the problem has not been detected professionally. When their learning disabilities have been detected and assessed, however, many individuals with learning disabilities have implemented various types of interventions that can diminish the impact of the disability and allow them to succeed.

Learning disabilities are relatively common conditions faced by millions of Americans. One can point to many examples of individuals with learning disabilities who have made significant contributions to society, however, includ-

* Corresponding author.
E-mail address: asiah.mason@gallaudet.edu (A. Mason).

ing scientist and inventor Thomas Edison, former president Woodrow Wilson, scientist Albert Einstein, and governor of New York and vice-president of the United States Nelson Rockefeller. Students with learning disabilities can lead productive, even distinguished, adult lives. The student from the above-quoted excerpt graduated from college and entered graduate school. With considerable effort and appropriate information and support, the future for people with learning disabilities can be promising.

Prevalence

The percentage of full-time college freshmen reporting disabilities at 4-year institutions has remained stable (6–8%) between 1988 and 2000. By 2000, two in five freshmen with disabilities (40%) reported having a learning disability [2]. In 2002, learning disabilities accounted for 51% of special education classifications [3]. The effects of chronic school failure frequently shape the experience of students with learning disabilities.

The proportion of students with learning disabilities planning to attend or entering college or university is growing [3,4]. There is little question that these students will encounter educational difficulties and that careful transition planning is essential for their success as students. College students with identified learning disabilities have higher dropout rates, and their academic performance indicators are lower than their counterparts without learning disabilities [5]. With some additional academic assistance, however, college students with learning disabilities not only survive, but also become competitive college students [4].

Transitioning to college

College-bound students with learning disabilities need substantial college preparatory counseling before they leave secondary school. There is a con- siderable difference in the relatively controlled setting of high school and the more unstructured environment of college. High school students can profit from planned intensive assistance in planning from their parents, teachers, and high school counselors to make this significant transition [6]. College-bound students with learning disabilities may find that many of their specific needs are related to basic survival skills in higher education.

At the college level, it is assumed that students already have adequate ability in taking notes, listening to and processing lecture information, writing skills, reading skills, and study habits. Transition programs must strengthen these abilities as much as possible and show the students how to compensate for deficits, using a range of perspectives and strategies to plan the student's pursuit of postsecondary education [7]. These strategies are summarized later in Tables 1 through 3. Perhaps the most helpful survival technique that can be taught to an adolescent with learning disabilities is more than a specific skill—it is a way of

Table 1
Characteristics and strategies of successful people with learning disabilities

Characteristic	Strategy
Self -aware	Aware of the problems they have, academic skill deficits, academic-related skills such as attention or organizational difficulties, and nonacademic difficulties such as motor deficits or emotional/behavioral problems
	Open and specific about their difficulties and understand how they affect their lives
	Able to see their learning difficulties as only one aspect of themselves
	Recognize their talents along with accepting their limitations
	Seek classes, professors, and jobs that provide the best fit or match with their abilities and needs
Proactive	Engaged in the world around them — politically, economically, socially
	Creative in their self-advocacy and problem solving
	Flexible, not rigid or passive, when coping with everyday problems
	Make decisions and act on those decisions
	Assume responsibility for their actions and resulting outcomes
	Show willingness to consult with others
Persevere	Keep pursuing their chosen path despite difficulties
	Know when to change their path to reach desired goal
Set goals	Set attainable goals that are specific, yet flexible so that they can be changed to adjust to specific circumstances and situations
	Understand step-by-step process for obtaining goals
Use support systems	Accept support from family members, friends, mentors, teachers, therapists, and coworkers
	During the transition into adulthood, attempt to reduce their dependence on others
	Often switch roles and help out others
Coping skills	Develop effective means of reducing and managing stress, frustration, and the emotional aspects of their learning disabilities
	Aware of situations that trigger stress
	Recognize stress as it is developing
	Ensure ready access to coping supports

From Raskind MH, Goldberg RI, Higgins EL, Herman KL. Life success for children with learning disabilities: A parent guide. Frostig Center (CA); 2003. Available at: www.LDsuccess.org; with permission.

thinking about survival, an overall attitude of resourcefulness and confident approach to solving problems.

Social and behavioral characteristics

Definitions and labels used for students with learning disabilities tend to focus on the academic perspective. Children, adolescents, and adults with learning disabilities often encounter emotional and interpersonal difficulties that are quite serious and highly resistant to treatment [8]. Because of their learning problems, students in all grades frequently experience low self-esteem and negative emotional consequences that present significant problems [9]. They may not be able to interact effectively with others because they misunderstand social cues or

Table 2
Techniques students can use to help themselves

Strategy	Description
Use your IEP	Many arriving college students with learning disabilities do not anticipate needing or having access to accommodations or support services
	Secure a copy of your most recent evaluation or Individualized Education Plan (IEP). You will need to provide this documentation or be reevaluated to be eligible for services
Use Section 504 law	Find out what accommodations and support services your college provides and, should you need them, where to find them
Learn about your disability	Increase your understanding of the nature of learning disabilities in general and specifically the type and severity of your own learning disability by discussing your test results with a disability specialist
Rehearse	Rehearse how to explain the nature and impact of your learning disability before you approach an instructor for accommodation requests
Classroom accommodations	If you require classroom accommodations of some kind, schedule an appointment with your instructor early in the semester
	Be specific about what you need, but reasonable about making accommodations practical
Tape recording lectures	If you need to tape record lectures, ask permission from the instructor before doing so as a courtesy
	Be sure to explain why you need this modification and how you will use the tape to enhance your learning
Learning strategies	Know the support techniques you need based on your learning style
	Meet with a learning disability specialist if you don't already know
Meet with instructors often	Make sure you understand assignments completely before starting them
	Schedule an appointment with your instructor before beginning major assignments
Proofread	Use a word processor with a spelling and grammar checker to identify misspelled words and incorrect grammar
	If your instructor agrees, request that a writing tutor, friend, roommate, or relative proofread your paper and assist you in error identification and correction as a final step
Seek help early	Schedule an appointment with your instructor at the beginning of the semester before getting confused or floundering
	Do not wait until you are in danger of failing the course to meet with your instructor
	Speak to the coordinator of the Office for Disabled Student Services and/or your advisor and find out what help is available
Drop-add and pass-fail	Be aware of drop-add and pass-fail options and deadlines to adjust your schedule. Use them to your advantage to enhance success
Be Active	Work with others to inform and sensitize the student body, faculty, administration, and staff about learning disabilities
	Organize public lectures, student panels, films, and videos
	Write articles for the student newspaper on your campus
	Become a student member of and/or provide input to policy-making university committees

(continued on next page)

Table 2 (*continued*)

Strategy	Description
Support groups	Find out if there is a support group for students with learning disabilities on your campus and become an active member in this group
	Seek peer counseling and support from other students with learning disabilities on an individual basis or through a support group on campus
	Join professional organizations as a student member to advocate for the rights of adults with learning disabilities and other persons with disabilities (e.g., Learning Disabilities Association, the Association of Higher Education and Disabilities, and the International Dyslexia Association)

From Vogel S. College students with learning disabilities: a handbook. 7th edition. Pittsburgh: LDA; 2000; with permission.

cannot discriminate among or interpret the subtleties of typical interpersonal associations. In some cases, the social dimensions of life present greater problems to students with learning disabilities than their specific academic deficits, yet this dynamic is essentially ignored in the definitions and labels related to learning disabilities.

Learning disabilities are unique to each individual, but professionals talk about them, particularly in the school setting, as if they are a one-size-fits-all type of condition. The message that seems to come through to so many children is one of disempowerment. They have or own a kind of illness that limits what they can do. So much of the focus tends to be on what they cannot do; what they can do usually receives less attention [10].

Children often learn much about their learning disabilities from their parents. Parents may communicate this information in positive or negative ways. Parents may not limit negative messages to the early years. In trying to help and advocate for their children, they unwittingly may become factors in reinforcing the perceptions that their children are not capable [10]. Late adolescence is typically the time that most individuals are able to assert independence from their parents. Ironically, for many adolescent students with learning disabilities, particularly students bound for or transitioning to college, parents become more rather than less involved, often to an excessive degree [11]. When parents assume the role of advocates for their college-age children, they may send a message that their children cannot advocate for, articulate, or even understand their own needs. This perception undoubtedly exacerbates the learned helplessness endemic to many students with learning disabilities, an attribution largely attributed to beliefs about the negative consequences of learning disabilities [12]. Opportunities for college students with learning disabilities to engage in a directed self-study program may increase a sense of autonomy, which is a crucial step in gaining the control described by Reif [10] that is crucial to successful adults with learning disabilities.

Table 3
Strategies to build self-confidence

Area	Strategy
What to tell yourself	After preparing as well as you could, tell yourself as you go into an exam or to make a presentation, you will succeed and you are well prepared, rather than you are going to fail
Set realistic goals	Identify a realistic goal and work toward it
	When you succeed in accomplishing a goal, identify the strategies that you developed that contributed to your success
Analyze and refine	If you don't achieve your goal on the first attempt, sit down with a family member, friend, teacher, or counselor, and analyze and refine your strategies
	Identify new strategies and intermediate goals that will prepare you better to achieve your final goal. Tell yourself, "Next time I know I'll do better"
Develop timelines	Develop a timeline to accomplish each goal, building in extra time for the unexpected
	There is no point rushing toward failure. Take a long range perspective on your life, rather than focusing on just one semester
List successes	Keep a list of your successes and accomplishments
	Review this list frequently
Take credit	Take credit for your achievements and work well done
	Accept compliments with a simple "thank you"
	If your performance did not meet your expectations, critique it at a later time with your teacher, coach, counselor, or friend
Identify your talents	Identify your strengths, and keep expanding the list of what you do well
	Identify your talents, develop and enjoy them
Keep perspective	Keep disappointments in perspective; a "D" on one quiz does not mean you will fail the course or be dismissed from college
Learn from mistakes	If you do poorly on a paper or exam, find out why rather than condemning yourself or rejecting the good along with the ineffective strategies that you may have used
	Mistakes are often the best teachers. By analyzing what went wrong, you will be better able to avoid such mistakes in the future
Admire and respect	What do you admire and respect about your friends? Because they also chose you as a friend, you share in their attributes and have other qualities that they admire and respect as well
	What teachers do you admire and respect? What qualities do they exhibit that you could emulate?
Dress for success	If you are not sure of the appropriate dress code for a specific occasion, setting, or social event, check ahead of time with a knowledgeable person
	A modest investment in your apparel leaves a lasting impression on others
Smile	People who smile send a message to others that they are comfortable with themselves and are self-confident
	Smiling is contagious. You will find people around you will reflect your facial expression, be much more pleasant, and have confidence in you when you smile
Remember others have confidence in you	Look at those who have expressed confidence in you, provided you with opportunities, and given you responsibilities. These people know you well, have observed your past performance, and have confidence in your abilities and potential to succeed
	As you accept new challenges, keep them and their confidence in you clearly in mind

From Vogel S. College students with learning disabilities: a handbook. 7th edition. Pittsburgh: LDA; 2000; with permission.

Defining learning disabilities

For the purpose of this article, the authors use the definition of *learning disabilities* provided by the American Psychiatric Association as written in the *Diagnostic and Statistical Manual of Mental Disorders, Fourth Edition* (DSM-IV) [13]. The DSM-IV states that learning disorders are diagnosed when:

> ... the individuals' achievement on individually administered, standardized tests in reading, mathematics, or written expression is substantially below that expected for age, schooling, and level of intelligence. The learning problems significantly interfere with academic achievement or activities of daily living that require reading, mathematical, or writing skills. ... Substantially below is usually defined as a discrepancy of more than two standard deviations between achievement and established intelligence quotient. ... If a sensory deficit is present, the learning difficulties must be in excess of those usually associated with the deficit. Learning Disorders may persist into adulthood. (pp. 46–47)

This definition and diagnostic approach of the DSM-IV is similar to the definition and approach described in the Individuals with Disabilities Education Act [3]. Also, many state departments of education incorporate a similar or consistent definition into their statutory regulations [14].

Common problems

Students with learning disabilities face academic and social-emotional challenges. This section summarizes the most common problems encountered to highlight how these problems affect the academic and social-emotional achievements of the students. All of these difficulties are unique to individual students and may appear in any combination. Reading, written language, math, memory, and metacognition are areas that affect every aspect of academic life. A student with difficulties in any of these crucial academic foundation areas struggles daily. Emotional, behavioral, and social characteristics, such as attribution of the learning disabilities experiences, also are significant areas affecting the lives of students with learning disabilities.

Reading

Although the term *learning disabilities* applies to a variety of functional characteristics, more than 80% of all identified learning disabilities are estimated to be reading related, influencing students' abilities to access and comprehend written material [15]. At the same time, most college courses transmit content primarily through reading and lecture [16]. These methods of transmission, coupled with particular students' neurologic and functional characteristics, can create barriers to learning for students with learning disabilities in the post-secondary setting. Often the goals of a course (eg, understanding of relationships in history) inadvertently are pursued in a manner (eg, via printed text) that make it difficult for students with learning disabilities to achieve the course goals [17].

Written language

For students with learning disabilities, problems of written language can occur in handwriting, spelling, sentence structure, vocabulary usage, volume of information produced, and organization of written ideas. Individuals who have difficulties in one area may show strengths in others. Many students with learning disabilities also have difficulty writing because both areas are language based (receptive and expressive). Difficulties with writing affect a student's achievement in virtually every content area. Students with writing difficulties may understand concepts in science or social studies, but be unable to express their understanding on an essay examination or in a laboratory report. They also may show considerable understanding in group or class discussions, but later turn in a homework assignment on the same material that lacks clarity or organization [18].

Mathematics

Poor math achievement may manifest in difficulties differentiating numbers and copying shapes (poor visual perception), recalling math facts (memory problems), writing numbers legibly or in small spaces (weak motor functions), and relating math terms to meaning (poor understanding of math-related vocabulary). Other weak areas may include abstract reasoning (solving word problems and making comparisons) and metacognition (including identifying, using, and monitoring the use of algorithms to solve math problems) [18].

Memory

Some people with learning disabilities have weaknesses in working memory. They have a difficult time processing information, interfering with translating recently presented information into long-term memory. Difficulties in working memory lead to poorly encoded long-term memory and are apparent when a person needs to search for and retrieve knowledge in a timely, organized manner. The length of time and effort required for an individual with deficits in working memory to acquire and store new or complex information are much greater [18].

Metacognition

Individuals with learning disabilities may display deficits in metacognition, the awareness of how one thinks and the monitoring of one's thinking. Weaknesses in metacognition affect the understanding of when, where, and why a person's known strategies are important and proficiency in selecting and monitoring the use of strategies. Many individuals with learning disabilities do not possess effective cognitive strategies for acquiring, processing, storing, and showing their understanding of information [18].

Attributions

Students who attribute their learning difficulties to factors beyond their control tend to avoid challenging tasks because they fear failure. The effects of chronic school failure frequently shape the attributions of students with learning disabilities. Such students may enter into a negative cycle of maladaptive attributions for success, which then contribute to future learning failures. A negative cycle of learned helplessness may inhibit adult learners with learning disabilities from most effectively seeking out and engaging with assistive technologies available to them at institutions of higher education, which could help them achieve college success [19].

Recommendations

Many effective strategies are available to help students with learning disabilities improve their study, memory, and test-taking abilities (Table 1) [20]. Table 2 summarizes techniques that college students with learning disabilities can teach themselves to help minimize the impact of their learning disabilities on their academic performance [21]. Table 3 summarizes strategies that students with learning disabilities can use to help support their continued development of self-confidence and esteem [21]. These strategies are not exhaustive, but are representative of many common approaches.

In a 20-year longitudinal study by Raskind et al [6], individuals with learning disabilities identified a set of personal attitudes and behaviors, the possession of which would predict success. Specifically the attributes of self-awareness, proactivity, perseverance, goal setting, use of effective support systems, and emotional stability were more powerful predictors of success than numerous other variables, including IQ, academic achievement, life stressors, age, gender, socioeconomic status, ethnicity, and many other background variables. These attributes and their relationship to college success are supported by other studies. [10,22].

Traditionally the study of learning disabilities has focused on developing strategies to improve only academic skills. The remediation of academic deficits should focus beyond classroom skills, however. This is not to suggest that efforts to enhance the academic abilities of individuals with learning disabilities are ill advised, but rather that a balanced emphasis on academic, interpersonal, self-management, and introspective skills should be pursued.

References

[1] Gelfand DM, Jenson WR, Drew CJ. Understanding child behavior disorders. 3rd edition. Fort Worth (TX): Harcourt Brace; 1997.

[2] Heath Resource Center, American Council on Education. College freshmen with disabilities: a biennial statistical profile. 2001. Available at: http.health-resource-center.org.

[3] US Department of Education, Office of Special Education Programs. Twenty-second annual report to Congress on the implementation of the Individuals with Disabilities Education Act. Washington (DC): US Department of Education; 2000.

[4] Jenkins YM. Diversity in college settings: directives for helping professionals. New York: Routledge; 1999.

[5] Sinclair ME, Christenson SL, Elevo DL, Hurley CM. Dropout prevention for youth with disabilities: efficacy of a sustained school engagement procedure. Except Child 1998;65:7–21.

[6] Raskind MH, Goldberg RJ, Higgins EL, Herman KL. Patterns of change and predictors of success in individuals with learning disabilities: results from a twenty-year longitudinal study. Learning Disabilities Research and Practice 1999;14:35–49.

[7] National Joint Committee on Learning Disabilities. Operationalizing the NJCLD definition of learning disabilities for ongoing assessment in schools. Learning Disability Quarterly 1998;21: 186–93.

[8] Persinger MA, Tiller SG. Personality, not intelligence or educational achievement, differentiate university students who access special needs for "learning disabilities." Soc Behav Pers 1999; 27:1–10.

[9] Bender WN. Learning disabilities: characteristics, identification, and teaching strategies. 3rd edition. Boston: Allyn & Bacon; 1998.

[10] Reif HB. Reframing the learning disabilities experience redux. Learning Disabilities Research and Practice 2004;19:185–98.

[11] Brinckerhoff LC, Shaw SF, McGuire JM. Promoting access, accommodations, and independence for college students with learning disabilities. J Learn Disabil 1992;25:417–29.

[12] Smith DD. Teaching students with learning and behavior problems. 2nd edition. Englewood Cliffs (NJ): Prentice Hall; 1989.

[13] American Psychiatric Association. Diagnostic and statistical manual of mental disorders. 4th edition. Washington (DC): American Psychiatric Association; 1994.

[14] Dombrowski SC, Reynolds CR, Kamphaus RW. After the demise of the discrepancy: proposed learning disabilities diagnostic criteria. Prof Psychol Res Pract 2004;35:364–72.

[15] Lyon RR, Moats LC. Critical conceptual and methodological considerations in reading intervention research. J Learn Disabil 1997;30:578–88.

[16] Pugh SL, Pawan F, Antommarchi C. Academic literacy and the new college learner. In: Flippo RF, Caverly DC, editors. Handbook of college reading and study strategy research. Mahwah (NJ): Lawrence Erlbaum Associates; 2000. p. 25–42.

[17] Torgesen JK, Wagner RK. Alternative diagnostic approaches for specific developmental reading disabilities. Learning Disabilities Research and Practice 1998;13:220–32.

[18] Boudah DJ, Weiss MP. Learning disabilities overview: update 2002. ERIC Clearing House on Disabilities and Gifted Education: ERIC EC Digest, #E624. 2000. Available at: http://ericec.org/digests/e624/.

[19] Raskind MH, Higgins EL. Assistive technology for postsecondary students with learning disabilities: an overview. J Learn Disabil 1998;31:27–40.

[20] Raskind MH, Goldberg RJ, Higgins EL, Herman KL. Life success for children with learning disabilities: a parent guide. Frostig Center (CA); 2003. Available at: www.LDsuccess.org.

[21] Vogel S. College students with learning disabilities: a handbook. 7th edition. Pittsburgh: LDA; 2000.

[22] Wehmeyer ML. Self-determination as an educational outcome: how does it relate to the educational needs of our children and youth? In: Sands DJ, Wehmeyer ML, editors. Self-determination across the life span: independence and choice for people with disabilities. Baltimore: Brookes; 1996. p. 17–36.

ELSEVIER
SAUNDERS

Pediatr Clin N Am 52 (2005) 71–84

Attention-Deficit/Hyperactivity Disorder Psychopharmacology for College Students

W. Bryan Staufer, MD[a],
Donald E. Greydanus, MD, FAAP, FSAM[a,b,c,*]

[a]Sindecuse Health Center, Western Michigan University, 1903 W. Michigan,
Kalamazoo, MI 49008-5445, USA
[b]Professor, Pediatrics & Human Development,
Michigan State University College of Human Medicine, 1000 Oakland Drive,
Kalamazoo, MI 49008-1284, USA
[c]Michigan State University/Kalamazoo Center for Medical Studies, 1000 Oakland Drive,
Kalamazoo, MI 49008-1284, USA

Attention-deficit/hyperactivity disorder (ADHD) is a descriptive term for the problems and behaviors described by the DSM-IV [1]. Although ADHD was once considered a pediatric disorder, it is now generally accepted that the symptoms and problems of ADHD often persist throughout one's lifetime [2,3] and that ADHD is problematic for a significant percentage of college students [4,5]. The college setting presents unique challenges to the student with ADHD. The structured days and smaller classes of elementary and secondary school are replaced by schedules that differ from day to day and didactic lecture classes of several hundred students. Students with ADHD who had satisfactory academic performance in elementary, middle, and high school under the close watch of teachers and parents are often unable to cope in the college setting. The sheer brain power and compensatory behavior acquired in the earlier years alone are not enough. The realization of the inability to satisfactorily meet the demands of college may come in the first semester of the first year, in later years when challenged by more advanced courses, or at the graduate level. Distractibility is the common denominator among college students with ADHD and is the primary

* Corresponding author. Sindecuse Health Center, Western Michigan University, 1903 W.
Michigan, Kalamazoo, MI 49008-5445.
E-mail address: greydanus@kcms.msu.edu (D.E. Greydanus).

reason students seek help from the primary care clinician or from clinicians at the college health service.

When the diagnosis of ADHD is established, the use of medications is the single most helpful strategy of treatment to help the student achieve his or her potential. Other aspects of management—coaching in studying and organization, counseling, academic accommodations, use of tutors, and behavior modification—are complementary. Many students come to the university with the diagnosis of ADHD already well established and managed by medication and academic accommodations. For them, adjustments often need to be made both to the accommodations and the medications that were helpful in the secondary school setting. This article is a practical guide to the use of medications for the treatment of ADHD in the college setting. It briefly reviews the most common medications and discusses the initiation and management of ADHD with those medications.

Psychopharmacology of attention-deficit/hyperactivity disorder

There are more than 1000 studies regarding the use of medications to treat children and adolescents with ADHD [6]. There are fewer articles about their use in adults, but clinical studies are ongoing. Recent articles provide summaries regarding management of ADHD in adults [7,8]. Even as the symptoms of ADHD may continue throughout one's lifetime, the medications that are useful in the earlier years continue to be helpful in the adult years.

The common classes of medications for treating ADHD are psychostimulants (methylphenidate, amphetamines), buproprion (Wellbutrin), and the norepinephrine reuptake inhibitor atomoxetine (Strattera) [9–11]. Other medications that have been tried in selected situations include tricyclic antidepressants, alpha-2 agonists, and pemoline (Cylert); however, these agents have limited use for the treatment of ADHD in college students and thus are not discussed in this article [9–12]. Pemoline has been a useful medication for managing ADHD in the past; however, it is now rarely used because of the potential for hepatic dysfunction, liver failure, and death. If used in selected circumstances, it must be done with informed consent and close monitoring of liver function. Modafinil (Provigil) has been approved by the US Food and Drug Administration (FDA) for the treatment of narcolepsy and daytime sleepiness; however, there are no studies to support its use for ADHD.

Psychostimulants

Psychostimulants are the most commonly used medications for the treatment of ADHD in college students and are helpful in greater than 70% of students with ADHD. About an equal percentage of students with ADHD will respond to medications in the methylphenidate group or the amphetamine group of drugs.

Some who do not tolerate or respond well to drugs from one group will do well when given a medication from the other class of psychostimulants.

Methylphenidate

Methylphenidate (MPH), a Schedule II medication, has been a standard part of ADHD treatment for the past four decades. MPH shares common effects and side effects with the other stimulant medications. The mechanism of action of MPH is believed to be its ability to increase the levels of both the norepinephrine and dopamine neurotransmitters by increasing release into the extraneural space and blocking uptake [13]. MPH is available in a variety of forms with different durations of action (Box 1, Table 1). The duration of clinical effects also varies among patients.

Clinical effects of immediate release forms of MPH may be noticed within 30 to 40 minutes, and maximum blood levels are reached in 1½ to 2 hours. Taking this medication with meals delays absorption slightly, which may mitigate some of the side effects. Absorption from the regular tablets is maximized when

---

Box 1. Available methylphenidate medications

Ritalin (Novartis): MPH, immediate release; 5-mg, 10-mg, 20-mg tablets; 3 to 6 hours duration

Ritalin SR (Novartis): MPH, sustained release; 20-mg tablets; 6 to 8 hours duration

Generic MPH (Geneva): immediate release and sustained-release tablets (see Ritalin)

Ritalin LA (Novartis): MPH, extended release; 20-mg, 30-mg, 40-mg capsules; 8 + hours duration

Metadate ER (Celltech): MPH, sustained release; 20-mg tablets; 6 to 8 hours duration

Metadate CD (Celltech): MPH, extended release; 20-mg capsules; 8 + hours duration

Methylin ER (Mallinckrodt): MPH, sustained release; 10-mg, 20-mg tablets; 6 to 8 hours duration

Concerta (Alza-McNeil): MPH, extended release; 18-mg, 36-mg, 54-mg tablets; up to 12 hours duration

Focalin (Novartis): dexmethylphenidate, immediate release; 2.5-mg, 5-mg, 10-mg tablets; 4 to 6 hours duration

Modified from Greydanus DE, Pratt HD, Rappley M. Attention-deficit/hyperactivity disorder in children and adolescents: interventions for a complex costly clinical condundrum. Pediatr Clin N Am 2003;50:1063; with permission.

Table 1
Medication release from extended-release formulations

Formulation	Immediate release	Delayed release
Ritalin SR (Novartis)	50%	50%
Metadate ER (Celltech)	50%	50%
Methylin ER (Mallinckrodt)	50%	50%
Metadate CD (Celltech)	30%	70%
Ritalin LA (Novartis)	50%	50%
Concerta (Alza-McNeil)	22%	78%
Dexedrine Spansules (Glaxo-Smith-Kline)	50%	50%
Adderall-XR (Shire)	50%	50%

the medication is taken with a high-fat meal. Most of the drug is metabolized to ritalinic acid and excreted through the kidneys.

Special methylphenidate formulations

MPH has a trilayer core covered by a semipermeable membrane that results in gradual release of MPH. This osmotic time-release process allows immediate release of 22% of MPH in the overcoat leading to a plasma MPH peak in 1 to 2 hours. The balance of MPH is released over 10 to 16 hours with an ascending MPH profile. The tablet is nearly impossible to alter and thus it cannot be abused. The tablets are taken once or twice a day.

Focalin (dexmethylphenidate HCL) is the *d*-threo-enantiomer of racemic MPH; the effective dose is half the regular dose of MPH. The *d*-threo-enantiomer seems to be the most effective component of the four optical isomers of MPH in treatment of the symptoms of ADHD. Use of dexmethylphenidate decreases side effects associated with the other enantiomers of MPH [6]. Side effects of both MPH and the amphetamines are similar (Box 2).

Amphetamines

Amphetamines have been used as a medication since the late 1800s [4]. One of the earliest reports of the use of the amphetamines for behavior and learning in children was by Charles Bradley in 1937 [14]. He observed significant improvement in mood, behavior, and learning in response to the use of benzedrine in 30 children aged 5 to 14 years during a 30-day period of observation in a residential setting [14]. During the past several decades, amphetamines have been used for the treatment of ADHD; initially they were used primarily for the hyperkinetic behavior of minimal brain dysfunction, but were later used to help with the full ADHD spectrum of distractibility, hyperactivity, and impulsivity.

As with MPH, amphetamines are believed to have a clinical benefit primarily because they increase levels of the neurotransmitters dopamine and norepinephrine, block their uptake, and increase their release [15]. The clinical effects of

> **Box 2. More common side effects of methylphenidate and amphetamines in adults**
>
> Abdominal pain
> Dry mouth
> Insomnia (delayed onset of sleep)
> Increase in heart rate, blood pressure, and palpitations
> Moodiness (irritability)
> Anorexia
> Weight loss (due to decreased appetite)
> Jitteriness
> Increased hyperactivity
> Constipation/diarrhea
> Headache
> Altered sexual interest or function
>
> *Modified from* Greydanus DE, Sloane MA, Rappley MD. Psychopharmacology of ADHD in adolescents. Adolesc Med 2002;13: 607; with permission.

amphetamines are slightly stronger per milligram dose than those of MPH; side effects are similar for both (Box 2). Amphetamines are available in several different formulations and approximate durations of action (Table 1, Box 3). Adderall is a mixture of salts of both *d* and *l* amphetamine in a 75%:25% ratio. It is not known if this mixture of *d* and *l* enantiomers is superior to the *d* enantiomer dextroamphetamine alone. The onset of clinical effects from Adderall tends to be less abrupt than with MPH, and the effects are of slightly longer duration.

Methamphetamine (Desoxyn) is a psychostimulant approved for the management of ADHD, but it is considered to be less effective behaviorally in ADHD than the *d* and *l-* amphetamine preparations [6]. It is also considered to have a higher risk for abuse than the other psychostimulants [16]. It is not recommended for use in the college setting or for other adults.

Bupropion

Bupropion is an antidepressant medication of racemic mixture that is sometimes used for ADHD. It has been approved by the FDA for use as an antidepressant in children, adolescents, and adults; it is not classed as a psychostimulant. Postulated pharmacologic mechanisms of action include the inhibition of the uptake of neurotransmitters serotonin, dopamine, and norepinephrine. The effects may be weaker than those from the psychostimulants [17]. Bupropion is available as Wellbutrin in 75-mg and 100-mg tablets; sustained release forms are Wellbutrin SR in 100-mg and 150-mg tablets given twice a day and Wellbutrin

---

Box 3. Available amphetamine stimulant medications

Dexedrine (GlaxoSmithKline): dextroamphetamine; 5-mg tablets;
    4 to 5 hours duration
Dexedrine Spansule (GlaxoSmithKline): dextroamphetamine, long-
    acting; 5-mg, 10-mg, and 15-mg capsules; 8 + hours duration
Dextroamphetamine, generic (Barr): see Dexedrine
Dextrostat (Shire US): dextroamphetamine; 5-mg and 10-mg
    tablets; 4 to 5 hours duration
Adderall (Shire US): amphetamine mixed salts; 5-mg, 7.5-mg,
    10-mg, 12.5-mg, 15-mg, 20-mg, and 30-mg tablets; 4 to
    6 hours duration
Adderall XR (Shire US): amphetamine mixed-salts; 5-mg, 10-mg,
    15-mg, 20-mg, 25-mg, and 30-mg capsules; 8 + hours duration
Desoxyn (Abbott): methamphetamine; not recommended (see
    later discussion)

Modified from Greydanus DE, Pratt HD, Rappley M. Attention-
deficit/hyperactivity disorder in children and adolescents: interventions for a complex costly clinical condundrum. Pediatr Clin N
Am 2003;50:1075; with permission.

XL given once a day as 150-mg or 300-mg tablets. Bupropion is usually well tolerated, but a variety of side effects may occur; some bupropion side effects are listed in Box 4.

Although it is not usually the first choice for treatment of ADHD, bupropion may be the ideal medication for some, whether alone or in combination with one of the psychostimulants. It can be considered in the presence of depression, heavy smoking, or a history of undesirable side effects from caffeine. Some individuals who do not tolerate any of the psychostimulants do well when treated with bupropion. Many college students have an improved sense of well-being apart from the effects on ADHD symptoms.

The usual therapeutic dose of bupropion is 150 mg of the SR formulation twice a day or 300 mg of the XL preparation once a day. Transient nausea or other gastrointestinal discomfort is common during the first few days of treatment. Symptoms are minimized by starting therapy with the 100-mg SR tablet. Approximately 25% of students who take bupropion will do well at 100 mg SR twice a day and do not need to increase to the 150-mg SR dose. The clinician should not exceed 450 mg/d in three divided doses.

There is an increased risk of seizure among people who use bupropion. The risk is approximately 0.1% at doses up to 300 mg/d and approximately 0.4% above 400 mg/d [17]. Doses should be increased incrementally to minimize the risk of seizure. It is recommended that bupropion not be used if an individual has

---

Box 4. Common side effects of bupropion

Dry mouth
Anorexia
Agitation
Tachycardia
Nausea
Restlessness
Insomnia
Drowsiness
Dizziness
Headache
Increased sweating
Constipation
Seizures (see discussion of precautions elsewhere in the text)

---

a history of seizures, serious cranial injury, bulimia, or anorexia nervosa. High doses of sedatives, anxiolytics, and alcohol or their abrupt discontinuation, may trigger seizures while taking bupropion.

Two absolute reasons that a student will be unable to use bupropion are dysphoria and allergic reaction. With dysphoria, the student may be in a bad mood or "the worst mood of my life" after one or two doses. This feeling is not usually dose-related and occurs in spite of efforts to titrate to tolerance from a very low dose. If the bad mood occurs, discontinue the trial and try an alternate medication. With an allergic reaction, generalized pruritis may develop about 4 to 6 weeks after beginning therapy. The allergic reaction progresses to generalized urticaria within 1 to 2 days unless the medication is discontinued.

Atomoxetine

Atomoxetine (Strattera) was released in January of 2003 and has been approved by the FDA for clinical use in the treatment of ADHD in children (6 years and up), adolescents, and adults [18–20]. It is considered to be a nonstimulant medication that acts as a norepinephrine reuptake inhibitor to raise the level of the neurotransmitter norepinephrine; it does not primarily affect the level of dopamine. It is available as 10-mg, 18-mg, 25-mg, 40-mg, and 60-mg capsules. There is a wide variety of possible side effects (Box 5). Atomoxetine must be used with caution when the patient is also using paroxetine, fluoxetine, or quinidine because of their inhibitory effect on the CYP2D6 enzyme receptors [18].

In our practice, atomoxetine is the preferred medication for only about 10% of college students. During the first 18 months of the use of atomoxetine for ADHD in our university health center, less than 10% of the students who tried it continued to use it. Reasons for discontinuation included multiple side effects

Box 5. Atomoxetine side effects (partial list)

Anorexia
Dry mouth
Nausea (may last for weeks)
Drowsiness
Insomnia
Dysphoria/mood swings
Fatigue/lethargy
Increased heart rate and blood pressure/palpitations
Constipation
Dizziness
Difficulty voiding
Altered sexual interest or function

and lack of efficacy. A period of 2 to 3 weeks is usually necessary to establish the optimal dose, achieve a tolerance to side effects, and evaluate the therapeutic effects. Because of significant side effects and weaker clinical benefits, atomoxetine is a medication to be tried last in the algorithm of treatment for ADHD [18].

The usual therapeutic dose range for college students is 80 to 100 mg/d as a single morning dose or in two divided doses. For optimal effect, it should be taken every day. A single morning dose sometimes does not provide coverage for the entire day; for this reason, it is recommended that two divided doses be given in the morning and at noon. Although it may be taken without food, administration of the medication with meals (breakfast and lunch) helps to minimize gastrointestinal side effects.

Atomoxetine may be the preferred medication in selected situations. For example, it can be tried if the response to psychostimulants or bupropion is unsatisfactory or the side effects to the psychostimulants or bupropion are too severe. It may also be tried if a student specifically requests it or if a student's career choice prohibits the use of a psychostimulant other than caffeine (eg, a commercial airplane pilot).

Principles in the management of medication for college students with attention-deficit/hyperactivity disorder

Having the diagnosis of ADHD is not an excuse for college students to perform poorly in their studies. They are still responsible for their performance in the academic environment, the social setting, and in the workplace. Medication can help with concentration and reduce hyperactivity and distractibility, but will not do the work that is necessary. In providing medication and related guidance, the clinician serves a role similar to that of a coach for the college athlete. In this regard, there are two important axioms:

1. *Each student is uniquely different.* Each student has a distinctive personal history and psychologic construct. Daily schedules and patterns of work, study, and play differ, while each student has a unique physiologic response to and tolerance of ADHD medications. Therapy must be tailored specifically for each student.
2. *Each clinician develops his or her own personal style and preferences in working with students who have ADHD.* In addition to information acquired through residency, attendance at conferences, medical literature, and the experiences of others treating college students and adults with ADHD, a clinician's skills in managing ADHD are honed by the feedback from each student that is followed. This feedback continuously modifies a clinician's approach and skill in the management of ADHD.

The following basic principles for the use of medications in the college setting can be adapted to one's own clinical situation.

Algorithm of treatment: a general guide

The initial medication trial for a college student with ADHD is usually with a psychostimulant (eg, methylphenidate or amphetamine). If this is not tolerated or is not helpful, a trial with a medication from the other class of stimulants is suggested. If there is a favorable response with MPH, but adverse effects are noted, consider a trial with dexmethylphenidate. If there is unsatisfactory effect or undesirable side effects from stimulants, begin a trial with buproprion. If there is an unsatisfactory response to bupropion and stimulants, begin a trial with atomoxetine, a trail of a combination of bupropion and a psychostimulant, or other ADHD medication.

A majority of students with ADHD do well with one of the psychostimulants. Comorbid conditions such as anxiety, depression, and bipolar disorders are often present with ADHD; these conditions need to be addressed concurrently. A clinical decision must be made in each situation whether to treat the ADHD or the comorbid conditions primarily. Treatment of one condition does not preclude treatment of the others.

Practical aphorisms about the use of psychostimulants

Methylphenidate and amphetamines are each helpful for about 70% of students with ADHD. A single initial dose of a psychostimulant allows one to begin to evaluate for desirable effects, tolerability, and side effects. When the optimal dosage is reached, it may take several days or weeks to determine the best timing and number of doses throughout the day; it is a learning process for both the student and the clinician. After the optimal dosage has been established, it usually does not change over time. A student may come to college using the same dosage of medication used since middle school and continue on the same dosage throughout the college years.

The frequency and timing of doses may change in response to changes in the life of the student; there may be longer days due to increased number of classes or credit hours, added commitments from work or extracurricular activities, or increased stress related to work, family, school, and other psychosocial stressors. Students who have a favorable response to methylphenidate but undesirable side effects may do well with the *d*-threo isomer dexmethylphenidate (Focalin); the dose of dexmethylphenidate is half of the dose of methylphenidate. The optimal dose of psychostimulants is unpredictable and is not related to age, sex, weight, or degree of impairment from the symptoms of ADHD. Most students do well with individual doses of psychostimulants in the range of 10 mg to 20 mg per dose. A few find that 5 mg per dose or 30 mg to 40 mg per dose is optimal for them. Also, most students find two or three doses a day satisfactory; some do well with a single dose per day. Occasionally, a student will prefer five or more small doses throughout the day to provide the smoothest effect and flexibility.

A majority of students have varied schedules—for classes, work, and extra-curricular activities. They often prefer regular tablets, which give them more flexibility in managing the ADHD. Students with routine schedules may find an extended release preparation convenient. Students using extended release medications often need a second dose or a regular tablet later in the day to complement the effects of the earlier dose. About half of the students need medication only for academic pursuits, such as classes, examinations, study, and projects, and their employment. The others (about half) find that, when medications are used daily, life is improved in all aspects, including academic, employment, personal, and social activities.

Management of common side effects of psychostimulants

Irritability sometimes occurs at the peak blood level or as the medication effect wears off. Tapering the medication with a smaller dose at the end of the day may be helpful. Some students report that the irritability is minimized if they eat something; for some, the irritability is transient and occurs only during the first days of treatment. Students who are smokers may feel an urge to smoke more when taking the psychostimulants. This effect is variable and many who have that feeling are subsequently able to quit smoking while continuing the medication. Regular exercise is helpful is this regard, and bupropion may be helpful for quitting smoking and management of the ADHD.

Headaches do not commonly cause students to discontinue the use of psychostimulants. Headaches often clear after the first few days of accommodation to the medication. Students who have a history of headaches are more likely to report headaches when taking psychostimulants. For some, headaches do not occur every time the psychostimulants are used or are not temporally related to the dose of medication. Stomachache and decreased appetite are minimized by taking the psychostimulant medication with meals or after meals. Most students eat enough to maintain their usual weight. As one of our students noted, "I'm not as hungry, but I eat because it's time." Checking weight at the periodic follow-up visits is helpful (if this is a concern). Occasionally a student experiences persistent weight loss, which requires a change in medication.

Increased pulse rate and blood pressure are problems that do occur with the use of the psychostimulants and atomoxetine. Pulse and blood pressure must be monitored at each visit. The increases that occur are rarely physiologically problematic in the short term. However, having ADHD is a lifelong situation, and treatment may be continued for many years. Any higher pulse rate or blood pressure is less desirable compared with pretreatment values and must be addressed as one would for patients who do not have ADHD. It is difficult to evaluate the causes of pulse and blood pressure elevations in college students and specifically the relationship, if any, to taking the medication. A detailed history of their activities and current life circumstances is necessary in this regard.

The response of feeling wired is usually evident after the initial one or two doses. It may be also be precipitated by the concomitant use of caffeine or a decongestant, such as pseudoephedrine. If the effect occurs with subsequent doses, a trial with a different psychostimulant or a different type of medication is indicated. Sleep concerns may also arise while on psychostimulants. If taken too late in the day, the psychostimulants may delay the onset of sleep; this effect varies among students. Some can fall asleep within a few hours of the last dose, while others must allow 6 or 8 hours between the last dose and expected time of sleeping. Many who had difficulty falling asleep before they were treated with psychostimulants for ADHD report that they sleep much better when they are using a psychostimulant.

Occasionally a student reports feeling tired when the effect of the medication wears off. The feeling may be minimized by tapering the dosage at the end of the day. However, most students using psychostimulants sleep well (see earlier discussion). If psychostimulants are discontinued after being used regularly for an extended period, it may be 1 to 2 weeks until these students feel that they are functioning as they did before any treatment. A similar phenomenon may occur when coffee consumption is discontinued after prolonged, regular use.

Concerns regarding abuse of psychostimulants

Although psychostimulants are substances of potential abuse, their use in the treatment of ADHD rarely leads to the addictive behavior associated with abuse of narcotics and other illicit drugs. Many studies suggest that treatment of adolescents who have ADHD is associated with decreased use of illicit substances, compared with those who have ADHD who are untreated [21,22]. The frequency of abuse among individuals who have ADHD and who are treated is similar to the substance abuse rate among those who do not have ADHD.

It must be acknowledged, however, that in the college setting psychostimulants are sometimes diverted from students with legitimate prescriptions for the treatment of ADHD. Students may manipulate the system and may attempt to obtain medication by presenting clinicians with a fraudulent history of ADHD or by getting the diagnosis through an inadequate evaluation. A detailed initial history and careful evaluation will minimize this possibility. Also, some obtain medications at examination time from friends or roommates who legitimately have the medications for treatment of their ADHD.

Medications are sometimes stolen—from a car, a backpack, a drawer, or a medicine cabinet. The entire vial or just some of the tablets may be taken. Thefts may happen during parties, when roommates have visitors, or when the roommate who has ADHD is not present. Besides reporting stolen medication, students present a variety of explanations when they run short of medication before the predicted time of renewal: the medication fell out of the car, backpack, or pocket; spilled into the sink; or was left in the hotel or at home on the weekend. Students may say, "I lost it," and this is indeed characteristic of students with ADHD—they lose things. However, most students are protective. As one student said, "I'm not going to give them away. I need them."

Out of concern that students might conspire to "beat" the college health system, an informal study was done to see if there were any similarities among the histories and evaluations of students getting medication for ADHD who lived at the same address. The review was done in our student health service for a university of 26,000 to 27,000 students (Sindecuse Health Center); in this health center, approximately 375 students who have ADHD are followed each year. During 2 consecutive years, individual records of students receiving stimulants were compared when two or more lived at a given address. The records were examined with regard to details of initial history, responses to standardized testing, evidence of impairment, date of initial evaluation, time of year when first seen, and academic year at the university. No similarities or patterns were found among the records of students receiving treatment for ADHD at any given address. The study was somewhat reassuring, and we conclude that it is appropriate to provide optimal treatment for students with ADHD, and that often includes psychostimulants, even though some of the medication may be diverted as previously discussed.

Summary

ADHD is a problem that often persists throughout one's lifetime, and it is problematic for many college students who have this condition. The use of medications is the single most helpful approach to enable these students with ADHD to realize their potential in the college setting along with academic accommodations and other supports. This article has provided a practical guide to the use of medication in the management of ADHD in the college student. It is helpful for an individual clinician to follow a student with ADHD over time to select the optimal medication, dose, and schedule, as well as make modifications in response to changes in the student's life as previously discussed. The references provide some resources for questions and problems beyond the scope of this article. Having ADHD does not preclude the presence of other psychologic, mood, or learning disorders; these must be addressed concurrently with management of ADHD. Working with students with ADHD and related disorders helps them succeed in the college setting—and this, indeed, is a gratifying experience.

References

[1] American Psychiatric Association. Diagnostic and statistical manual of mental disorders. 4th edition. Washington, DC: American Psychiatric Association; 1994.

[2] Wender PH. ADHD in adults. Psychiatric Times 1996;13:2. Available at http://www. psychiatrictimes.com/p960741.html. Accessed June, 2004.

[3] Biederman J. Attention-deficit/hyperactivity disorder: a life-span perspective. J Clin Psychiatr 1998;59(Suppl):4–16.

[4] Jaffe P. History and overview of adulthood ADD. In: Nadeau KG, editor. A comprehensive guide to attention deficit disorder in adults. New York: Brunner/Mazel; 1995. p. 3–17.

[5] Quinn PO. What is attention deficit disorder? In: Quinn PO, editor. ADD and the college student. New York: Brunner/Mazel; 1993. p. 1–5.

[6] Wilens TE, Spencer TJ. The stimulants revisited. Child Adolesc Psychiatr Clin N Am 2003;9: 573–603.

[7] Adler LA, Chua HC. Management of ADHD in adults. J Clin Psychiatr 2002;63(Suppl 12):29–35.

[8] Wilens TE, Faraone SV, Biederman J. Attention-deficit/hyperactivity disorder in adults. JAMA 2004;292:619–23.

[9] Greydanus DE, Sloane MA, Rappley MD. Psychopharmacology of ADHD in adolescents. Adol Med 2002;13:599–624.

[10] Greydanus DE, Pratt HD, Rappley M, et al. Attention-deficit/hyperactivity disorder in children and adolescents: interventions for a complex costly clinical conundrum. Pediatr Clin North Am 2003;50:1049–92.

[11] Greydanus DE. Psychopharmacology of ADHD in adolescents: Quo vadis? Psychiatric Times 2003;20:5–9.

[12] Spencer TJ, Biederman J, Wilens TE. Nonstimulant treatment of adult attention-deficit/hyperactivity disorder. Psychiatr Clin North Am 2004;27:373–83.

[13] Solanto MV, Arnsten AFT, Castellanos FX. Stimulant drugs and ADHD: basic and clinical neuroscience. In: Solanto MV, Arnsten AFT, Castellanos FX, editors. London: Oxford University Press; 2001. p. 134–5.

[14] Bradley C. The behavior of children receiving Benzedrine. Am J Psychiatry 1937;94:577–85.

[15] Amphetamines. Mosby's drug consult 2004. St. Louis (MO): Mosby, Inc.; 2004. Available at http://home.mdconsult.com/das/drug/view/43049176-2. Accessed August 2004.

[16] Anonymous. Methamphetamine abuse. Med Lett 2004;46:62–3.

[17] Bupropion. Mosby's drug consult 2004. St. Louis (MO): Mosby, Inc.; 2004. Available at http://home.mdconsult.com/das/drug/view/43049176-2. Accessed August 2004.

[18] Anonymous. Atomoxetine. Strattera revisited. Med Lett 2004;46:65.

[19] Atomoxetine. Mosby's drug consult 2004. St. Louis (MO): Mosby, Inc.; 2004. Available at http://home.mdconsult.com/das/drug/view/43049176-2. Accessed August 2004.

[20] Anonymous. Atomoxetine. Strattera for ADHD. Med Lett 2003;45:11–2.

[21] Biederman J, Wilens TE, Mick E, et al. Pharmacotherapy of attention-deficit/hyperactivity disorder reduces risk for substance abuse disorder. Pediatrics 1999;104:E20.

[22] Wilens TE, Faraone SV, Biederman J, et al. Does stimulant therapy of attention-deficit/hyperactivity disorder beget later substance abuse? A meta-analytic review of the literature. Pediatrics 2003;111:179–85

Further readings

Allen AJ, Spencer TJ, Heiligenstein JH, et al. Safety and efficacy of atomoxetine for AHDH in two double-blind, placebo-controlled trials. Biol Psychiatry 2001;49(Suppl 8):32S–3S.

Barkley RA. Attention-deficit/hyperactivity disorder. Sci Amer 1998;279:66–71.

Dimaio S, Gruzenko K, Joober R. Dopamine genes and attention-deficit hyperactivity disorder. J Psychiatr Neurscience 2003;28:27–38.

Fleming H, editor. Physicians desk reference 2004. Montvale (NJ): Thompson PDR; 2004.

Michelson D, Allen AJ, Busner J, et al. Once-daily atomoxetine treatment for children and adolescents with ADHD: a randomized, placebo-controlled study. Am J Psychiatry 2002;159:1896–901.

National Institute of Mental Health. NIMH research on treatment for attention deficit hyperactivity disorder (ADHD): the multimodal treatment study—questions and answers. Washington, DC: National Institute of Mental Health; 2000. Available at: http://www.nimh.nih.gov/events/mtaqa.cfm. Accessed December 1, 2004.

National Institute of Mental Health. Attention deficit hyperactivity disorder. NIH publication no. 01–4589. Washington, DC: National Institute of Mental Health; 2001. Available at: http://www.nimh.nih.gov/publicat/helpchild.cfm.

Parmet S, Glass RM. Attention-deficit/hyperactivity disorder. JAMA 2002;288:1804.

Spencer TJ, Biederman J, Wilens TE, et al. Pharmacotherapy of attention-deficit hyperactivity disorder across the life cycle. J Am Acad Child Adolesc Psychiatry 1996;35:409–32.

Spencer TJ, Biederman J, Wilens TE, et al. Effectiveness and tolerability of atomoxetine in adults with attention-deficit hyperactivity disorder. Am J Psychiatry 1998;155:693–5.

Weiss M, Murray C. Assessment and management of attention-deficit hyperactivity disorder in adults. Can Med Assoc 2003;168:715–722.

ELSEVIER
SAUNDERS

PEDIATRIC CLINICS
OF NORTH AMERICA

Pediatr Clin N Am 52 (2005) 85–96

Eating Disorders in College

Elaine L. Phillips, PhD[a],*, Helen D. Pratt, PhD[b]

[a]University Counseling and Testing Center, 2513 Faunce Student Services Building,
Western Michigan University, Kalamazoo, MI 49008-5323, USA
[b]Pediatrics and Human Development, Michigan State University, Kalamazoo Campus,
East Lansing, MI 48824-1317, USA

Although anorexia nervosa and bulimia nervosa are typically characterized as psychiatric disorders involving severe disturbances in eating patterns and behaviors [1], both are multifaceted psychiatric disorders affecting the emotions, thinking, behavior, and physical health of afflicted individuals [2]. As such, the college-age patient may initially present with concerns other than eating behaviors. Typical concerns may involve low energy, difficulty concentrating, moodiness, blood in the stool, swollen parotid glands, or broken blood vessels in the eyes. These complaints may be reported with no mention of disturbed eating behaviors. The patient may desire treatment for the physical sequelae of the eating disorder but may be resistant to treatment for the eating disorder itself, once identified, due to fears of weight gain if behavior change occurs and fears of inability to cope with feelings and situations if these coping behaviors are removed. Treatment is typically time consuming and involves psychologic, nutritional, and physical evaluation and monitoring. The treating physician must be thorough, alert, and sensitive at intake, in the hopes of accurate diagnosis and engaging the college patient in an appropriate course of treatment.

Eating disorder categories and diagnostic criteria

Anorexia nervosa (AN) and bulimia nervosa (BN) involve excessive concern with body weight and shape and the use of inappropriate or extreme behaviors to control weight [1]. The hallmark of AN is the individual's refusal to maintain or

---

* Corresponding author.
E-mail address: elaine.phillips@wmich.edu (E.L. Phillips).

attain a normal body weight. Suggested guidelines are a body mass index (BMI) of 17.5 or less or body weight less than 85% of that expected [1,3]. The guidelines are offered with the understanding that the physician will consider body build, age, height, and weight history when determining if an individual meets the criterion [1]. Other diagnostic criteria include: fear of obesity even though the individual is underweight, amenorrhea, and disturbance in body shape and size perception [1]. The American Psychiatric Association identifies two subtypes of AN: restricting type and binge-eating purging type. In the former, a low BMI is attained or maintained through dieting, fasting, or excessive exercise; in the latter, binge eating or purging is present [1].

In BN, the individual may be slightly underweight, of normal weight, overweight, or obese [1]. The primary criteria for a diagnosis of BN are behavioral: the individual binges and engages in compensatory methods to prevent weight gain at least twice a week for a 3-month period on average [1]. Other criteria include: excessive influence of body weight and shape on self-evaluation and bingeing and purging does not occur only during episodes of AN [1]. Two subtypes of BN are identified: purging type, in which the individual uses laxative, vomiting, diuretics, or enemas to prevent weight gain; and nonpurging type in which the individual fasts or engages in excessive exercise as the regular method of preventing weight gain.

Eating disorder not otherwise specified (EDNOS) is used for diagnostic purposes when the disorder does not meet the all of the criteria for AN or BN [1]. Specific examples are given in the Diagnostic and Statistical Manual–Revised. Simple obesity is classified as a medical condition and is not included in the DSM-IV [1]. Binge eating disorder (BED) is a research category in the DSM-IV [1]. These two categories are, therefore, beyond the scope of this article.

Demographics

Anorexia and bulimia are most frequently reported in industrialized, Westernized societies, with rare occurrence in developing or third world nations [1]. Researchers speculate that as more nations become Westernized, this disorder will increase [4]. Approximately 90% of those diagnosed with AN or BN are female, with only 10% of males currently diagnosed with either disorder [1]. The American Psychiatric Association estimates that in the general female population, approximately 0.5% of women will be diagnosed with AN and 1% to 3% will be diagnosed with BN [1].

Certain groups within the general population have higher rates of eating disorders and subthreshold eating disorders. These include college students, athletes (both student and professional), dancers, dietetics students, and models [5–9]. For example, in a review of empirical research, Stein [5] reported that 7.7% to 19% of college women were identified as having a diagnosable or subthreshold bulimia. He speculated that differences in reported prevalence in this group had more to do with research methods (confidentiality assurances, interview versus paper and pencil evaluations, broad versus restrictive diagnostic adherence) than with actual differences between the subjects at various colleges [5].

Eating disorders historically have been thought to afflict white women. Several researchers have questioned this assumption and have called attention to the lack of inclusion of women of color in research studies [10–14]. Although studies have now been conducted to assess the prevalence of AN and BN in women of color, Gilbert [10] states that the reported prevalence rates vary. Walcott, Pratt, and Patel [11] reported in their literature review that AN occurs with approximately the same frequency among the Asian American, Native American, and Hispanic female populations as among the white female population but occurs with less frequency among the African American female population. They cite research that reports that African American women who develop BN often use laxatives, rather than vomiting, to purge [11].

Problems in the research on women of color include: use of assessment measures that are standardized only on white populations, bias, unclear definitions regarding the ethnicity of the sample, and ethnic variations in presentation [10]. Regardless, diagnosable eating disorders and disturbed body image are present in women of color [10,11]. Physicians, psychologists, nutritionists, and others need to screen for eating disorders in the college population, regardless of ethnicity.

Etiology

AN and BN evolve from a complex interaction of biologic, psychologic, and sociologic phenomena. Several studies have identified a familial or genetic predisposition for eating disorders. In a recent study of AN and major depression among twins, researchers concluded that that genetic factors appeared to be significant in the risk for AN and also contributed to the risk of co-morbidity between AN and major depression [15]. Numerous studies have reported that the incidence of AN among first-degree relatives of those diagnosed with AN is higher than would be expected to occur by chance [1,16]. In the case of those diagnosed with BN, more first-degree biologic relatives report a history of BN than the general population [1,16,17]. First-degree biologic relatives of those diagnosed with AN or BN report an increased incidence of mood disorders [1]. In the case of BN, there also are increased reports of family members with substance abuse and dependence disorders [1].

Psychologic and behavioral constructs related to eating disorders have been well documented and are incorporated into a widely used assessment instrument, the Eating Disorders Inventory–2 [18]. Constructs such as ineffectiveness, asceticism, poor impulse regulation, perfectionism, interpersonal distrust, lack of interoceptive awareness, social insecurity, and maturity fears are frequently reported by those with AN or BN [19]. Perfectionism in particular is highly correlated with a diagnosis of AN. In an international multiple site study of those diagnosed with AN, perfectionism was found to be a discriminating characteristic of this disorder [20].

Family interactions have long been of interest to eating disorders researchers. Although the search for a prototypical family that produces offspring diagnosed with AN or BN has been unsuccessful (there does not appear to be one family style, system, or dynamic), researchers do state that subjects with eating disorders tend to describe their families as disorganized and critical, filled with conflict, mistrusting, not nurturing, and lacking in cohesiveness (subjective reports). These descriptions are also given in observational studies [21]. Therefore, some researchers speculate that eating disorders may be a method by which adolescents cope with the loneliness and alienation they feel in their families [21].

The eating disorder literature is filled with reviews of cultural (sociologic) changes and the impact of the development of AN and BN. The disparity between the number of men and women exhibiting bulimic or anorexic symptoms and the fact that these disorders are prevalent in industrialized societies but rare in the developing world have led researchers to a careful examination of cultural expectations and ideals for women.

For at least the past 30 years, Western cultures have valued and idealized youthfulness and slimness in women. Researchers point to the number of low-calorie diets, the many weight loss programs, and the increase in articles and advertisements on dieting in women's magazines and the media as evidence of this [22]. In classic studies researchers have found that over the past 30 years magazines have shown slimmer female models and centerfolds [22–24]. Other researchers have studied television as a purveyor of cultural standards of beauty and have found that the female characters portrayed are thinner and younger than the male characters [25]. By 1990, researchers had concluded that the emphasis by Western culture on slimness in women was related to the development of eating disorders [26].

Onset

The onset of AN is often identified as occurring in mid to late adolescence ages 14 to 18 [1].Although rare, onset can occur in the mid-adult years [1]. The course of this disorder can be chronic, especially if untreated, and can result in numerous medical complications including death [1]. BN most often begins in late adolescence through young adulthood with a course that may be chronic or intermittent and lead to a variety of physiologic problems [1].

Treatment

AN and BN affect all aspects of a patient's functioning. Given this, a multidimensional, multidisciplinary team approach to treatment is recommended.

Such teams typically include physicians or psychiatrists, psychologists or social workers, and dietitians. Monitoring and management of medical needs are primary, but treatment must also include attention to nutritional, psychologic, social, emotional, and familial functioning.

Treatment settings

In colleges located within large metropolitan communities, treatment sites are plentiful and include: outpatient treatment, intensive outpatient hospitalization, partial hospitalization/day treatment programs, residential care, and inpatient (hospital-based) treatment. Many colleges, however, are not located in large metropolitan communities, and treatment site choices are limited. In this article, the investigators discuss outpatient, intensive outpatient, and inpatient sites. The American Psychiatric Association Practice Guidelines for Treatment of Patients with Eating Disorders [27] includes a discussion of the full range of treatment sites.

Patients who are referred to hospital, residential, or intensive outpatient treatment programs are first evaluated by the referring therapist who identifies the preferable treatment program setting. Patients are referred to the program for an evaluation. Staff members of the intensive outpatient treatment program, residential, or hospital program determine if their site is the best choice or if referral to another setting would be more appropriate. The final decision for inclusion or rejection is made by the evaluating treatment team and the patient. If the patient is a minor, the parents make the final decision.

In the college community, most eating disordered students are psychologically and medically stable enough to show symptom reduction or remission through weekly psychologic treatment combined with some form of nutritional counseling, medical monitoring, and when warranted, psychotropic medication. Campus communities also often offer outpatient group treatment for those with BN, but usually this is an adjunct to individual treatment rather than the primary treatment modality. Outpatient group treatment with AN students is contraindicated.

On campuses that have psychiatric hospitals located in the larger community, intensive outpatient programs may be an option. Intensive outpatient treatment programs for eating disorders allow students to continue with their college courses but receive intensive treatment approximately 4 hours per day for 8 to 14 weeks [28]. This type of treatment is beneficial for students whose symptoms are severe enough to limit the success of weekly outpatient therapy sessions but not severe enough to require hospitalization. Unfortunately, intensive outpatient programs are not widely available.

Hospitalization (inpatient treatment) must be an option for students who are medically or psychologically unstable, even if this requires sending the student to a hospital some hours distant from campus. Most colleges will work with students and their families when hospitalization necessitates a temporary withdrawal from school or a temporary schedule and workload adjustment. On many campuses a dean of students, housed in the division of student affairs, will facilitate a student's transition from college to the hospital and return to campus with the least amount of disruption to the college career as possible.

Hospitalization is expensive, restrictive, and stigmatizing. When hospitalization is necessary, a hospital program that specializes in eating disorders is the preferred site. Staff in these programs are experienced in dealing with patients with eating disorders and offer individualized, well-defined treatment plans.

Typical reasons for hospitalization of a college student with an eating disorder are medical instability or psychiatric instability [29–32]. Physiologic problems such as electrolyte imbalance, abnormal cardiac rhythms, or dehydration may prompt a referral to a hospital-based treatment program [29,31,32]. Psychiatric instability involving psychosis, suicidal ideation or suicidal attempts, other self-harming behaviors, alcohol or substance abuse, severe depression, or severe obsessive-compulsive disorder result in the physician recommending hospital-based treatment [32].

Psychologic issues and treatment

Psychologists and psychiatrists have written extensively on the symbolic meaning of food. Hilde Burch, one of the earliest and most widely respected psychiatrists to specialize in the area of eating disorders, identified many emotion-based food and eating (or refusing to eat) associations in her anorexic patients. Some of these associations included expressions of anger, rage, hatred, aesthetic denial, rejection, power, and sexual gratification [33,34]. It is clear from this partial list that the act of eating represents much more than calories in and energy out.

Students who are diagnosed with AN or BN often have a long history of ignoring body cues of hunger and satiety. They have regularly experienced not eating when hungry and continuing to eat even when eating is painful. Therefore, they often report they can no longer clearly identify feelings of hunger or satiety.

The ability to distinguish physical hunger or satiety from emotional states is greatly diminished or not present at all. Eating or not eating often becomes the person's main way of coping with frightening, painful, intense, or unacceptable emotions. Patients often describe a paucity of skills in coping with uncomfortable emotions, thoughts, and situations and a general inability to tolerate intense emotions. They often describe feelings of worthlessness and strong identification with the intellectual and physical side of the self, with little emphasis on the self as a spiritual, social, or emotional being. Body image issues often involve seeing oneself as a physical being who attracts or deserves love only if she looks a certain way.

A variety of psychologic treatment approaches is used in the treatment of patients diagnosed with AN or BN. In the clinical setting, psychodynamic, psychoanalytic, behavioral, cognitive, interpersonal, and family approaches are used with anecdotal reports of positive outcomes. However, most of the research literature focuses on the cognitive-behavioral model of treatment (CBT) with fewer reported studies on interpersonal therapy (ITP) and even fewer controlled studies using other modalities.

Cognitive behavior therapy

Positive outcomes using cognitive behavior therapy (CBT) for the treatment of BN have been well documented. Literature reviews of this psychologic treatment technique report 50% of clients eliminate bingeing and purging at the end of treatment [35]. Agras and Apple [35] also assert that 5-year follow-up studies indicate that the improvements achieved continue to be maintained. They do indicate that some of the subjects in these studies report a periodic return of bingeing and purging [35].

There are three major components of CBT: psychoeducation, cognitive restructuring, and relapse prevention [35–37].The psychoeducational phase involves transmission of information regarding BN, the role cognition in maintaining the disorder, and nutritional information. Phase two involves nutritional and cognitive behaviors. The last component focuses on relapse and prevention activities.

Interpersonal psychotherapy

Interpersonal psychotherapy (IPT) has also been demonstrated to be successful in the treatment of bulimia nervosa [36].The IPT approach was originally developed for treatment of depression [37]. In this approach, the focus is on current difficult interpersonal relationships [35,36,38].

IPT has three phases. The first phase involves development of a positive relationship between therapist and client, sharing information regarding the treatment approach and eating disorders, and assessment of interpersonal difficulties [36]. Categories of interpersonal difficulties targeted for treatment include: grief, interpersonal disputes, role transitions, and interpersonal deficits [37].Phase two consists of weekly sessions that focus on the interpersonal difficulties that were identified in the assessment phase [36]. Role playing is used and problem-solving strategies implemented. In the final phase of treatment, therapist and client review progress and focus on coping with problems that may arise.

Research results with IPT are promising. A controlled study comparing IPT with CBT resulted in clients in both groups showing significant improvement at 12 month follow-up [38]. In the CBT group, clients made positive gains that were maintained at follow-up. In the IPT group, symptom improvement continued after the treatment ended [38]. Other research on the efficacy of ITP found at a 5-year follow-up, in clients who had received IPT or focal interpersonal therapy (focal interpersonal therapy and interpersonal therapy were combined given their similarities) only 28% of the subjects had a diagnosable eating disorder [39].

Family therapy

Family therapy is often difficult to arrange for the college student due to geographic distance. In the college setting, some therapists do arrange one family session per semester with outpatient clients.

Even if the family is not able to attend sessions, there will typically be some focus on family of origin issues. Sometimes these sessions take the form of Bowen's family therapy work with adults; sometimes the sessions are part of developmental work; and sometimes part of the IPT focus on grief, role transitions, and interpersonal disputes. Focus on the family of origin will usually occur in some manner as the underlying processes or the overt behaviors of AN and BN most often developed within the family context and most students will be residing with their families during holiday and summer breaks. Additionally, given the age of the typical college student, developmental issues that deal with emancipation and individuation are bound to involve some discussion of family relationships.

The numerous positive clinical reports regarding family therapy for the treatment of AN and BN have not yet evolved into a body of controlled studies of the type that would be required for inclusion on a list of empirically validated treatments [2]. This does not mean that physicians should hesitate to recommend family treatment when feasible. Especially in the case of AN, numerous empirical studies support the treatment using this model [40]. Additionally, the American Psychiatric Association has long recommended family therapy for those with BN, if such therapy is possible [41].

Self-help groups

Self-help groups (sometimes called support groups) may serve as a useful adjunct to individual or family therapy. These groups have not been developed to serve as the primary treatment modality, and physicians should express concern when patients state they are pursuing self-help treatment only.

In the college setting, it can be useful to give patients who are going home for the summer the names and addresses of support groups in their area. The purpose is to assist them in maintaining progress they have made during the school year and to provide them with added support as they transition from working with a therapist in the college community to working with a therapist in their home community. Contact people for support groups in a patient's home community can often be located by a phone call to the national headquarters of the support group.

Nutritional consultation

Nutritional consultation can be beneficial to many clients as part of their outpatient treatment program. It is important to remember, however, that preoccupation with food, weight, and eating habits are only components of the problem. Nutritional information alone will not resolve underlying issues or the distorted eating behaviors.

In the outpatient setting, nutritional consultation is a helpful adjunct when clients are expressing a lack of information or confusion about nutritional requirements and healthy food intake. It is counter-therapeutic for anorexic or bulimic clients to work with a nutritionist toward a goal of weight loss. In the inpatient setting, nutritional consultation and treatment are necessary, especially in the case of AN where setting and adjusting re-feeding and weight goals are used to establish physiologic stability.

Medical management

Evaluation and management of students who present with symptoms of diagnosable or subclinical eating disorders require a careful assessment. As reported earlier, this multidisciplinary assessment should include examination of nutritional, medical, and psychologic aspects of this condition [42,43].

In severe cases of AN, medical management is usually the first priority. Some students who are seen in the physician's office will present late in the course of the disease. These students will usually have significant loss of weight and nutritional and metabolic disturbances. Many youth who present in university medical clinics may present with milder symptoms which may allow for the effective use of preventative techniques.

For those students who present with chronic or more severe symptoms, greater care must be taken. A number of acute and chronic complications result from starvation and unhealthy dietary habits. Acute medical complications such as dehydration, fluid and electrolyte disturbances, cardiac dysrhythmias, hypotension, syncope, and seizures should be managed according to standard medical care on an urgent basis [42,43]. The physician's role in evaluating the student will focus on medical management, nutritional rehabilitation, and psychopharmacologic management of the many potential co-morbidities of eating disorders, such as mood disorders, anxiety disorders (obsessive-compulsive disorder, panic disorder, general anxiety disorder, post-traumatic stress disorder), substance abuse (for BN), kleptomania [42,43]. The priority for the physician will be directed toward general medical care and interventions that will stabilize the physiologic aspects of the disorder (ie, for the anorexic, weight restoration, management of menstrual disorders. and prevention or stabilization of bone loss).

Researchers have concluded that psychopharmacology has not been proven to be helpful for most youth with AN [42,43]. They did find that fluoxetine (Prozac, Dista, Indianapolis, Indiana) used with some adults with AN prevented relapses in subjects within 85% of expected body weight, even those without overt major depressive disorder.

More success has been reported with adults diagnosed with BN. Research on the use of selective seratonin reuptake inhibitors (SSRIs) in the treatment of bulimia has demonstrated decreased binge eating and decreased emesis with the use of fluoxetine (Prozac) especially at a daily dose of 60 mg [2]. Similar benefits have not been reported with fluvoxamine (Luvox, Solvay, Brussels, Belgium) or paroxetine (Paxil, SmithKline Beecham, Wilmington, Delaware) [44,45]. The impact on eating disorders of other SSRIs (such as sertraline [Zoloft, Pfizer, New York, New York] and citalopram [Celexa, Forest Pharmaceuticals, Inc., St. Louis, Missouri]) is currently being investigated [42].

More than 20 years of controlled, double-blind research has demonstrated that subjects diagnosed with BN benefit from tricyclic antidepressants (imipramine, amitriptyline, desipramine) [2]. However, their many well-known side effects limit their use in bulimics, especially adolescents [2].

Summary

College students with AN and BN benefit most from a multidisciplinary treatment team approach in which members of the team remain objective and focused on treatment goals and coordination of treatment interventions. The ability to establish and maintain trusting relationships with young adults requires that clinicians remain reliable, consistent, flexible, and tolerant.

References

[1] American Psychiatric Association. Diagnostic and statistical manual of mental disorders. 4th edition, text revision. Washington, DC: American Psychiatric Association; 2000.

[2] Phillips EL, Pratt HD, Greydanous DE, Patel DR. Treatment of bulimia nervosa: psychological and psychopharmacolgic considerations. J Adolesc Res 2003;18(3):261–79.

[3] World Health Organization. International classification of diseases. 10th edition. Geneva, Switzerland: World Health Organization; 1993.

[4] Patel DR, Phillips EL, Pratt DR. Eating disorders. Indian J Peds 1998;65:487–94.

[5] Stein DM. The prevalence of bulimia: a review of the empirical research. J Nutr Educ 1991; 23(5):205–13.

[6] Johnson C, Powers PS, Dick R. Athletes and eating disorders: The National Collegiate Athletic Association Study. Int J Eat Disord 1999;6:179–88.

[7] Sudgot-Borgen J. Risk and trigger factors for the development of eating disorders in female athletes. Med Sci Sports Exerc 1994;26(4):414–9.

[8] Garner DM, Garfinkel PE. Sociocultural factors in the development of anorexia nervosa. Psychol Med 1980;10:647–57.

[9] Garner DM, Garfinkel PE, Rockert W, Olmsted MP. A prospective study of eating disturbances in the ballet. Psychother Psychosom 1987;48:170–5.

[10] Gilbert SC. Eating disorders in women of color. Clinical Psych Sci Prac 2003;10(4):444–55.

[11] Walcott D, Pratt HD, Patel DR. Adolescents and eating disorders: gender, racial, ethnic, sociocultural and socioeconomic Issues. J Adolesc Res 2003;18(3):223–43.

[12] Striegel-Moore R, Smolak L. The influence of ethnicity on eating disorders in women. In: Eisler R, Herson M, editors. Handbook of gender, culture, and health. Mahwah, NJ: Erlbaum; 2000. p. 227–54.

[13] Lester R, Petrie TA. Personality and physical correlates of bulimic symptomatology among Mexian American female college students. J Coun Psych 1995;42(2):199–203.

[14] Mulholland AM, Mintz LB. Prevalence of eating disorders among African American women. J Coun Psych 2001;48(1):111–6.

[15] Wade TD, Bulik CM, Neale M, Kendler KS. Anorexia nervosa and bulimia nervosa: shared genetic and environmental risk factors. Am J Psychiatry 2000;157:469–71.

[16] Kendler KS, MacLean C, Neale M, et al. The genetic epidemiology of bulimia nervosa. Am J Psychiatry 1991;148:1627–37.

[17] Leung F, Geller J, Katzman M. Issues and concerns associated with different risk models for eating disorders. Int J Eat Disord 1996;19(3):249–56.

[18] Garner DM. Eating disorder inventory-2. Odessa, FL: Psychological Assessment Resources, Inc; 1991.

[19] Garner DM. Measurement of eating disorder psychopathology. In: Brownell DK, Fairburn CG, editors. Eating disorders and obesity: A comprehensive handbook. New York, NY: Guilford Press; 1995. p. 117–21.

[20] Halmi KA, Sunday SR, Strober M, et al. Perfectionism in AN: variation by clinical subtype, obsessionality, and pathological eating behavior. Am J Psychiatry 2000;157:1799–805.

[21] Pike KM, Rodin J. Mothers, daughters, and disordered eating. J Abnorm Psychol 1991;100(2): 198–204.

[22] Nasser M. Culture, weight, and consciousness. J Psychosom Res 1980;32(6):573–7.

[23] Adams LB, Shafer MB. Early manifestations of eating disorders in adolescents: defining those at risk. J Nutr Ed 1988;20(6):309–12.

[24] Garner DM, Garfinkel PE, Shwartz D, Thompson M. Cultural expectations of thinness in women. Psychol Rep 1980;47:483–91.

[25] Perdue L, Silverstein B. A comparison of the weights and ages of women and men on television. Paper presented at the annual Meeting of the Eastern Psychological Association, Boston, MA, 1985.

[26] Anderson AE, DiDomenico L. Diet vs. shape content of popular male and female magazines: a dose response relationship to the incidence of eating disorders? Int J Eating Dis 1992;11: 283–7.

[27] American Psychiatric Association. Practice guidelines for the treatment of eating disorders. Am J Psychiatry 2000;157(1):1–84.

[28] Woodside DB, Kaplan AS. Day hospital treatment in males with eating disorders—response and comparison to females. J Psychosom Res 1994;38(5):471–5.

[29] Becker AE, Grinspoon SK, Klibanski A, Herzog DB. Eating disorders. N Engl J Med 1999;340: 1092–8.

[30] Hill K, Maloney M. Anorexia nervosa and bulimia nervosa. In: Klykylo WM, Kay JG, Rube D, editors. Clinical child psychiatry. Philadelphia: W.B. Saunders; 1998. p. 279–88.

[31] Piran N. Treatment model and program overview. In: Piran N, Kaplan AS, editors. A day hospital group treatment program for anorexia nervosa and bulimia nervosa. New York: Brunner/Mazel; 1990. p. 3–19.

[32] Robin AL, Gilroy M, Dennis AB. Treatment of eating disorders in children and adolescents. Clin Psychol Rev 1998;18(4):421–46.

[33] Bruch H. Eating disorders, obeseity, anorexia nervosa, and the person within. New York: Basic Books; 1973.

[34] Bruch H. Four decades of eating disorders. In: Garner DM, Garfinkle PE, editors. Handbook of psychotherapy for anorexia nervosa and bulimia. New York: Guilford Press; 1985. p. 3–18.

[35] Agras WS, Apple RF. Overcoming eating disorders. San Antonio, TX: Graywind Publications. Psychological Corp; 1997.

[36] Fairburn CG. Interpersonal psychotherapy for bulimia nervosa. In: Klerman GL, Weissman MM, editors. New applications of interpersonal psychotherapy. Washington, DC: American Psychiatric Press; 1993. p. 353–78.

[37] Klerman GI, Weissman MM, Rounsaville BJ, Chevron ES. Interpersonal therapy for depression. New York, NY: Basic Books; 1984.

[38] Fairburn CG, Jones R, Peveler RC, et al. Psychotherapy and bulimia nervosa: longer-term effects of interpersonal psychotherapy, behavior therapy, and cognitive behavior therapy. Arch Gen Psychiatry 1993;50:419–28.

[39] Fairburn CG, Norman PA, Welch SL, et al. A prospective study of outcome in bulimia nervosa and the long-term effects of three psychological treatments. Arch Gen Psychiatry 1995;52: 304–12.

[40] Dare C, Eisler I. Family therapy in eating disorders. In: Brownell KD, Fairburn CG, editors. Eating disorders and obesity: a comprehensive handbook. New York: Guildford Press; 1995. p. 318–23.

[41] American Psychiatric Association. Practice guidelines for eating disorders. Am J Psychiatry 1993;150:207–28.
[42] Greydanus DE, Patel DR, Pratt HD. Female athlete triad Part I: abnormal eating patterns. Southwest Michigan Med Jl 2004;1(1):28.
[43] Patel DR, Pratt HD, Greydanus DE. Treatment of adolescents with anorexia nervosa. J Adolesc Res 2003;18(3):261–79.
[44] Freeman C. Drug treatment for bulimia nervosa. Neuropsychobiology 1998;37:72–9.
[45] Greydanous DE, Sloane MA. Psychopharmacology. In: Hofmann AD, Greydanus DE, editors. Adolescent medicine. 3rd edition. Stamford, CT: Appleton & Lange; 1997. p. 868–79.

ELSEVIER
SAUNDERS

Pediatr Clin N Am 52 (2005) 97–134

PEDIATRIC CLINICS
OF NORTH AMERICA

Anxiety and Depressive Disorders in College Youth

Swati Bhave, MD, DCH, FCPS[a],*,
Jitendra Nagpal, MD, DNB[b]

[a]Bombay Hospital & Medical Research Center, 302, Charleville Societey, "A" Road,
Churchgate Mumbai (Bombay), 400 020 India
[b]Child Development & Adolescent Health Centre, Vidyasagar Institute of Mental Health and
Neurosciences, No. 1, Institutional Area, Nehru Nagar, New Delhi 110065, India

Anxiety disorders are very common psychiatric conditions that very re-sponsive to treatment. At one time or another everyone has experienced anxiety or fear. Anxiety and fear are the same emotional condition, but they can be experienced in different ways. The feeling of anxiety generally is characterized as diffuse and unpleasant with a sense of apprehension or worry; physical symptoms may include headache, muscle tension, perspiration, restlessness, and chest as well as stomach discomfort. Anxiety can produce confusion, memory problems, and distortions of reality and the meaning of events. Anxiety becomes a disorder when the symptoms are severe, pervasive, and persistent, and when they interfere with normal life. Anxiety disorders can develop gradually over long periods of time or very quickly. These disorders can become disabling and interfere with school, relationships, social activities, and work.

Anxiety disorders are not rare and often mimic or are comorbid with other disorders. Youth need to be evaluated within a biopsychosocial framework; the anxiety disorder that exists in isolation, with a context, is extremely rare. Genetic vulnerability, biologic causes, life experiences, social and family con-texts, and developmental phases are interwoven to a greater or lesser extent in the expression of pathologic anxiety. The role of these interdependent factors requires clarification. The clinician must understand the inner experiential

* Corresponding author.
E-mail address: sbhave@bom7.vsnl.net.in (S. Bhave).

context and the external behavioral contingencies in which the anxious youth is operating. Given the uniqueness of each youth and the complex interplay among the internal and external variables that drive anxiety, a multi-modal approach to diagnosis and treatment is the rule rather than the exception [1].

How symptoms are reinforced

Once a fear or anxiety response has been elicited, the response tendency can be maintained in several ways. These include: self-talk or automatic thoughts (eg, I can't handle new situations. All dogs want to bite me.); avoidant behavior (eg, after a dog bites a person, he or he/she avoids dogs, but also avoids talking about the fear); inappropriate response (fear of being ridiculed in potentially harmless situations).

Symptoms and behaviors associated with anxiety

Box 1 lists various symptoms and behavioral associated with anxiety, while Box 2 provides diagnostic categories of anxiety disorders. There is much research regarding the biological and psychological basis of anxiety disorders. Anxiety disorders occur in 10% to 15% of the population. Panic disorder occurs in approximately 2% to 4% of the population. Approximately 50% of all patients with panic disorder have an immediate blood relative with panic disorder. Studies of identical twins have shown that panic disorder may occur with one twin but not the other. Most people experience an anxiety disorder purely on the basis of psychological, social, and environmental influences. Anxiety disorders are not necessarily inherited, although some people appear to inherit a risk or vulnerability for an anxiety disorder.

Box 1. Symptoms and behaviors associated with anxiety

Excessive or unreasonable fears

Recurrent memories and feelings about a traumatic event

Persistent avoidance of a feared situation, object, or situation associated with a previous trauma

Physiological reactivity associated with feared situations, objects, or previous trauma

Recurrent or persistent ideas, thoughts, impulses, or images that initially are experienced as intrusive or senseless

Repetitive, purposeful, and intentional behavior designed to minimize discomfort or prevent some feared event. The behavior is excessive or not connected to the situation or feared object.

Box 2. Diagnostic categories associated with anxiety disorders

Separation anxiety disorder—Anxiety is the result of separation from a significant figure or person (usually a parent).

Avoidant disorder—Fear of social contact with others

Overanxious disorder—Persistent anxiety that is not linked to an identifiable situation

Generalized anxiety disorder (GAD)—Unrealistic or excessive anxiety or worry about two or more life circumstances

Agoraphobia without history of panic disorder—Fear and anxiety associated with being alone or in a public place from which escape or aid might be difficult

Panic disorder—Unexpected and immediate episodes of intense fear that are not linked to any specific situation

Panic disorder with agoraphobia—Same as a panic disorder but also an intense fear of situations in which escape or aid might be difficult

Obsessive–compulsive disorder (OCD)—Anxiety is related to recurrent obsessive thoughts, images, or impulses. Symptoms also may be tied to compulsive behavior in the form of regimented, rigid, or useless behavior that is excessive or unreasonable.

Post-traumatic stress disorder—Anxiety is related to a catastrophic event and repeatedly is relived symbolically through play, dreams, or flashbacks.

Social phobia—Fear associated with being scrutinized by others or appearing foolish

Simple phobia—A fear/anxiety response to any object or situation not mentioned in any of the other diagnostic categories

---

Comorbidity of anxiety disorders

Anxiety disorders are also frequent comorbid conditions in other psychiatric disorders. Depressive disorders co-occur with anxiety disorders in up to two thirds of patients with an anxiety disorder diagnosis. Older children who have separation anxiety disorder or multiple anxiety disorders are more likely to have comorbid depression. Anxiety disorders tend to precede the development of depression and often persist after remission of the depressive episode. From 20% to 40% of youngsters with conduct disorder (CD) and oppositional defiant disorder (ODD) have comorbid anxiety diagnoses, with higher comorbidity rates in the ODD youth. The rates for comorbid anxiety in youth with substance abuse disorders are unknown; estimates range from one fourth to one third of alcohol and polysubstance abusers. The choice of therapeutics and treatment targets in clinical work is influenced by the type and number of comorbid conditions. Anxiety disorders tend to be more silent than the outwardly problematic behaviors of externalizing disorders and hence can be overlooked easily. Clinicians are well advised to assess for anxiety symptoms in all students presenting for a behavioral, academic, or psychiatric problems.

Common treatment approaches

Several treatment strategies have been developed for treating anxiety-related disorders. Some of these include Prolonged Exposure, Modeling, Contingency Management, and Self-Management. With Prolonged Exposure, the patient is encouraged to confront the feared situation or object using real or imagined versions in conjunction with other supportive aids such as relaxation, hypnosis, or biofeedback. In Modeling, patients observe another person interacting with the feared situation or object. Adaptive responding is demonstrated with guided instruction, support, and feedback. In Contingency Management, external events that follow the patient's fear/anxiety reactions are manipulated using rewards for successful interaction and bolder steps. Rewards are rescinded for refusing to interact. Finally, with Self-Management, subjective and physiological reactions are altered or changed by teaching a patient adaptive ways of appraising an upcoming situation, adaptive ways of thinking, and deep muscle relaxation techniques.

In general, anxiety disorders are very responsive to psychotherapy. Panic disorder is one of the most responsive. Effective therapy must include evaluation of the student's entire biological, psychological, social, and cultural background. Medications can be helpful, but adverse effects must be considered. Psychotherapy can be a very effective alternative to the use of medications. In most cases, there must be changes in the student's environment and social support system for treatment to be successful. Families of people with anxiety disorders can fail to see how they reinforce the disorder. Families are often resistant to change despite expressed dedication of support and a desire to do whatever is necessary. Embarrassing or punishing an anxious person will only make the disorder worse. Competence, commitment, and outstanding interpersonal qualities in a therapist are crucial for treatment to be successful.

Psychotherapy requires significant commitment of time, while treatment of anxiety and panic disorders with medication requires less effort. Because normal anxiety can improve over time without therapy, a brief period of medication can relieve symptoms, restore functioning, and not necessarily require long-term or life-long reliance on medication. Use of medication in some cases can result in a dependence on that medication to manage anxiety. Psychotherapy is almost always the first treatment of choice except in cases where anxiety or panic is so severe that immediate relief is necessary to restore functioning and to prevent immediate and severe consequences. Medication is usually the second choice after a comprehensive and competent trial of psychotherapy.

Psychopharmacological management

Benzodiazepines

Box 3 and Table 1 review medications used for the treatment of anxiety disorders. In equipotent doses, all benzodiazepines have similar effects. The choice among benzodiazepines generally is based on differences in half-life, rapidity of onset, metabolism, and potency.

Box 3. Medications of choice for specific anxiety disorders

GAD

- Buspirone
- Benzodiazepines
- Venlafaxine
- Selective serotonin reuptake inhibitors (SSRIs)*

OCD

- Clomipramine
- SSRIs

Panic disorder

- SSRIs
- Tricyclic antidepressants (TCAs)
- Monoamine oxidase inhibitors (MAOIs)
- Benzodiazepines

Performance anxiety

- β-Blockers
- benzodiazepines

Social phobia

- SSRIs
- MAOIs
- Benzodiazepines
- Buspirone

* Paroxetine was recently approved for the treatment of GAD, but other SSRIs are probably also effective.

Table 1
Commonly used anxiolytic and hypnotic medications

Generic (trade) name	Single-dose (mg)	Usual therapeutic dosage (mg/d)	Approximate dose equivalent (mg)	Methods of administration and supplied form	Approximate elimination half-life including metabolites*
Benzodiazepines					
Alprazolam (Xanax and generics)	0.25–1	1–4	0.5	Oral, 0.25/0.5 mg	12 hours
Chlordiazepoxide (Librium and generics)	5–25	15–100	10	Oral, 5/10/25 mg; iv, im**	1–4 days
Clonazepam (Klonopin)	0.5–2	1–4	0.25	Oral, 0.5/2 mg	1–2 days
Clorazepate (Tranxene and generics)	3.75–22.5	15–60	7.5	Oral, 3.75/7.5/30 mg	2–4 days
Diazepam (Valium and generics)	2–10	4–40	5	Oral, 2/5/10 mg; intravenous; intramuscular**	2–4 days
Lorazepam (Ativan and generics)	0.5–2	1–6	1	Oral, s/1:0.5/1/2 mg; intravenous; intramuscular**	12 hours
Oxazepam (Serax and generics)	10–30	30–120	15	Oral, 10/15/30 mg	12 hours
Nonbenzodiazepines					
Buspirone (BuSpar)	10.30	30–60	NA	Oral, 5/10/15 mg	2–3 hours

Abbreviation: NA, not applicable.

  * The clinical duration of action for the benzodiazepines does not correlate with the elimination half-life; ** Lorazepam im is well absorbed. We do not recommend chlordiazepoxide or diazepam.

Adapted from Teboul E, Chouinard G. A guide to benzodiazepine selection, part I: pharmacological aspects. Can J Psychiatry 1990;35:700–10.

Risks, adverse effects, and their management.   Benzodiazepine-induced sedation may be considered either a therapeutic action or an adverse effect. Residual daytime somnolence is a function of two variables: drug half-life and dosage [2]. With longer-acting agents, such as flurazepam and quazepam, a morning-after hangover is common, although some tolerance to this effect may develop with time. On the other hand, any benzodiazepine, short- or long-acting, can cause daytime drowsiness if the night-time dose is too great. In general, it is clinically unclear and theoretically uncertain whether sedation is a desirable component of anxiolytic activity. Many patients both expect and desire some degree of sedation when they are intensely anxious. Anxious patients who have received chronic treatment with benzodiazepines rarely complain about daytime sedation, even when compared with drug-free anxious subjects [3]. Regardless of whether sedation is desired, patients must be warned that driving, engaging in dangerous physical activities, and using hazardous machinery should be avoided during the acute stages, and possibly during the later stages, of treatment with benzodiazepines.

Concerns about physical and psychological dependence on benzodiazepines are raised frequently by patients and often affect a clinician's choice of treatment. On the basis of the criterion of self-reinforcement, however, most of the benzodiazepines, with the possible exception of diazepam, have low abuse potential when properly prescribed and supervised [4,5]. Physical dependence often occurs when benzodiazepines are taken in higher than usual dosages or for prolonged periods of time [6–8].

If benzodiazepines are discontinued precipitously, withdrawal effects may occur, including hyperpyrexia, seizures, psychosis, and even death. Several studies also suggest that physical dependence may occur even when benzodiazepines are taken in usual clinical doses for prolonged periods beyond several weeks and that the symptoms of withdrawal may arise even when drug discontinuation is not abrupt [9,10]. The signs and symptoms of withdrawal may include tachycardia, increased blood pressure, muscle cramps, anxiety, insomnia, panic attacks, impairment of memory and concentration, and perceptual disturbances. These withdrawal symptoms may begin as soon as the day after discontinuation of benzodiazepines and may continue for weeks to months. Evidence indicates that withdrawal reactions peak more rapidly and more intensely with the benzodiazepines that have a briefer half-life [6]. These withdrawal effects are reversed rapidly with the readministration of benzodiazepines. Although it generally is believed that there is cross-tolerance for all benzodiazepines, there has been a report of withdrawal symptoms from alprazolam that were not reversed with diazepam [11].

Rebound anxiety is defined as the return, on discontinuation of a benzodiazepine, of the anxiety signs and symptoms with greater intensity than existed before treatment. For this diagnosis, accurate documentation of specific symptoms and measures of the severity of preexisting anxiety are required. A general principle for most psychoactive medications is that discontinuation should be accomplished gradually. For patients taking benzodiazepines for longer than 2 to

3 months, it is suggested that the dosage be decreased by approximately 10% per week. Therefore, for a patient receiving 4 mg per day of alprazolam, the dosage should be tapered by 0.5 mg per week for 8 weeks. The last few dosage levels may be the most difficult to discontinue, and the patient will require increased attention and support from the physician during this time [12].

Intravenous use of the benzodiazepines is associated with significant anterograde amnesia [13,14]. The degree of anterograde amnesia appears to be related to dosage, and the amnesia may occur in the first several hours after each dose of benzodiazepine is taken, even after repeated use. An area of controversy is the allegation that benzodiazepines may, in some instances, cause behavioral disinhibition, leading to acts of aggression. Some caution should be exercised when benzodiazepines are prescribed to patients with a history of poor impulse control and aggression. The possibility of acts of aggression should be communicated to patients and documented in the medical record [12].

Benzodiazepines are remarkably safe when taken in overdose. Dangerous effects occur when the overdose includes several sedative drugs, especially when alcohol is included; this is because of synergistic effects at the chloride ion site and resultant membrane hyperpolarization. The diagnosis of possible overdose usually is made on the basis of questioning by the clinician of the patient, family, or friends about what drugs were ingested. The result is confirmed by physical examination finding signs and symptoms of toxicity with a central nervous system (CNS) depressant (eg, sedation, mental confusion, reduced respiration) and by urine or blood drug screens. The standard during drug screen assay may not detect the presence of many commonly prescribed benzodiazepines, including lorazepam, alprazolam, clonazepam, temazepam, and triazolam; thus, the clinician should research the presence and accuracy of these tests in the laboratory being used. A safe and effective benzodiazepine antagonist, flumazenil, now exists that may be used by means of intravenous injection in an emergency setting to reverse the effects of any potential overdose with a benzodiazepine [15].

Buspirone

Buspirone is effective in the treatment of generalized anxiety (Box 4). Although it has a longer onset of action, its efficacy is not statistically different from that of the benzodiazepines [16,17]. Despite its successes in the treatment of GAD, buspirone does not appear to be effective in the treatment of panic disorder [18], except perhaps in an auxiliary role for the treatment of anticipatory anxiety [19]. Buspirone also is used as an augmenting agent for treating OCD [20,21]. Some evidence suggests that buspirone may be an effective treatment for social phobia [22,23].

It is recommended at an initial dosage of 7.5 mg twice a day, increased after 1 week to 15 mg twice a day. The dosage then may be increased as needed to achieve optimal therapeutic response. The usual recommended maximum daily dosage is 60 mg, but many patients safely tolerate and benefit from

Box 4. Benzodiazepine versus buspirone for treating anxiety disorders

Benzodiazepines

Rapid onset of therapeutic effect
Effective in many anxiety disorders
May be particularly effective for somatic symptoms
May cause sedation
May impair performance
Additive effects with alcohol
May cause dependence and withdrawal
Low abuse potential
Higher plasma levels and extended half-life in elderly persons
Associated with falls in elderly persons (long half-life agents only)

Buspirone

Delayed onset of therapeutic effect
Proven effective in GADs only
May be particularly effective for psychic symptoms
No sedation
No effect on performance
Does not cause dependence or withdrawal
No abuse potential
Pharmacokinetics same in young and old
Does not increase number of falls

90 mg per day. Because buspirone is metabolized by the liver and excreted by the kidneys, it should not be administered to patients with severe hepatic or renal impairment.

The adverse effects that are more common with buspirone than with the benzodiazepines are nausea, headache, nervousness, insomnia, dizziness, and light-headedness [24]. Restlessness also has been reported, which theoretically may be related to the activity of this drug at the dopamine receptor. Buspirone does not appear to interact with alcohol or other CNS depressants to increase sedation and motor impairment [25]. When administered to subjects who had histories of recreational sedative abuse, buspirone showed no abuse potential [26], a finding confirmed by subsequent studies [5]. As mentioned previously, buspirone is not sedating and does not impair mechanical performance, such as driving [26]. Because adverse effects in any individual patient cannot be predicted, however, these activities should be avoided during the initial stages of buspirone therapy. No fatal outcomes of buspirone overdose have been reported. Overdose of buspirone with other drugs, however, may result in more serious outcomes.

Pharmacotherapy for generalized anxiety disorders

Generalized anxiety disorder can be treated with benzodiazepines, buspirone, and certain antidepressants. Benzodiazepines have the advantage of being rapidly effective and the obvious disadvantages of abuse potential and sedation. Although benzodiazepines are indicative for relatively short-term use only (1 to 2 months), they are, in general, safe and effective for long-term use for the minority of patients who require such medication [27,28]. Whereas tolerance to sedation often develops, the same is not true of the anxiolytic effects of these agents.

All benzodiazepines indicated for the treatment of anxiety are equally efficacious. It is advocated to start with 0.25 mg of alprazolam two or three times a day or an equivalent dosage of another benzodiazepine (Table 1). Titration of the dose is according to anxiolysis versus sedation. Benzodiazepines should be avoided in patients with a history of recent or significant substance abuse; also, all patients should be advised to take their first dose at home in a situation that would not be dangerous in the event of greater than expected sedation. For anxious patients taking a benzodiazepine who require a switch to buspirone, the benzodiazepine must be tapered gradually to avoid withdrawal symptoms, despite the fact that the patient is receiving buspirone.

Patients with GAD also respond to antidepressant treatment [29,30]. In studies comparing benzodiazepines, MAOIs, SSRIs, and TCAs in the treatment of concurrent anxiety and depression, all had some measure of success, depending on the degree of depression and the type of anxiety disorder [31]. The duration of pharmacotherapy for GAD is controversial. Psychotherapy is recommended for most patients with this disorder, and it may facilitate the tapering of medication. Generalized anxiety is often a chronic condition, however, and some patients require long-term pharmacotherapy. As in other anxiety disorders, the need for ongoing treatment should be reassessed every 6 to 12 months.

Pharmacotherapy for panic disorder

Benzodiazepines, TCAs, MAOIs, and SSRIs are all effective for treating panic disorder. Among the benzodiazepines, the higher-potency agents (alprazolam and clonazepam) are preferred, because they are tolerated well in the higher dose ranges often required to treat panic disorder [32,33]. For the treatment of panic disorder, clonazepam is started at 0.5 mg twice a day and increased to a total of 1 to 2 mg per day in two divided doses. Higher dosage levels may be necessary to completely relieve symptoms. The starting dosage alprazolam is usually 0.25 or 0.5 mg three times a day [33].

Because long-term exposure to high-dose benzodiazepines may place some patients at risk for physical or psychological dependence, the use of antidepressants for the treatment of panic disorder is recommended. Many antidepressants have been shown to be effective in this setting, including TCAs [34,35], MAOIs [36,37], and SSRIs [38–42]. For most patients, the SSRIs should be considered first-line agents. For highly anxious patients with panic disorder, initiate treatment with clonazepam or alprazolam and add a low-dose antidepressant, which is then increased slowly. The rapid onset of action of the benzodiazepine is helpful to the patient until the antidepressant becomes effective. When panic symptoms have not been present for several weeks, the benzodiazepine may be tapered slowly. In patients with marked residual anticipatory anxiety, longer-term use of a benzodiazepine or buspirone should be considered as an adjunct to the antidepressant. Although some patients respond to lower doses, standard to high-standard antidepressant doses generally are used to treat panic disorder.

For most patients, pharmacotherapy combined with time-limited cognitive–behavioral therapy is highly effective in reducing panic attacks, but possibly less effective in attenuating avoidance behavior. Unfortunately, there are no guidelines for the duration of pharmacotherapy. It is recommended to taper medication every 6 to 12 months if the patient has been relatively symptom-free. Many patients, however, require longer-term pharmacotherapy.

Pharmacotherapy for social phobia

Social phobia responds to several medications, including SSRIs [38,42–44], MAOIs [45,46], benzodiazepines [47–49], and buspirone [22,23]. Dosages for the treatment of social phobia are similar to dosages of these medications for other disorders. TCAs, although highly effective in the treatment of panic disorder, appear to be ineffective for most patients with social phobia. Similarly, β-blockers, although effective in treating performance anxiety, are not effective in treating generalized social phobia [49]. The high-potency agents, alprazolam [48] and clonazepam [47,49], appear to be the most effective benzodiazepines for treating social phobia. Although the MAOIs are highly effective in reducing social anxiety and social avoidance, these drugs are not first-line agents, as they are not in the treatment of depression, because of their increased risks compared with other available agents.

Pharmacotherapy for performance anxiety

Several studies have shown the efficacy of β-blockers in the treatment of performance anxiety. Taken within 2 hours of the stressor, propranolol, in doses ranging from 20 to 80 mg, may improve performance on examinations [50], in public speaking [51], and in musical performances [52]. A trial dose of 40 mg of propranolol (eg, during a vacation day) should be administered before the specific performance situation in which the patient anticipates anxiety. This initial dose should not be taken in a high-risk or critical situation in which any unexpected adverse effect could result in serious consequences. Subsequently, doses of propranolol should be administered approximately 2 hours before the situation in which disabling performance anxiety is expected. The dose may be increased gradually by 20-mg increments during successive performances until adequate relief of performance distress is achieved [53].

Pharmacotherapy of obsessive–compulsive disorder

The discovery of the SSRIs brought about a revolution in the treatment of OCD. As a consequence of these drugs, the understanding of OCD and related conditions multiplied manifold. Clomipramine, a tricyclic with potent serotonin reuptake inhibition, was the first medication with established efficacy for treatment of OCD [54]. Currently, clomipramine and the SSRIs provide the foundation of pharmacological treatment of OCD.

Before initiating clomipramine treatment, the clinician must heed all the precautions associated with the use of any TCA. Initial dosing and titration of clomipramine also must follow the guidelines for TCAs, with the additional caveat that 250 mg is the maximum recommended dosage because of an increased risk of seizures above this level. Most patients with OCD respond to dosages of clomipramine between 150 mg and 200 mg per day. Because adverse effects associated with the anticholinergic, antihistaminic, and α_2-adrenergic actions of clomipramine may occur, patients must be monitored for and made aware of the potential for symptoms. These include constipation, dry mouth, urinary hesitancy, sedation, and orthostatic hypotension.

The SSRIs are also effective treatments for OCD. Therapeutic dosages of fluvoxamine range from 100 to 300 mg per day in divided doses [55–58]. The recommended dosage range for paroxetine in the treatment of OCD is 40 to 60 mg per day [12]. As in the treatment of depression, the SSRIs tend to be tolerated better than the TCAs. It has been suggested that an effective antiobsessional dosage of fluoxetine may be higher than its usual antidepressant dosage. Many clinicians seek to establish a daily dose of 60 to 80 mg in treating OCD [59]. OCD is often a lifelong disorder with a waxing and waning course, for which many patients require prolonged pharmacotherapy. Although relatively high dosages of SSRIs are recommended for the acute treatment, lower dosages may be effective for maintenance treatment [60]. Finally, Box 5 provides general advice for college students experiencing anxiety.

Understanding and dealing with depression in college youth

Depression is a feeling of sadness and gloom, often with reduced activity. Self-injurious behavior occurs when people damage or hurt themselves. Suicide

---

Box 5. Information and steps a college youth can take for anxiety

- Seek advice and consultation from a qualified mental health professional if you experience symptoms of anxiety and panic that are either recurrent, severe, debilitating, or seem unusual or unrelated to an existing health problem.
- Seek medical advice if you have health problems, or if you have not had a medical evaluation for your symptoms.
- Recognize the biological effects of alcohol. Alcohol is a depressant in which prolonged or excessive use will increase and deepen symptoms associated with anxiety. Withdrawal from alcohol and certain drugs can produce symptoms of anxiety and panic.
- Avoid drugs that are not medically appropriate or approved by your physician. Some symptoms of anxiety and panic are associated with certain medications.
- When anxious or panicked, remember to breathe fully and calmly and at normal regular intervals. An occasional slow deep breath can help you relax and can prevent symptoms of panic. Avoid rapid short breaths.
- Maintain regular physical activity. Physical activity can be an effective way to relieve symptoms and build strength to resist stress.
- Do not fight your symptoms of anxiety by trying to wish the feelings away. Will power is not a solution.
- Do not focus or dwell on how it might get worse. Negative predictions can result in panic.
- It can help to focus on and do simple, fun, interesting, and safe, manageable activities or tasks.
- Notice that when you eventually stop thinking frightening thoughts your symptoms tend to fade in time.
- Humor and laughter are good best ways to reduce and prevent symptoms of anxiety and panic.
- Notice if there is a relationship between what you are doing and your symptoms. This can help during an evaluation and in treatment of these disorders.

---

is an extreme form of self-injurious behavior that often occurs in depressed individuals. Approximately half of the adolescents in trouble with the law are depressed; this situation is called a masked depression. Depression is one of the most common psychological/psychiatric disorders. Feeling sad or depressed is a normal reaction to a tragedy, change, or a significant loss in peoples' lives. For most people, the symptoms of depression are only temporary. Depression is

---

Box 6. Symptoms of depression in older children and adults

Too much or too little sleep
Significant increase or decrease in appetite
Loss of interest or pleasure in others or most activities
Feeling discouraged or worthless
A significant drop in performance in school or at work
Fatigue or loss of energy most of the time
Restlessness, fidgeting, or pacing
Crying or feeling sad, helpless, or hopeless
Episodes of fear, tension, or anxiety
Frustration, irritability, emotional outbursts
Excessive guilt or inappropriate self-blame
Repeated medical complaints without a known medical cause
(headaches, stomach aches, pain in arms or legs)

Serious and critical symptoms

Suicidal thoughts or feelings or self-harming behavior
Aggressive, destructive, threatening, or violent behavior
Abuse or prolonged use of alcohol or other drugs
Symptoms of depression combined with strange, bizarre, or
unusual behavior

---

described in terms of the severity, duration, and type of symptoms. The general feeling of depression is characterized by diminished motivation, low self-esteem, low energy, and impaired thinking and emotional well-being. Depression affects a person's overall energy, mood, expressions of emotion, and behavior. Box 6 lists symptoms of depression.

Diagnosis

The correct diagnosis of depression is complicated, and there are many alternative diagnostic systems and criteria for depressive syndromes. The *Diagnostic and Statistical Manual of Mental Disorders (DSM)* of the American Psychiatric Association often is used to diagnose depression. The fourth edition of this manual (*DSM-IV*) lists three depression categories: Major Depression, Dysthymia, and Adjustment Disorder with depressed mood. Major Depression is a severe form of depression that may involve disturbed sleep, appetite, suicidal thinking or self-harming behavior, loss of interest, problems thinking or concentrating, fatigue or loss of energy, restlessness or lethargy, and lowered self-esteem. Dysthymia is a less severe form of major depression in which symptoms are less evident and may appear chronic and last more than 2 years.

In Adjustment Disorder with depressed mood, depressive symptoms emerge as a reaction to an identifiable psychosocial stress. The reaction is viewed as mal-adaptive, and the symptoms are considered in excess of what usually is expected.

There has been much research regarding the biological and psychological basis of depressive disorders. Depressive disorders occur in approximately 15% to 25% of the population. Studies have found that 30% to 70% of all medical patients seen by physicians have depressive disorders in addition to their medical problems. Medical outcome studies have found that more than 50% of these patients will not make significant improvement until their depression is recognized and treated. Depression appears to be inherited, although most people appear to inherit vulnerability for depression. Approximately 50% of all patients with depressive disorder have a close blood relative with depression. Studies of identical twins have shown that depressive disorder may occur with one twin but not the other. Most people become depressed purely from the impact of psychological, social, or environmental influences. When people are overwhelmed and subjected to significant stress or loss, they can become depressed and stay depressed until they are treated.

Dealing with symptoms of depression requires an understanding as to whether the symptoms are a normal reaction, the result of a psychological disorder, or the result of a medical problem or condition. There are several medical conditions that can look and feel like depression. The symptoms associated with a psychological disorder or a medical condition are usually severe, unexplained, and interfere with one's ability to function.

Some common features of depressed youth
Guilt.   Youth who believe that they are basically rotten or bad want to be punished. They think that they deserve to be hurt because of their bad thoughts or behaviors. Guilt feelings come from having committed a breach of conduct, from feelings responsible for imagined offenses, or from a general sense of inadequacy. "I am so bad no one could possibly love me." With this feeling, expressions of love and acceptance are not believed. The situation becomes more serious when others actually like these youth. Their behavior may be such that they appear to ask for rejection. Others say, "How can you like him when he acts as if he didn't deserve to be liked?" Youth who feel guilty blame themselves for any problems or failure and often talk to themselves in very negative terms. "I'm such a jerk, no wonder my parents can't stand me." When these youth are told that something is not their fault, they do not believe it. They feel that others are just trying to be nice. Because they already feel guilty, words do not affect their negative self-concept.

Anger turned inward.   The patients who feel guilty may become angry at themselves and become depressed or hurt themselves in some way. This is a straightforward way of punishing oneself for being bad. Even more typical is the situation where youth become very angry at the unfairness of others. They see their parents, professors, peers, or siblings as unfair, mean, and insensitive to them. Usually, there is some combination of truth and imagination of exaggeration to their feelings. Normal events become blown up more than usual, and temporary anger may result. Because of their dependence upon adults for physical support and psychological approval, direct expression is unlikely.

Feeling helpless.   Depression usually follows a conviction that one just cannot cope with everyday problems. Prolonged helplessness and despair may lead to suicidal thoughts as a means of escaping a hopeless situation. At times, helplessness is combated by some types of self-injurious behavior. It is as if causing self-stimulation or pain means that one is not totally helpless. Young people are vulnerable if their feelings of self-esteem all depend upon one external source. If that source is no longer available, depression is very likely. Youth may be very attached to one friend, teacher, or relative. The point is that youth feel devastated if that all-important supply of acceptance vanishes. Some youth are more sensitive and vulnerable than others.

Reaction to tension.   Tension may be defined as opposition or hostility between individuals and an inner feeling of unrest, often accompanied by physical indications of emotion (sweating, muscle tightness, and increased pulse). Youth who frequently experience negative feelings in interaction with others develop a need to relieve tension.

Family context.   More than half the parents of depressed youth are depressed themselves. It is always difficult to assess how much of a disposition is inherited and how much is learned from living with people who often are depressed. There is evidence that suggests that proneness to depression is an inherited characteristic. Living with a parent who is a model for a depressed approach to life certainly would bring out this proneness. Youth learn to be pessimistic, sad, worried, and not easily aroused to joy or pleasure. Depressed or withdrawn parents do not easily arouse to joy or pleasure. Depressed or withdrawn parents do not communicate well with their children. This lack of communication directly contributes to isolated, helpless, and depressed feelings in these children when they grow up.

What help can be given

Open communication and expression of feelings
   Respecting and listening to students promotes basic warmth and acceptance. It is crucial that youth feel that adults take them seriously and can be turned to for support and guidance. An essential aspect is that adults allow open expression

of all genuine feelings, especially anger. In this atmosphere, anger does not have to be expressed in other ways such as gaining revenge by self-destructive acts. Communication has been defined as any behavior, verbal or nonverbal, that carries a message that is perceived by someone else. Several helpful rules of communication have been spelled out. These include:

- Action speaks louder than words. It is what you do rather than what you say you do that counts.
- Be clear, specific, and positive when communicating. The meaning of a communication depends upon the experiences and perception of each person.
- Be honest, fair, considerate, and tactful.
- Do not lecture, nag, or make excuses. Sensitive and constructive communication fosters a caring and optimistic family setting.

Promote adequacy and effectiveness

Individuals who do not feel a general sense of helplessness do not lapse into hopelessness and depression. It is essential to promote feelings of adequacy and independence. Active problem solving and gaining personal satisfaction prevents helplessness. Youth should be given choices, and their sense of having good judgments should be reinforced continuously. This is accomplished by setting challenging but reachable goals and expecting youth to master most tasks.

Promote many sources of self-esteem

"Having all your eggs in one basket" is not a good idea. Students are especially vulnerable to depression if their self-worth basically depends upon one or two sources. This is similar to people whose main attraction are good looks.

Model optimism and flexibility

By imitating parents, youth can learn to count their blessings, not their misfortunes. People must be aware of their direct influences in promoting optimism or pessimism by their own example. Parents who focus on the problems and tragedies in life usually have youth who do the same. The best indicator is to be aware of the amount of time spent on positive versus negative topics. If much of the conversation is dominated by worry and concern about the future, a negative atmosphere is generated. Instead, the future should be viewed with interest and excited anticipation. An optimistic attitude can be worked at and developed.

Be alert to warning signs

There is no substitute to being sensitive to, youth's feelings and behavior. Be aware of any signs of continuing feelings of helplessness or depression. Take student's complaints seriously and with respect. Pay attention to their comments and nonverbal behavior. Making light of someone's complaints may lead to depression or self-injurious acts as a means of gaining attention or respect. Any sudden change in behavior is good warning and indicator of a need for professional evaluation and intervention.

Common treatment approaches

Several treatment strategies have been developed for treating depression. Many can be implemented individually, in groups, or in a family therapy environment. Much evidence suggests that interventions, which emphasize treatment of the family, and not the identified patient, are critical to positive treatment outcome. Managing depression in youth involves psychotherapeutic and pharmacological management.

Psychotherapeutic approaches
Cognitive. Cognitive approaches use specific strategies that are designed to alter negatively based cognitions. Depressed patients are trained to recognize the connections between their thoughts, feelings, and behavior; to monitor their negative thoughts; to challenge their negative thoughts with evidence; to substitute more reality-based interpretations for their usual interpretations; and to focus on new behaviors outside treatment.

Behavioral. Behavioral approaches designed to increase pleasant activities include several components such as self-monitoring of activities and mood, identifying positively reinforcing activities that are associated with positive feelings, increasing positive activities, and decreasing negative activities.

Social skills. Social skills training consists of teaching youth how to engage in several concrete behaviors with others (eg, initiating conversations, responding to others, refusing requests, making requests). Patients are provided with instructions, modeling by an individual or peer group, opportunities for role-playing, and feedback. The object of this approach is to provide the patient with an ability to obtain reinforcement from others.

Self-control. Self-control approaches are designed to provide the self-control strategies, including self-monitoring, self-evaluation, and self- reinforcement. Depressive symptoms are considered to be the result of deficits from one or more areas and are reflected in attending to negative events, setting unreasonable self-evaluation criteria for performance, setting unrealistic expectations, providing insufficient reinforcement, and too much self-punishment.

Interpersonal. Interpersonal approaches focus on relationships, social adjustment, and mastery of social roles. Treatment usually includes nonjudgmental exploration of feelings, elicitation and active questioning on the part of the

Box 7. Indications for antidepressant use

Major depression

    Acute depression
    Prevention of relapse
    Other depressive syndromes
    Bipolar depression atypical depression
    Dysthymic disorder

Other indications

TCAs
    Strong evidence
    Panic disorder (most)
    OCD (clomipramine)
    Bulimia nervosa (imipramine, desipramine)
    Enuresis (imipramine)
    Moderate evidence
    Separation anxiety
    Attention-deficit hyperactivity disorder (ADHD)
    Phobias
    Generalized anxiety disorder
    Anorexia nervosa
    Body dysmorphic disorder
    Migraine (amitriptyline)
    Other headaches
    Diabetic neuropathy, other pain syndromes (amitriptyline, doxepin)
    Sleep apnea (protriptyline)
    Cocaine abuse (desipramine)
    Tinnitus
    Evidence for but rarely used for these disorders
    Peptic ulcer disease
    Arrhythmias

Atypical agents
    Trazodone
    Insomnia
    Dementia with agitation
    Minor sedative-hypnotic withdrawal
    Bupropion
    ADHD

MAOIs
  Strong evidence
  Panic disorder (most)
  Bulimia nervosa
  Moderate evidence
  Other anxiety disorders
  Anorexia nervosa
  Body dysmorphic disorder
  Serotonin Reuptake Inhibitors
  Strong evidence
  Obsessive-compulsive disorder (high-dose fluoxetine, sertraline)
  Bulimia nervosa (fluoxetine)
  Moderate evidence
  Panic disorder
  Obesity (high-dose fluoxetine)
  Substance abuse
  Impulsivity, anger associated with personality disorders
  Pain syndromes
  Preliminary evidence
  Obsessive jealousy
  Body dysmorphic disorder

Serotonin reuptake inhibitors
  Strong evidence
  OCD (high-dose fluoxetine, sertraline)
  Bulimia nervosa (fluoxetine)
  Moderate evidence
  Panic disorder
  Obesity (high-dose fluoxetine)
  Substance abuse
  Impulsivity, anger associated with personality disorders
  Pain syndromes
  Preliminary evidence
  Obsessive jealousy
  Body dysmorphic disorder
  Hypochondriasis
  Behavioral abnormalities associated with autism and mental retardation
  Anger attacks associated with depression
  Hypochondriasis
  Behavioral abnormalities associated with autism and mental retardation
  Anger attacks associated with depression

Depersonalization disorder
Social phobia
ADHD (as an adjunct)
Chronic enuresis
Paraphiliac sexual disorders
Nonparaphiliac sexual disorders

therapist, reflective listening, development of insight, exploration and discussion of emotionally laden issues, and direct advice.

Psychopharmacology

Box 7 lists indications for the use of antidepressants in depression, and Box 8 lists questions to ask about the use of medications to treat depression. Table 2 lists key features for use of antidepressants along with adverse effects. Antidepressants of all groups are indicated for treating major depression. An initial choice in a treatment paradigm is often an SSRI, venlafaxine, or a TCA. SSRIs offer easy titration, single daily dosing, and an excellent adverse effect profile. As an initial choice of antidepressant, the TCAs offer years of

Box 8. Drug selection for treating depression

- Is there a history of antidepressant response?
- How well was the antidepressant tolerated?
- Is there a family member with a history of antidepressant response and to what medication?
- If there is a history of antidepressant failure, were the trials of an adequate dose and of an adequate duration?
- Are there melancholic, atypical, or psychotic features present?
- Does the patient have a history of sensitivity to anticholinergic, histaminic α-adrenergic, serotonergic, or noradrenergic adverse effects?
- Does the patient have a history of a cardiac conduction delay or recent myocardial infarction (which would contraindicate the use of TCAs)?
- Does the patient presently take or need sympathomimetics (which would contraindicate the use of MAOIs)?
- If an antidepressant trial has failed, was the patient a partial responder or a nonresponder?
- Were any augmentation strategies employed?

Table 2
Summary of key features and adverse effects of antidepressant medications

| Medication | Key features | | | | | | |
	Proposed mechanism/receptor effects	Dosing	Titration required	Sedation	Weight gain	Sexual dysfunction	Other key adverse effects
TCAs	5-HT + NT reuptake inhibition	Once daily	Yes	Most, yes	Yes	Yes	Anticholinergic*, orthostasis, quinidine-like effects on cardiac condition, lethal in overdose
SSRIs	5-HT reuptake inhibition	Once daily	Minimal	Minimal	Rare	Yes	Initial: nausea, loose bowel movements, headache, insomnia
Bupropion SR	DA + NE reuptake inhibition	Multiple, if dose > 200 mg	Some	Rare	Rare	Rare	Initial: nausea, headache, insomnia, anxiety/agitation; seizure risk
Venlafaxine XR	5-HT + NE > DA reuptake inhibition	Once daily	Some	Minimal	Rare	Yes	Similar to SSRIs; dose-dependent hypertension
Nefazodone	5-HT$_2$ antagonist + week 5-HT+NE reuptake inhibition	Twice daily	Yes	Yes	Rare	Rare	Initial: nausea, dizziness, confusion, visual changes, sedation
Trazodone	5-HT$_2$ antagonist + week 5-HT$_2$ reuptake inhibition	Twice daily	Yes	Yes	Rare	Rare	Initial sedation, priapism, dizziness, orthostasis
Mirtazapine	α_2-Adrenergic + 5-HT$_2$ antagonism	Once daily	Minimal	Yes	Yes	Rare	Anticholinergic*; may increase serum lipids; rare: orthostasis hypertension, peripheral edema, agranulocytosis
MAOIs	Inhibit monoamine oxidase	Two or three times a day	Yes	Rare	Yes	Yes	Orthostatic hypotension, insomnia, peripheral edema; avoid in patients with congestive heart failure, avoid phenelzine in patients with hepatic impairment; potentially life-threatening drug interactions; dietary restrictions

Abbreviations: DA, dopamine; 5-HT, serotonin; NE, norepinephrine.
* Anticholinergic adverse effects include dry mouth, blurred vision, constipation, urinary retention, tachycardia, and possible confusion.

demonstrated efficacy, clinician familiarity, and the capacity for therapeutic blood level monitoring. Another advantage of the TCAs is their cost. A balancing disadvantage for the TCAs is their narrow therapeutic index and potential lethality in overdose.

There is evidence, some of it anecdotal, to suggest that subtypes of major depression respond preferentially to specific groups of antidepressants. Atypical depression is a subtype characterized by mood reactivity, overeating, hypersomnia, and chronic rejection hypersensitivity. There is evidence that MAOIs and SSRIs are most effective in this disorder. All effective antidepressants can induce mania. Accordingly, the treatment of choice for bipolar patients in a depressive phase is a mood stabilizer alone. Recently, there has been the suggestion that severe depressions respond preferentially to agents with multiple neurotransmitter blockade (eg, TCAs, MAOIs, and venlafaxine). Dysthymia has also shown clinical efficacy in controlled trials. With this group of patients, activating agents such as the SSRIs, venlafaxine, and bupropion may be the drugs of choice [61].

Tricyclic and heterocyclic antidepressants

Clinical use

These agents often are used as a second line of defense for treating depression, after the SSRIs. Before starting treatment with TCAs, the physician must obtain a comprehensive cardiovascular history and review of symptoms. Because TCAs often cause orthostasis, other potential risk factors for hypotension should be considered, and patients should be instructed to change from sitting or lying to the standing position slowly. Patients with significant anxiety, panic, or a tendency to be sensitive to adverse effects should receive initial dosages that are 50% lower.

Imipramine, amitriptyline, doxepin, desipramine, clomipramine, and trimipramine can be initiated at 25 to 50 mg per day. Divided dosing may be used initially to minimize adverse effects, but eventually the entire dosage can be given at bedtime. The dosage can be increased to 150 mg per day the second week, 225 mg per day the third week, and 300 mg per day the fourth week. The dosage of clomipramine should not exceed 250 mg per day because of an increased risk of seizures at higher dosages.

Nortriptyline should be initiated at 25 mg per day and increased to 75 mg per day over 1 to 2 weeks depending on tolerability and clinical response. Some patients require dosages up to 150 mg per day. Amoxapine should be started at 50 mg per day and titrated up to 400 mg per day; it has a short half-life and should be given in divided doses. Protriptyline can be started at 10 mg per day and increased to 60 mg per day. Maprotiline should be started at 50 mg per day and maintained at that dosage for 2 weeks because of an increased risk of seizure if the dosage is raised too quickly. The dosage can be increased over 4 weeks to 225 mg to day.

Adverse effects of tricyclic antidepressants

Anticholinergic effects

The most common anticholinergic adverse effects are dry mouth, constipation, urinary retention, blurred vision, and tachycardia. Cholinergic medications have been reported to relieve some of the anticholinergic adverse effects [62,63]. Bethanechol chloride may alleviate dry mouth, constipation, urinary hesitancy and retention, and erectile and ejaculatory dysfunction. The addition of a medication to treat adverse effects should be considered only after dosage reduction and alternative antidepressants with fewer anticholinergic adverse effects have been attempted.

Sedation

The relative sedating properties of the TCAs appear to parallel their respective histamine receptor-binding affinities. Trimipramine, amitriptyline, and doxepin are the most sedating TCAs; desipramine and protriptyline are less sedating.

Cardiac effects

Many of the TCAs have cardiovascular effects, including orthostatic hypotension and cardiac conduction delays. Increases in heart rate that occur with TCAs rarely result in morbidity or morality [64]; however, patients often find tachycardia frightening or distracting. Antidepressants with greater anticholinergic properties are associated with a higher incidence of this effect, which may be quite troublesome to patients with panic disorder.

Weight gain

Patients treated with TCAs may experience undesirable weight gain. This appears to be unrelated to improvement in the patient's mood [65,66].

Neurological effects

Dose-related seizures have been found with clomipramine, which has led to the recommendation that the daily dosage of this drug should not exceed 250 mg [54]. Overdoses of TCAs, particularly amoxapine and desipramine, are associated with seizures [67]. Whether therapeutic dosages of TCAs lower the seizure threshold is controversial [68]. Nonetheless, other classes may be safer for individuals will epilepsy [69]. Amoxapine, which has a mild neuroleptic effect, can cause extrapyramidal syndrome (EPS), akathisia, and even tardive dyskinesia [70–72]. For this reason, the authors do not recommend prescribing amoxapine as a first-line treatment for depression.

Overdose

The major complications from overdose with TCAs include those that arise from neuropsychiatric impairment, hypotension, cardiac arrhythmias, and seizures.

Allergic reactions

Allergic and hypersensitivity reactions may occur with TCAs, as they may with most drugs. If a mild rash develops, the drug may be continued and symptomatic treatment instituted. For more serious skin eruptions, the drug should be discontinued, preferably over several days to reduce the possibility of cholinergic rebound symptoms. Elevated temperature or signs of infection associated with the rash necessitate a complete medical evaluation, including complete blood count and liver function tests.

Selective serotonin reuptake inhibitors

Clinical use

Selective serotonin reuptake inhibitors are the antidepressants of choice for patients with depression who are placed on medications. Although all patients with depression should receive a thorough medical evaluation, no specific tests are required before treatment is initiated with an SSRI. Patients with panic disorder or significant anxiety symptoms are often intolerant of the initial stimulating effects that commonly occur with SSRIs. In these cases, the initial dosage also should be decreased by 50% (or more) and then increased as tolerated to the usual therapeutic dosage. It is often advantageous to apply this approach to patients who generally tend to be sensitive to adverse effects. A liquid preparation of fluoxetine is available for patients who require doses of less than 10 mg or who have difficulty swallowing pills. The other SSRIs are available in scored tablets.

The usual therapeutic dosages for the treatment of depression are citalopram 20 mg, fluoxetine 20 mg, paroxetine 20 mg, and sertraline 50 to 150 mg. For the treatment of depression, the SSRIs' higher dosages tend not to be more effective than standard dosages, although isolated patients respond better to higher dosages. Premature escalation of the SSRI dosage when treating a patient with depression is most likely to add adverse effects without improved antidepressant efficacy. Therefore, it is recommended to maintain the usual therapeutic dosage for 4 weeks. If there is no improvement at that time, a trial of a higher dose may be warranted. If a partial response is evident at 4 weeks, the dosage should remain constant for an additional 2 weeks, because improvement may continue.

Common adverse effects

Mild nausea, loose bowel movements, anxiety, headache, insomnia, and increased sweating are frequent initial adverse effects of SSRI treatment. They are usually dose-related and may be minimized with low initial dosing and gradual titration. These early adverse effects almost always attenuate after the first few weeks of treatment. Sexual dysfunction, discussed later, is the most common longer-term adverse effect of the SSRIs.

Neurological effects

Tension headaches are common early in treatment. These usually can be managed with over-the-counter pain relief preparations. SSRIs initially may worsen migraine headaches, but if the patient can tolerate the first few weeks of treatment with symptomatic relief, SSRIs are often effective in reducing the severity and frequency of migraines [73–75].

Stimulation/insomnia

Some patients complain of jitteriness, restlessness, muscle tension, and disturbed sleep. These effects typically occur early in treatment, before the antidepressant effect. All patients should be informed of the possibility of these adverse effects and reassured that if they develop, they tend to be transient. Patients with pre-existing anxiety should be started at low dosages with subsequent titration as tolerated. In this way, if overstimulation occurs, it will be less likely to be severe enough to result in a lack of compliance with medication. The short-term use of a benzodiazepine also may help the patient cope with overstimulation in the early stages of treatment, until tolerance to this effect occurs. Despite these common transient stimulating effects, SSRIs are effective for patients with anxiety or agitated depression. Similarly, insomnia that commonly occurs early in treatment may be tolerable if the patient is reassured that it will be transient. Symptomatic treatment with short-term use of benzodiazepines or low-dose trazodone (eg, 50 to 150 mg) at bedtime is reasonable [76,77].

Sedation

Despite occasional stimulating effects, SSRIs may induce sedation in some patients. Patients who experience significant treatment-emergent sedation with these medications often require lower dosages of the medication.

Weight gain or loss

All the SSRIs have the potential to cause weight gain in some individuals [78,79].

Gastrointestinal symptoms

Nausea and diarrhea may occur after treatment with an SSRI. This effect is dose-dependent and often transient.

Sexual dysfunction

Decreased libido, anorgasmia, and delayed ejaculation are common adverse effects of SSRIs. When possible, the management of sexual adverse effects should be postponed until the patient has completed an adequate trial of the antidepressant.

Vivid dreams

Reports of vivid dreams, distinct from nightmares, are common with SSRIs. The mechanism is unknown.

Rash

If a mild develops, the drug may be continued and symptomatic treatment instituted. Severe rashes require discontinuation of medication. Because the SSRIs share a similar mechanism but not similar structures, an allergy to one agent does not predict an allergy to another.

Serotonin syndrome

Affected individuals have the constellation of lethargy, restlessness, confusion, flushing, diaphoresis, tremor, and myoclonic jerks. As the condition progresses, hyperthermia, hypertonicity, rhabdomyolysis, renal failure, and death may occur [80]. The syndrome must be identified as rapidly as possible, because discontinuation of the serotonergic medications is the first step in treatment, followed by emergency medical treatment, as required. Life-threatening serotonin syndrome is fortunately rare and most often occurs with medication combinations that involve MAOIs.

Discontinuation syndromes

Several reports have described a series of symptoms following discontinuation or dose reduction of serotonergic antidepressant medications. The most common symptoms include dizziness, headache, paresthesia, nausea, diarrhea, insomnia and irritability. Of note, these symptoms also are seen when a patient misses doses [81].

Apathy syndromes

The authors and others have noted an apathy syndrome in some patients after months or years of successful treatment with SSRIs. Patients often confuse this syndrome with a recurrence of depression, but the two conditions are distinct. The syndrome is characterized by a loss of motivation, increased passivity, and often feelings of lethargy and flatness. There is no associated sadness, tearfulness, emotional angst, decreased concentration, or thoughts of hopelessness, worthlessness, or suicide, however. If specifically asked, patients often remark that the symptoms are not experientially similar to their original depressive symptoms. This syndrome has not been adequately studied, and the pathophysiology is not known. The syndrome appears to be dose-dependent and reversible. Mistakenly interpreting the apathy and lethargy for a relapse of depression and hence increasing the dose of medication will worsen the symptoms.

Drug interactions

Several deaths have been reported in patients taking a combination of SSRIs and MAOIs, presumably resulting from the serotonin syndrome [82–84]. Because of the potential lethality of this interaction, when it is necessary to switch from an SSRI to an MAOI, the patient must remain off the SSRI for a long enough time to ensure that it has been eliminated from the body fully. This time frame is the equivalent of five times the half-life of the SSRI. Therefore, at least 5 weeks are required between the discontinuation of fluoxetine and the institution of an MAOI [85] and about 1 week between other SSRIs and an MAOI. A 2-week waiting period is required when switching from an MAOI to an SSRI to allow resynthesis of the enzyme.

Bupropion

Clinical use

The sustained-release preparation is recommended over the original preparation because of increased tolerability and decreased seizure risk. The sustained-release preparation is initiated at 150 mg, preferably taken in the morning. After 4 days, the dosage may be increased to 150 mg twice a day. For the short-acting preparation, bupropion is initiated at 75 mg twice a day and increased as tolerated to a total daily dosage of 300 mg. Patients who do not respond after 4 weeks may warrant a trial of 450 mg per day. No single dose should exceed 200 mg. Gradual dose titration helps to minimize initial anxiety and insomnia. The temporary use of anxiolytic or hypnotic agents is reasonable in some patients, but generally this should be limited to the first few weeks of treatment.

Contraindications

Patients with seizure disorders should not use bupropion. Similarly, alternative treatment should be considered for patients with a history of significant head trauma, CNS tumor, or an active eating disorder.

Risks, adverse effects and their management

The most common adverse effects of bupropion are initial headache, anxiety, insomnia, increased sweating, and gastrointestinal upset. Tremor and akathisia also may occur.

Overdose

Much more is known about overdose with the immediate-release formulation of bupropion than with the newer, sustained-release formulation. Reported reactions with the immediate-release form include seizures, hallucinations, loss of consciousness, and sinus tachycardia. Treatment of overdose should include induction of vomiting, administration of activated charcoal, and ECG and electroencephalographic (EEG) monitoring. For seizures, an intravenous benzo-diazepine preparation is recommended [86]. The danger of bupropion overdose is, for the most part, limited to the risk of seizures.

Drug interactions

Combination with an MAOI is potentially dangerous, but less so than the combination of serotonergic drugs and MAOIs. Although the practice is not recommended, there are reports of combining MAOIs and bupropion in patients with refractory depression.

Monoamine oxidase inhibitors

Clinical use

The MAOIs are not used as first- or second-line agents because of the improved tolerability and safety of the newer antidepressants. They continue to be excellent medications for a subset of patients who do not respond to the other antidepressants, however. Patients with a depressive syndrome charac-terized by mood reactivity (ie, mood that is responsive acutely to favorable and unfavorable life experiences), oversleeping, overeating, extreme lethargy, and extreme sensitivity to rejection—the so-called atypical subtype—may show a preferential response to MAOI therapy [87–90]. These atypical symptoms may, in fact, provide a marker for patients who are likely to respond to MAOIs.

Phenelzine is initiated with 15 mg in the morning. If no response occurs within 2 weeks, the dosage may be increased in 15 mg increments to a usual maximum of 90 mg per day. Higher dosages are sometimes used, if tolerated, in patients with severe and refractory depression. Tranylcypromine is initiated at 10 mg and then increased every other day to 30 mg per day. As with phe-nelzine, higher doses may be necessary when the condition is refractory to treatment [91]. After tolerance to the hypotensive effects has developed, usually after 1 or 2 weeks, the patient may take the medication as a single daily dose in the morning. Morning dosing is preferred, because these medications tend to be activating, especially tranylcypromine, which is released to amphetamine. Some data suggest that once-daily dosing of the MAOIs may be therapeutically superior to multiple dosing [92].

More so than with other medications, it is imperative to review the patient's medical status and current medications before prescribing an MAOI. The importance of following the dietary and medication restrictions, as outlined in

Box 9. Instructions for patients taking monoamine oxidase inhibitors

- Avoid all the foods and drugs indicated on the list.
- In general, all the foods you should avoid are decayed, fermented, or aged in some way. Avoid any spoiled food even if it is not on the list.
- If you get a cold or influenza, you may use aspirin or acetaminophen. For a cough, glycerin cough drops or cough syrup without dextromethorphan may be used.
- All laxatives or stool softeners for constipation may be used.
- For infections, all antibiotics may be prescribed, such as penicillin, tetracycline, or erythromycin.
- Do not take any other medications without first checking with your doctor. These include any over-the-counter medicines bought without prescription, such as cold tablets, nose drops, cough medicine, and diet pills.
- Eating one of the restricted foods may cause a sudden elevation of your blood pressure. If this occurs, you will get an explosive headache, particularly in the back of your head and in your temples. Your head and face will feel flushed and full; your heart may pound, and you may perspire heavily and feel nauseated. If this rare reaction occurs, do not lie down, because this elevates your blood pressure further. If your blood pressure is high, go to the nearest emergency center for evaluation and treatment.
- If you need medical or dental care while taking this medication, show these restrictions and instructions to the doctor or dentist. Have the doctor or dentist call your doctor if he or she has any question or needs further clarification or information.
- Adverse effects such as postural light-headedness, constipation, delay in urination, delay in ejaculation and orgasm, muscle twitching, sedation, fluid retention, insomnia, and excess sweating are quite common. Many of these effects lessen after the third week.
- Light-headedness may occur after sudden changes in position. This can be avoided by getting up slowly. If tablets are taken with meals, this and the other adverse effects are lessened.
- The medication is rarely effective in less than 3 weeks.
- Care should be taken while operating any machinery or driving; some patients have episodes of sleepiness in the early phase of treatment.

> - Take the medication precisely as directed. Do not regulate the number of pills without first consulting the doctor.
> - In spite of the adverse effects and special dietary restrictions, your medication (an MAOI) is safe and effective when taken as directed.
> - If any special problems arise, call your doctor.

Box 9, should be discussed with the patient, and the discussion should be supplemented with written instructions. Patients also should be warned against gaining a false sense of confidence if dietary guidelines are broken without consequences. The current use of MAOIs is predominantly in patients with refractory depression, patients who are often suicidal. It often is emphasized to the patient that failure to adhere to the instructions is more likely to cause cerebral hemorrhage and disability than to cause death.

The following risks and adverse effects apply to the irreversible, nonselective MAOI antidepressants (phenelzine and tranylcypromine). The most common adverse effects are orthostatic hypotension, headache, insomnia, weight gain, sexual dysfunction, peripheral edema, and afternoon somnolence. Although the MAOIs do not have significant affinity for muscarinic receptors, anticholinergic-like adverse effects are present at the start of treatment. Dry mouth is common but not as marked as with the TCAs. Fortunately, the more serious risks, such as hypertensive crisis and serotonin syndrome, are not common.

Antidepressant medication discontinuation

Discontinuation of antidepressant medication should be concordant with the guidelines for treatment duration. It is advisable to taper the medication while monitoring for signs and symptoms of relapse. Abrupt discontinuation is also more likely to lead to antidepressant discontinuation symptoms, which often are referred to as withdrawal symptoms. The occurrence of these symptoms following medication discontinuation does not imply that antidepressants are addictive.

Abrupt discontinuation of TCAs commonly results in diarrhea, increased sweating, anxiety, and dizziness, symptoms previously attributed to cholinergic rebound. Among the SSRIs, withdrawal symptoms appear to occur most commonly following the discontinuation of short half-life serotonergic drugs [93], such as fluvoxamine, paroxetine, and venlafaxine. Patients describe symptoms as flulike, and they include nausea, diarrhea, insomnia, malaise, muscle aches, anxiety irritability, dizziness, vertigo, and vivid dreams [93]. Often and for unknown reasons, patients who experience this constellation of symptoms have transient electric shock sensations. This unique symptom is diagnostically useful and strongly suggests to the clinician that the patient is in fact experiencing withdrawal, because the symptom rarely occurs in other conditions such as viral infections or as an effect of a new medication.

Programs and interventions

Outpatient counseling or psychotherapy

This usually involves hourly appointment for 1 or 2 days a week. Duration of treatment can last 3 months to several years depending on the problem and treatment approach used.

Medications

A minimum of 6 to 9 months are required for medications. Long-term reliance on that medication is often the result. Adverse effects from medications can be substantial. Fig. 1 provides an algorithm for the use of antidepressant medications.

Short-term Admission to a Psychiatric Hospital

Brief stays normally are focused on stabilizing severe problems and crises. Programs almost never address underlying problems or long-term treatment issues that may be necessary for lasting or complete recovery.

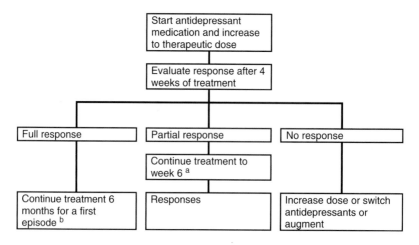

Fig. 1. Acute treatment for major depression. [a] If no further response is seen at week 5, it is not necessary to wait until week 6. [b] See text for maintenance treatment guidelines for patients with recurrent depression.

Outpatient day treatment program

This involves participation from 1 to 3 days a week in a program that usually is affiliated with a psychiatric hospital. Day treatment programs are usually a step down from a hospital and more intensive than outpatient counseling or psychotherapy.

Residential inpatient treatment

This involves living in a home or dormitory facility that may or may not be locked. The programs can have minimal structure or be highly structured. Residential programs normally include routines that involve daily living activities, an educational or occupational program, and individual and group therapy.

Outdoor therapeutic programs

This involves short-term or longer-term participation in wilderness and other outdoor settings that provide a variety of experiential and personal growth opportunities. These include personal and group challenges, activities that require initiative, outdoor sports, wilderness or survival education, exercise, nutrition, and separation from unhealthy environments. Healthy and therapeutic group interactions are facilitated and practiced. Individual counseling and therapy are often a component of these programs.

Summary

Recognition and treatment of anxiety and depression in adolescents and college students remain a major concern for physicians, educators and parents. The morbidity and mortality associated with these disorders can be decreased by increasing public awareness of the seriousness of these disorders and the need for timely assessment and intervention. It is important to keep in mind the developmental course of anxiety, including the boundaries between normal and pathological anxiety and continuity with adult disorders. Also important are the various biological, psychological, and social determinants that both protect against and lead to the development of pathological anxiety and feelings of depression in children and youth. Multi-modal treatment approaches combining cognitive, behavioral, and pharmacological should be used in managing anxiety and depression in adolescents and college students.

References

[1] Parmelee Dean X, David Ronald B. Child and adolescent psychiatry. In: Mosby's neurology psychiatry access series. St. Louis: Mosby; 1996.

[2] Roth T, Roehrs TA. Issues in the use of benzodiazepine therapy. J Clin Psychiatry 1992;53: 14–8.

[3] Lucki I, Rickels K, Geller AM. Chronic use of benzodiazepines and psychomotor and cognitive test performance. Psychopharmacology (Berl) 1986;88:426–33.

[4] American Psychiatric Association. Benzodiazepine dependence, toxicity and abuse: a task force report of the American Psychiatric Association. Washington (DC): American Psychiatric Association; 1990.

[5] Sellers EM, Schneiderman JF, Romach MK, et al. Comparative drug effects and abuse liability of lorazepam, buspirone, and secobarbital in nondependent subjects. J Clin Psychopharmacol 1992;12:79–85.

[6] Busto U, Sellers EM, Naranjo CA, et al. Withdrawal reactions after long-term therapeutic use of benzodiazepines. N Engl J Med 1986;315:854–7.

[7] Schopf J. Withdrawal phenomena after long-term administration of benzodiazepines: a review of recent investigations. Pharmacopsychiatrie Neuro- Psychopharmakologie 1983;16:1–8.

[8] Tyrer PJ, Own R, Dawling S. Gradual withdrawal of diazepam after long-term therapy. Lancet 1983;1:1402–6.

[9] Ashton H. Protracted withdrawal syndromes from benzodiazepines. J Subst Abuse Treat 1991;8:19–28.

[10] Noyes Jr R, Gravey MJ, Cook BL, et al. Benzodiazepine withdrawal: a review of evidence. J Clin Psychiatry 1988;49:382–9.

[11] Zipursky RB, Baker RW, Zimmer B. Alprazolam withdrawal delirium unresponsive to diazepam: case report. J Clin Psychiatry 1985;46:344–5.

[12] Marangell LB, Silver MJ, Gauff DC, et al. Pharmacology and electro convulsive therapy. Textbook of clinical psychiatry. Washington, DC: American Psychiatric Publishing; 2003.

[13] Dixon J, Power SJ, Grundy EM, et al. Sedation for local anaesthesia: comparison of intravenous midazolam and diazepam. Anaesthesia 1984;39:372–8.

[14] Reitan JA, Porter W, Braunstein M. Comparison of psychomotor skills and amnesia after induction of anesthesia with midazolam or thiopental. Anesth Analg 1986;65:933–7.

[15] Votey SR, Bosse GM, Bayer MJ, et al. Flumazenil: a new benzodiazepine antagonist. Ann Emerg Med 1991;20:181–8.

[16] Cohn J, Wilcox CS. Low-sedation potential of buspirone compared with alprazolam and lorazepam in the treatment of anxious patients: a double-blind study. J Clin Psychiatry 1986; 47:409–12.

[17] Goldberg HL, Finnerty RJ. The comparative efficacy of buspirone and diazepam in the treatment of anxiety. Am J Psychiatry 1979;136:1184–7.

[18] Sheehan DV, Raj AB, Sheehan KH, et al. Is buspirone effective for panic disorder? J Clin Psychopharmacol 1990;10:3–11.

[19] Gastfried DR, Rosenbaum JF. Adjunctive buspirone in benzodiazepine treatment of four patients with panic disorder. Am J Psychiatry 1989;146:914–6.

[20] Harvey KV, Balon R. Augmentation with buspirone: a review. Ann Clin Psychiatry 1995;7: 143–7.

[21] Laird LK. Issues in the monopharmacotherapy and polypharmacotherapy of obsessive-compulsive disorder. Psychopharmacol Bull 1996;32:569–78.

[22] Munjack DJ, Bruns J, Baltazar PL, et al. A pilot study of buspirone in the treatment o social phobia. J Anxiety Disorder 1991;5:87–98.

[23] Schneier FR, Saoud JB, Campeas RC, et al. Buspirone in social phobia. J Clin Psychopharmacol 1992;13:251–6.

[24] Rakel RE. Long-term buspirone therapy for chronic anxiety: a multicenter international study to determine safety. South Med J 1990;83:194–8.

[25] Moskowitz H, Smiley A. Effects of chronically administered buspirone and diazepam on driving-related skills and performance. J Clin Psychiatry 1982;43:45–55.

[26] Cole JO, Orzak MG, Beake B, et al. Assessment of the abuse liability of buspirone in recreational sedative users. J Clin Psychiatry 1982;43:69–74.

[27] Greenblatt DJ, Shader RI, Abernethy DR. Drug therapy: current status of benzodiazepines. N Engl J Med 1983;309:410–6.

[28] Rickels K, Case WG, Downing RW, et al. Long-term diazepam therapy and clinical outcome. JAMA 1983;250:767–71.

[29] Hoehn-Saric R, McLeod DR, Zimmerli WD. Differential effects of alprazolam and imipramine in generalized anxiety disorder: somatic vs psychic symptoms. J Clin Psychiatry 1988; 49:293–301.

[30] Kahn RJ, Menair D, Lipman RS, et al. Imipramine and chlordiazepoxide in depressive and anxiety disorders: efficacy in anxious outpatients. Arch Gen Psychiatry 1986;43:79–85.

[31] Keller MB, Hanks DL. Anxiety symptom relief in depression treatment outcomes. J Clin Psychiatry 1995;56:22–9.

[32] Spier SA, Tesar GE, Rosenbaum JF, et al. Treatment of panic disorder and agoraphobia with clonazepam. J Clin Psychiatry 1986;47:238–42.

[33] Tesar GE. High-potency benzodiazepines for short-term management of panic disorder: the US evidence. J Clin Psychiatry 1990;15:4–10.

[34] Klein DF, Ross DC, Cohen P. Panic and avoidance in agoraphobia; application of path analysis of treatment studies. Arch Gen Psychiatry 1987;44:377–85.

[35] Zitrin CM, Klein DF, Woerner MG, et al. Treatment of phobias: comparison of imipramine and placebo. Arch Gen Psychiatry 1983;40:125–38.

[36] Sheehan DV, Ballenger J, Jacobsen G. Treatment of endogenous anxiety with phobic, hysterical, and hypochondrial symptoms. Arch Gen Psychiatry 1980;39:51–9.

[37] van Vlient IM, Westenberg HG, Den Boer JA. MAO inhibitors in panic disorder: clinical effects of treatment with brofaromine: a double blind-blind placebo controlled study. Psychopharmacology (Berl) 1993;112:483–9.

[38] den Boer JA, van Vliet IM, Westenberg HG. Recent developments in the psychopharmacology of social phobia. Eur Arch Psychiatry Clin Neurosci 1995;244:309–16.

[39] Oehrberg S, Christiansen PE, Behnke K, et al. Paroxetine in the treatment of panic disorder: a randomized, double-blind, placebo-controlled study. Br J Psychiatry 1995;167:374–9.

[40] Schenier FR, Liebowitz MR, Davies SO, et al. Fluoxetine in panic disorder. J Clin Psychopharmacol 1990;10:119–21.

[41] Westenberg HGM, den Boer JA. Clinical and biochemical effects of selective serotonin-uptake inhibitors in anxiety disorders. In: Gastpar M, Wakelin JS, editors. Selective serotonin reuptake inhibitors: novel or commonplace agents? 1988. Basel (Switzerland): S KIarger; 1988. p. 84–99.

[42] Black B, Uhde TW, Tancer ME. Fluoxetine for the treatment of social phobia [letter]. J Clin Psychopharmacol 1992;12:293–5.

[43] Van Ameringen M, Mancini C, Streiner DL. Fluoxetine efficacy in social phobia. J Clin Psychiatry 1993;54:27–32.

[44] Westernberg HG, den Boer JA. New findings in the treatment of panic disorder. Pharmacopsychiatry 1993;26:30–3.

[45] Liebowitz MA, Gorman JM, Fyer AJ, et al. Pharmacotherapy of social phobia: an interim report of a placebo-controlled comparison of phenelzine and atenolol. J Clin Psychiatry 1988;49:252–7.

[46] Marshall RD, Schneier FR, Fallon BA, et al. Medication therapy for social phobia. J Clin Psychiatry 1994;55:33–7.

[47] Davidson JRT, Fort SM, Smith RD, et al. Long-term treatment of social phobia with clonazepam. J Clin Psychiatry 1991;52:16–20.

[48] Gelernter CS, Uhde TW, Climbolic P, et al. Cognitive-behavioural and pharmacologic treatment for social phobia: a preliminary study. Arch Gen Psychiatry 1991;48:938–45.

[49] Jefferson JW. Social phobia: a pharmacologic treatment overview. J Clin Psychiatry 1995; 56:18–24.

[50] Drew PJ, Barnes JN, Evans SJ. The effect of acute beta-adrenoceptor blockade on examination performance. Br J Clin Pharmacol 1985;19:783–6.

[51] Hertely LR, Unagapen S, Davie I, et al. The effect of beta-adrenergic blocking drugs on speakers' performance and memory. Br J Psychiatry 1983;142:512–7.

[52] Brantigan CO, Brantigan TA, Joseph N. Effect of beta blockade and beta stimulation on stage fright. Am J Med 1982;72:88–94.

[53] Yudofsky SC, Silver JM. Beta-blockers in the treatment of performance anxiety. Harvard Mental Health Letter 1987;4:8.

[54] Clomipramine Collaborative Study Group. Clomipramine in the treatment of patients with obsessive–compulsive disorder. Arch Gen Psychiatry 1991;48:730–8.

[55] Freeman CP, Trimble MR, Deakin JF, et al. Fluvoxamine versus clomipramine in the treatment of obsessive-compulsive disorder: a multi-center, randomized, double-blind parallel group. J Clin Psychiatry 1994;55:301–5.

[56] Goodman WK, Price LH, Delgado PL, et al. Specificity of serotonin reuptake inhibitors in the treatment of obsessive–compulsive disorder: comparison of luvoxamine and desipramine. Arch Gen Psychiatry 1990;47:577–85.

[57] Goodman WK, Kozak MJ, Liebowitz M, et al. Treatment of obsessive- compulsive disorder with fluvoxamine: a multi-centre, double-blind, placebo-controlled trial. Int Clin Psychopharmacol 1996;11:21–9.

[58] Perse TL, Greist JH, Jefferson JW, et al. Fluvoxamine treatment of obsessive–compulsive disorder. Am J Psychiatry 1988;144:1543–8.

[59] Mundo E, Bareggi SR, Pirola R, et al. Long-term pharmacotherapy of obsessive–compulsive disorder: a double-blind controlled study. J Clin Psychopharmacol 1997;17:4–10.

[60] American Psychiatric Association. Diagnostic and statistical manual of mental disorders. 4th edition. Washington (DC): American Psychiatric Association; 1994.

[61] Liberman JA, Tasman A. Antidepressant medication. In: Psychiatrist drugs. Philadelphia: WB Saunders Company; 2000. p. 53–6.

[62] Everett HC. The use of bethanechol chloride with tricyclic antidepressants. Am J Psychiatry 1976;132:1202–4.

[63] Yager J. Bethanecol chloride can reverse erectile and ejaculatory dysfunction induced by tricyclic antidepressants and mazindol: case report. J Clin Psychiatry 1986;47:210–1.

[64] Glassman AH. The newer antidepressant drugs and their cardiovascular effects. Psychopharmacol Bull 1984;20:272–9.

[65] Fernstrom MH, Krowinksi RL, Kupfer DJ. Chronic imipramine treatment weight gain. Psychiatry Res 1986;17:269–73.

[66] Kupfer DJ, Coble PA, Rubinstein MS. Changes in weight during treatment for depression. Psychosom Med 1979;41:535–44.

[67] Wedin GP, Oderda GM, Klein-Schwartz W, et al. Relative toxicity of cyclic antidepressants. Ann Emerg Med 1986;15:797–804.

[68] Daily JW, Naritoku DK. Antidepressants and seizures: clinical anecdotes overshadow neuroscience. Biochem Pharmacol 1996;52:1323–9.

[69] Rosenstein DL, Nelson JC, Jacobs SC. Seizures associated with antidepressants: a review. J Clin Psychiatry 1993;54:289–99.

[70] Gammon GD, Hansen C. A case of akinesia induced by amoxapine. Am J Psychiatry 1984; 141:283–4.

[71] Ross DR, Walker JI, Paterson J. Akathisia induced by amoxapine. Am J Psychiatry 1983; 140:115–6.

[72] Thornton JE, Stahl SM. Case report of tardive dyskinesia and parkinsonism associated with amoxapine therapy. Am J Psychiatry 1984;141:704–5.

[73] Doughty MJ, Lyle WM. Medications used to prevent migraine headaches and their potential ocular adverse effects. Optom Vis Sci 1995;72:879–91.

[74] Hamilton JA, Halbreich U. Special aspects of neuropsychiatric illness I women: with a focus on depression. Annu Rev Med 1993;44:355–64.

[75] Manna V, Bolino F, Di Cicco L. Chronic tension-type headache, mood depression and serotonin: therapeutic effects of fluvoxamine and mianserine. Headache 1994;34:44–9.

[76] Jacobsen FM. Low-dose trazodone as a hypnotic in patients treated with MAOIs and other psychotropics: a pilot study. J Clin Psychiatry 1990;51:298–302.
[77] Nierenberg AA, Keck Jr PE. Management of monoamine oxidase inhibitor-associated insomnia with trazodone. J Clin Psychopharmacol 1989;9:42–5.
[78] Bouwer CD, Harvey BH. Phasic craving for carbohydrate observed with citalopram. Int Clin Psychopharmacol 1996;11:273–8.
[79] Fisher S, Kent TA, Bryant SG. Postmarketing surveillance by patient self-monitoring: preliminary data for sertraline versus fluoxetine. J Clin Psychiatry 1995;56:288–96.
[80] Metz A, Shader RI. Adverse interactions encountered when using trazodone to treat insomnia associated with fluoxetine. Int Clin Psychopharmacol 1990;5:191–4.
[81] Marangell LB, Silver MJ, Gauff DC, et al. Pharmacology and electro convulsive therapy. In: Hales RE, Yudofsky SC, editors. Textbook of clinical psychiatry. 4th edition. Washington, DC: American Psychiatric Publishing; 2003. p. 1057–9.
[82] Francois B, Marquet P, Roustan J, et al. Serotonin syndrome due to an overdose of moclobemide and clomipramine: a potentially life-threatening association. Intensive Care Med 1997; 23:122–4.
[83] Hodgman MJ, Martin TG, Krenzelok EP. Serotonin syndrome due to venlafaxine and maintenance tranylcypromine therapy. Hum Exp Toxicol 1997;16:14–7.
[84] Kolecki P. Venlafaxine induced serotonin syndrome occurring after abstinence from phenelzine for more than two weeks [letter]. J Toxicol Clin Toxicol 1997;35:211–2.
[85] Beasley Jr CM, Masica DN, Heiligenstein JH, et al. Possible monoamine oxidase inhibitor–serotonin uptake inhibitor interaction: fluoxetine clinical data and preclinical findings. J Clin Psychopharmacol 1993;13:312–20.
[86] Marangell LB, Silver MJ, Gauff DC, et al. Pharmacology and electro convulsive therapy. In: Hales RE, Yudofsky SC, editors. Textbook of clinical psychiatry. 4th edition. Washington, DC: American Psychiatric Publishing; 2003. p. 1059–61.
[87] Liebowitz MR, Quitkin FM, Steward JW, et al. Phenelzine vs imipramine in atypical depression: a preliminary report. Arch Gen Psychiatry 1984;41:669–77.
[88] Qitkin F, Rifkin A, Klein DF. Monoamine oxidase inhibitors: a review of antidepressant effectiveness. Arch Gen Psychiatry 1979;35:749–60.
[89] Ravaris CL, Robinson DS, Ives JO, et al. Phenelzine and amitriptyline in the treatment of depression: a comparison of present and past studies. Arch Gen Psychiatry 1980;37:1075–80.
[90] Zisook S. A clinical overview of monoamine oxidase inhibitors. Psychosomatics 1985;26: 240–6.
[91] Amsterdam J, Berwish NJ. High-dose tranylcypromine therapy for refractory depression. Pharmacopsychiatry 1989;22:21–5.
[92] Weise CC, Stein MK, Pereira-Ogan J, et al. Amitriptyline once daily versus three times daily in depressed outpatients. Arch Gen Psychiatry 1980;37:555–60.
[93] Coupland NJ, Bell CJ, Potokar JP. Serotonin reuptake inhibitor withdrawal. J Clin Psychopharmacol 1996;16:356–62

Further readings

Bakshi I. Understanding children and their problems. Mumbai, India: Vakils, Feffer and Simons; 1999.

Durlak AJ. School-based prevention program for children and adolescents. London: SAGE Publications; 1995.

Gelder MG, Lopez-lbor Jr JJ, Andreasen NC. New Oxford textbook of psychiatry. New York: Oxford University Press; 2000.

Hurlock EB. Child development. Singapore: McGraw Hill; 1985.

Jacobson JL, Jacobson AM. Psychiatrist secrets. New Delhi: Jaypee Brothers; 1996.

Klykylo WM, Kay J, Rube D. Clinical child psychiatry. Philadelphia: WB Saunders Company; 1998.

Lewis L. Child and adolescent psychiatry—a comprehensive textbook. 2nd edition. Baltimore: Williams & Wilkins; 1991.

Singhal PK, Bhatia MS. Problem of behavior in children. Delhi: CBS Publishers; 1994.

Weissman MM. Treatment of depression. Washington, DC: American Psychiatry Press; 2003.

PEDIATRIC CLINICS
OF NORTH AMERICA

Pediatr Clin N Am 52 (2005) 135–161

Contraception for College Students

Donald E. Greydanus, MD, FAAP, FSAM[a,b,]*,
Mary Ellen Rimsza, MD, FAAP[c,d],
Lyubov Matytsina, MD, PhD[e,f]

[a]*Sindecuse Health Center, Western Michigan University, Kalamazoo, MI, USA*
[b]*College of Human Medicine, Michigan State University, East Lansing, MI, USA*
[c]*School of Health Management and Policy, W.P. Carey School of Business, Arizona State University, ASU Main Campus BA 318, P.O. Box 874506, Tempe, AZ 85287, USA*
[d]*Mayo Clinic College of Medicine, Rochester, MN, USA*
[e]*Department of Obstetrics, Gynecology, and Perinatology, Donetsk Medical University, Ukraine*
[f]*Pediatric and Adolescent Gynecology Department,
Donetsk Regional Centre of Maternal and Childhood Care, Donetsk, Ukraine*

Reproductive health and contraception

An important issue for human beings is the acquisition of normal sexual health, including the understanding and application of reproductive health when needed [1–5]. Comprehensive sexuality education is not a topic provided to many children, adolescents, or college students in the United States, however [6]. Students who were sexually active in high school may continue to be at risk for pregnancy and sexually transmitted diseases (STDs) in their college life; those who chose abstinence in high school may abandon this concept in college, choosing coital behavior at all levels of university life—freshman through graduate levels [7–12]. One study noted that 35% of students in college reported having six or more lifetime coital partners [13]. There are more than 15 million cases of STDs in the United States, and more than 60% of these occur in young people younger than 25 years [14].

Approximately 50% to 57% of pregnancies (90% in adolescents) in the United States are unintended (>3 million) and, in adolescents, approximately 35% of

* Corresponding author. Kalamazoo Center for Medical Studies, Michigan State University, 1000 Oakland Drive, Kalamazoo, MI 49008-1284.
E-mail address: greydanus@kcms.msu.edu (D.E. Greydanus).

0031-3955/05/$ – see front matter © 2005 Elsevier Inc. All rights reserved.
doi:10.1016/j.pcl.2004.11.005
pediatric.theclinics.com

these end in abortion [4,14–17]. Despite slight reductions in birth rates in the 1990s, increasing contraceptive prevalence, and condom use among adolescent girls [18], approximately 900,000 adolescent females aged 12 to 19 years in the United States become pregnant each year.

The median age at first intercourse of 16 years [19] is comparable to the age of coital initiation in other developed countries, such as Canada, countries of Western Europe (eg, France, Great Britain), countries of Eastern Europe (eg, Ukraine) [3] and Eurasia (eg, Russia). The birth, pregnancy, and abortion rates are significantly higher among adolescents in the United States in contrast to such countries as the Netherlands and Sweden [20].

Box 1. Contraceptive methods

Abstinence
Rhythm method of contraception (periodic abstinence)
    Calendar
    Ovulation method
    Symptothermal
    Postovulation
OCPs (combined)
Minipills (progestin-only pills [POPs])
Emergency contraceptives
Vaginal barrier contraceptives
    Diaphragm
    Vaginal contraceptive sponge
    Cervical cap (Prentif Cavity-rim)
    Female condom (Reality)
    Vaginal spermicides
    Male condoms
Injectable contraceptives
    Depo-Provera
    Lunelle
Intrauterine devices
    Progestasert IUD (with progesterone)
    ParaGard (Copper T380A IUD)
    Mirena (IUD with levonorgestrel)
Implants
    Norplant (six capsules)
    Norplant-2 (two rods)
Sterilization
    Female
    Male (vasectomy)
Coitus interruptus

Table 1
Contraceptive efficacy: first-year failure rate (per 100 women years of use)

Contraceptive method	Typical use	Perfect use
Combined OCPs	3–8	0.1
Progesterone IUD	2.0	1.5
Copper T IUD	0.8	0.6
Mirena IUD	0.2	0.1
Depo-medroxyprogesterone acetate (DMPA)	0.3	0.3
Norplant	0.05	0.05

Because 80% of college women are sexually active, it is important that clinicians caring for them provide appropriate contraceptive counseling, covering such topics as safe sex, contraception, and STD and AIDS prevention [9,11, 14,21–26]. Several safe and effective contraceptive methods are available (Box 1) [1–5,15,16,20,27,28]. The most effective contraceptive methods are as follows: abstinence; combined oral contraceptives, or oral contraceptive pills (OCPs); and intramuscular medroxy-progesterone acetate (Depo-Provera). These methods have pregnancy rates of less than 1 per 100 women-years of use (Table 1). The gap between the efficacy of the perfect use of contraceptives (eg, correct, consistent, and continued use of a chosen contraceptive method) and the typical use leads to millions of unintended pregnancies each year [29]. The barrier methods (eg, condoms, diaphragms, cervical caps, vaginal sponges, female condoms, and vaginal spermicides) can be used effectively by motivated college students who are taught how to use them; periodic abstinence has higher pregnancy rates but is a potentially effective contraceptive method. Norplant, an effective method in which six progesterone capsules are inserted subcutaneously into the upper arm, was removed from the US market in 2000. The intrauterine device (IUD) is an excellent contraceptive but has been tainted with the image of inducing pelvic inflammatory disease (PID) [1,30].

Approximately 5% of the 16 million women in the United States who take oral contraceptives experience an unintended pregnancy. Thus, new methods for hormonal contraception are needed [31]. The choice of currently available contraceptive methods has increased considerably in recent years, offering girls and women of reproductive age various methods depending on their needs and lifestyle. Several contraceptive methods have received US Food and Drug Administration (FDA) approval over the past two decades, including the following methods: emergency contraceptives (Preven, Plan B), Depo-Provera, the cervical cap, Lunelle (injectable contraceptive with estrogen), Mirena (an IUD with levonorgestrel), a contraceptive patch (Ortho Evra), and an intravaginal ring (NuvaRing) [15,16,28,31–33]. The FDA approval history for contraceptives is as follows:

December 1990: Norplant (withdrawn from US market in 2000)
October 1992: Depo-Provera

September 1998: Preven Kit
July 1999: Plan B
October 2000: Lunelle ("injectable pill")
December 2000: Mirena IUD
October 2001: NuvaRing (vaginal ring)
November 2001: Evra patch
Pending: Implanon (single rod)

Technology has expanded over the past decade to include the following forms of contraceptive steroid release: pills, patch, injectables, hormone-releasing IUDs, implants, and vaginal rings. This development has led to several potential advantages:

- An increased range of new contraceptive methods
- Methods that are very effective and easy to use
- Methods that offer reversible, but not daily hormonal effects with better compliance
- Methods with low-hormone doses available
- Methods that offer continuous low-hormone levels

Since the development of OCPs more than 40 years ago, the emphasis has been on having newer pill formulations with lower doses of estrogens and various progestins and developing phasic dosing regimens [34]. Recently, newer delivery systems of hormones have been developed to help decrease contraceptive failure rate associated with incorrect use of contraceptives. For example, the patch and ring are user-controlled and easy to discontinue—thus more appealing to some women.

To determine the pattern of contraception use, a survey was conducted in a large population of women drawn from five European countries (France, Germany, Italy, Spain, and the United Kingdom) [35]. More than 12,000 randomly selected women, aged 15 to 49 years, were interviewed using a standardized questionnaire which addressed the use of current methods of contraception [35]. The responses were analyzed for the total study population and, where appropriate, by country and age. An oral contraceptive was confirmed as the most widely used method of contraception for women in this European study population, with an estimated 22 million users in the five countries. Reasons for not using contraception included not being sexually active, wishing to become pregnant, concluding they or their partners were sterile, fear of contraceptive side effects (as breast cancer), religious grounds, and others. Despite good access to effective contraception and knowledge about condoms, many people, including college students, put themselves at risk for unwanted consequences of sexual activity. There are many strong feelings and emotions associated with individuals' sexual selves. They need better methods of prevention but also need greater understanding of why and how people of all ages use or do not use contraception.

Box 2. Combined oral contraceptive hormones

Hormones

Estrogen
  EE
  Mestranol (three brands)

Progestins
  Norgestrel
  Norethindrone
  Norethindrone acetate
  Ethynodiol acetate
  Gestodene (not available in United States)
  Levonorgestrel
  Norgestimate
  Desogestrel
  Drospirenone
  Ciproterone acetate

Oral contraceptives

One of the most popular contraceptives on the college campus is the OCP, and use of this method increases from freshman to senior years [11]. There are more than 145 brands of OCPs available; most OCPs contain both a synthetic estrogen and synthetic progestogen [1,2]. The estrogen is usually ethinyl estradiol (EE), but a few brands contain mestranol. In general, it is believed that 30 to 35 μg of EE is equivalent to 50 μg of mestranol (Box 2). There are many progestogens available, including norethindrone, levonorgestrel, gestodene, desogestrel, norgestimate, ciproterone acetate, and drospirenone. Drospirenone is a new synthetic progestin chemically related to spironolactone [36]. Estrogen may lead to nausea, breast tenderness, and breast enlargement; progestins may lead to unfavorable changes in low-density lipoprotein (LDL) and high-density lipoprotein cholesterol. Other adverse effects (eg, weight gain or depression) are difficult to link to either hormone class alone. The following questions should be posed to the student interested in oral contraceptives:

1. What methods have you used before?
2. What are your worries about this method?
3. What method do your friends use? What did they say?
4. Do you think you can use this method correctly?
5. Do you worry about your weight? Are you dieting?
6. Do you have questions I have not answered?

7. Can you deal with unexpected bleeding?
8. Have you heard of some negative comments about OCP use (eg, weight gain and infertility)?
9. Do you know the minor OCP side effects?

OCPs prevent pregnancy by inhibiting ovulation, increasing cervical mucus viscosity, causing endometrial atrophy, and changing tubal transport mechanisms [1]. Benefits of the oral contraceptive are listed in Box 3. A 50-μg estrogen pill may be used to treat such conditions as dysfunctional uterine bleeding, ovarian cyst disease, and endometriosis; it is also used to overcome a conflicting medication (eg, some antiepilepsy drugs). Most brands are manufactured as 21- or 28-day packs. The 20-day packs have 7 days of placebo pills so that the student continues to take a pill each day of the cycle. Newer variations include brands that have only 2 placebo days in each 28-day cycle. Also available is an OCP dial-pack dispenser with each pill numbered and a dial that only turns in one direction. There is no combined OCP brand shown to be more effective than any other brand in preventing pregnancy; thus, any brand the student wishes to take to prevent unwanted pregnancy is acceptable. Some OCPs can be counterfeit, and this possibility must be considered if pills are not obtained in pharmacies or other trusted places [37]. With OCPs, condoms are also recommended to reduce the risk for STDs [38,39].

Box 3. Noncontraceptive benefits of combined oral contraceptives

1. Treatment for dysmenorrhea
2. Treatment for dysfunctional uterine bleeding
3. Treatment for premenstrual syndrome
4. Decreased risk for ovarian and endometrial cancer
5. Decreased risk for symptomatic PID
6. Treatment for polycystic ovary syndrome
7. Treatment of acne vulgaris
8. Treatment for premature ovarian failure
9. Treatment for endometriosis
10. Treatment of hypothalamic amenorrhea caused by eating disorders, exercise, stress
11. Decreased mittelschmerz (pain associated with ovulation)
12. Prevention of ovarian cyst disease with 50-μg EE pill
13. Lower incidence of ectopic pregnancy (decreased risk by 90%)
14. Protective for rheumatoid arthritis
15. Possible benefit in prevention/treatment of disorders associated with decreased bone mineral density
16. Possible benefit in the prevention of the development of leiomyomata uteri

New OCP brands now available include the following: Alesse and Levlite (both with 20 µg of EE and 0.1 mg of levonorgestrel), Apri (with 30 µg of EE and 0.15 of desogestrel), Desogen (30 µg of EE with 0.15 of desogestrel), Estrostep (EE increasing from 20 to 35 µg over 3 wk with 1 mg of norethindone), Kariva (multiphasic: three levels of EE [20,0,10] and 0.15 mg of desogestrel), and Mircette (multiphasic: 3 wk of 20 µg of EE and 0.15 mg of desogestrel, then 2 placebo pills, then 5 days of 10 µg of EE alone). The two brands that are FDA-approved for treatment of acne vulgaris are Estro-step and Ortho Tri-Cyclen. Cyclessa is a new low-dose triphasic OCP that contains less estrogen than Tri-Cyclen and other triphasic pills; it contains 25 µg/day of EE plus desogestrel (0.1 mg/d, 0.125 mg/d, and 0.15 mg/d in each phase) [40].

Yasmin is a new OCP with 30 µg of EE and a new progestin, drospirenone. This progestin is a synthetic version of progesterone and a spironolactone analog that can lead to potassium retention; 3 mg of drospirenone is equivalent to 25 mg of spironolactone. This OCP is contraindicated in women with renal, hepatic, or adrenal insufficiency [36]. It is unclear if this OCP has any advantages over other OCPs, and its effect on acne is similar to other OCPs. A 2002 report noted 40 cases of venous thromboembolism with two deaths in Europe in women taking Yasmin [41].

Another new OCP is Seasonale, with 30 µg of EE and 0.15 mg of levonorgestrel [42]. It provides continuous combined estrogen plus progestin for 84 days followed by 7 days of placebo so that only four menses occur per year. This extended cycling (eg, absence of menses for several months) is especially helpful for adolescents who have medical problems that are worsened by menstruation or who have significant adverse symptoms caused by menstruation, such as dysmenorrhea or menorrhagia (Box 4) [43]. Extended cycling is associated with increased breakthrough bleeding, however, especially in the first year of use [42]. Some women also may be interested in extended cycling for lifestyle reasons. For example, an athlete may wish to extend her cycle to avoid menses during athletic competitions. Extended cycling can be accomplished

---

Box 4. Conditions that may benefit from extended cycling

Dysmenorrhea
Premenstrual tension syndrome
Menorrhagia
Iron-deficiency anemia
Endometriosis
Headaches
Epilepsy
Rheumatoid arthritis
Coagulapathies
Anticoagulation therapy

Box 5. World Health Organization medical eligibility categories for oral contraceptive pills

Category 1 (no restrictions)

  Antibiotics
  Benign breast disease
  Benign ovarian tumors
  Cervical ectropion
  Dysmenorrhea
  Endometriosis
  Epilepsy
  Family history of breast cancer
  Gestational trophoblastic disease (benign or malignant)
  Headaches (mild)
  History of ectopic pregnancy or abortion (postabortion after first
    or second trimester),
  History of gestational diabetes
  Increased STD risk
  Iron-deficiency anemia
  Irregular menstrual bleeding
  Obesity
  Ovarian or endometrial cancer
  Past pelvic surgery
  PID
  21 days or more after birth
  Thyroid disorders (hypo/hyperthyroidism, simple goiter)
  Varicose veins
  Various infections: malaria, tuberculosis, others
  STDs
  Viral hepatitis carrier

Category 2 (caution)

  Cervical cancer
  Diabetes mellitus (uncomplicated)
  Headaches (severe and if they start after beginning OCPs)
  Hypertension at 140–159/100–109 mm Hg
  Major surgery without prolonged immobilization
  Migraine headaches without focal neurologic involvement
  Patients who have a hard time taking the OCP correctly because
    of drug or alcohol abuse, mental retardation, persistent
    history as poor OCP takers, severe psychiatric disorders

Sickle cell disease or sickle C disease
Undiagnosed breast mass

Category 3 (usually no OCP given)

Gallbladder disease
Lactating (6 wk to 6 mo)
Less than 21 days post partum
Medications that interfere with OCP efficacy
Undiagnosed abnormal vaginal/uterine bleeding

Category 4 (OCP contraindicated)

Breast cancer
Cerebrovascular accident (active or history)
Complicated structural heart disease (with pulmonary hypertension, atrial fibrillation, or history of subacute bacterial endocarditis)
Coronary (or ischemic) heart disease (active or history)
Deep vein thrombosis or pulmonary embolism (active or history)
Diabetes mellitus (complicated with retinopathy, neuropathy, nephropathy)
Headaches (including migraine headaches) with focal neurologic symptoms
Hypertension (severe: 160+/110+ mm Hg, or with vascular complications)
Lactation under 6 weeks post partum
Liver disease (including liver cancer, benign hepatic adenoma, active viral hepatitis, severe cirrhosis)
Pregnancy, complicated
Surgery (involving the lower extremities or prolonged immobilization

Data from Greydanus DE. Contraception. In: Greydanus DE, Patel DR, Pratt H, Bhave S, editors. Course manual for adolescent health. Delhi, India: Cambridge Press; 2002. p. 309–24.

with any OCP by omitting the placebo pills and starting a new pack of OCPs after 21 days. The Ortho Evra patch and NuvaRing have not been studied for extended or continuous use regimens.

Contraindications to oral contraceptive pills

The World Health Organization (WHO) has published a list of medical eligibility guidelines to aid clinicians in prescribing OCPs (Box 5) [40,44–46].

Women in WHO category 1 have no restrictions to use of the OCP, whereas women in category 2 have some increased medical risk, although pregnancy risks typically exceed OCP risks. Those in category 3 are typically not prescribed the OCP unless the pregnancy risk is high and there is no other method of contraception that is acceptable to the patient. If a condition places the woman in category 4, the individual should not be placed on OCPs because of the high risks of significant OCP-induced adverse effects.

Cardiovascular risks and oral contraceptive pills

A past medical history of venous thrombosis (VT) is an absolute contra-indication to OCP use. The risk of VT is more significant for the adolescent and young adult female than the risk of arterial thrombosis. Although significant obesity is a known risk factor for VT, it is not known if OCPs are additive for VT risk in obese individuals. In general, most adolescents and young adults who develop a VT do not have recognizable VT risk factors. The number of deaths caused by cardiovascular disease (venous and arterial) among nonsmoking women aged 20 to 24 years is 2 to 6 per million per year [47]. Screening questions for students seeking OCPs are as follows:

Have you or a close family member (including uncles/aunts) had blood clots in legs or lungs?
Have you or a close family member been hospitalized for blood clots in legs/lungs?
Have you or a close family member taken blood thinners?
Under what circumstances did the clot form (eg, during air travel)?

If there is no clear family history of VT, there is no reason to screen for factor V Leiden or other prothrombotic mutations. OCPs should be discontinued before situations that will result in prolonged bed rest, such as some major surgeries. Smoking is not a major risk factor for cardiovascular disease in the healthy adolescent or young adult female. Because blood pressure (BP) may increase in susceptible women taking OCPs, BP should be checked before starting OCPs and monitored while on OCPs (Mottram Hall guidelines [48]). If there is a family or personal history of hyperlidemia, OCPs may still be prescribed if LDL remains lower than 160 mg/dL and triglycerides are lower than 250 mg/dL.

Miscellaneous illness risks and oral contraceptive pills

Low-dose OCPs are acceptable for adolescents and young adults who have diabetes mellitus unless they are poorly controlled or use tobacco. OCPs should not be used if diabetic complications are present, however, such as neuropathy, retinopathy, nephropathy, or hypertension. Some experts believe that OCPs should be avoided in women who have migraine headaches associated with auras (classic migraines). If OCPs are prescribed for women who have migraines, a change in the aura or worsening of the headache pattern should prompt re-evaluation and, potentially, discontinuation of OCPs. Women who have epilepsy may have reduced OCP efficacy if they are concomitantly taking anticonvulsants that induce hepatic enzymes (eg, barbiturates, phenytoin, carbamazepine, felbamate, topiramate, vigabatrin). Women with active liver disease should not be placed on OCPs. OCPs may be used in women who have cervical dysplasia and actually reduce the risk for ovarian and endometrial carcinoma [49]. Contrary to OCP package inserts, there is no pharmacokinetic interference with antibiotics except for rifampin that interferes with OCP efficacy [50]. Antacids and OCPs should be taken at least 3 hours apart.

Several minor side effects may occur with OCP use, including nausea, headaches, mood changes, and breast tenderness [51–53]. These side effects often disappear with increasing duration of OCP use. Although many women feel that OCPs are associated with weight gain, there is no convincing evidence that OCPs cause an increase in weight [51,54]. Breakthrough bleeding is a common side effect of OCP use and one of the most common reasons for OCP discontinuation [55]. In most patients, breakthrough bleeding decreases with consistent, continued use, and there is no need to change OCP brands because of this side effect. If breakthrough bleeding is severe or unrelenting, however, switching to an OCP containing norgestrel (eg, Lo/Ovral), norgestimate (eg, Ortho-Cyclen), or levo-norgestrel (eg, Nordette, Triphasil) may be helpful. The physician can also recommend taking 2 pills a day until the bleeding stops or adding 20 µg of EE for 7 to 10 days. It is rare that a pill with 50 µg of EE is needed to control bleeding.

Transdermal hormonal contraception

Transdermal mechanisms for delivery of medication became available in the early 1980s. Medications that are now available in transdermal formulations include the following: clonidine, estradiol, fentanyl, nicotine, nitroglycerin, scopolamine, and testosterone [56]. The FDA approved the first transdermal contraceptive patch in November 2001 [57,58]. This patch has similar side effects as OCPs with the addition of mild to moderate application site reactions and increased incidence of breast symptoms [59]. It is not yet clear if the patch offers any significant increase in efficacy or safety advantages over OCPs [59]. This method may improve compliance in some women, however.

The contraceptive patch is a matchbook-size device placed on the skin (abdomen, upper outer arm, buttocks, upper torso [not the breasts]). It consists of a three-layer matrix with an outer polyester protective layer (light tan), a middle layer that contains adhesive and contraceptive steroids, and a clear polyester liner that is removed before skin application [60,61]. The patch results in a daily hormone release of 20 µg of EE and 150 µg of norelgestromin, the primary active metabolite of norgestimate [16,40,58,62–64]. The hormones are rapidly absorbed into the blood and a steady state is reached in 2 days, similar to that noted with the oral contraceptive Ortho-Cyclen. The patch is started on day 1 of menses, replaced weekly for 3 weeks, and week 4 is patch-free. Each patch should be placed at a different site [58].

Pregnancy rates in adult women are similar when comparing the OCP and the patch, with pregnancy rates of 0.7 to 1.24 per 100 women-years reported with the patch versus 2.18 for OCPs [34,58,60,61]. Adequate steroid levels are maintained for 2 days past the manufacturer's recommended 7-day application. The efficacy is similar with various application sites. This rate is not affected by warm, humid climates, vigorous exercise, or exposure to saunas or water baths [60,61,65–67] .

Of the 15 pregnancies reported during clinical trials of the patch, five were in women who weighed more than 90 kg (198 pounds) [58]. This finding led to a warning from the manufacturer that the patch may not be as effective in obese women. There has been little research on the efficacy of other hormonal contraceptives in obese women, however, so this finding may not be limited to the patch. Causes of increased risk of contraceptive failure include the following: wearing the patch for more than 7 days, patch detachment, and failure to start a new patch after 7 days of being off the patch. Of more than 70,000 patches that were used in women during clinical trials, only 4.7% were replaced because they fell off (1.8%) or were partially detached (2.9%) [58]. One study of adolescents aged 15 to 18 years, however, noted a complete or partial detachment rate of 35.5% [63].

If the patch is off for more than 24 hours, there is a need for back-up contraception for the next 7 days.

In general, the adverse effects of the patch are similar to the OCPs, with the exception of potential site reactions (1.9%), a transient increase in breast tenderness, and an increase in dysmenorrhea [58,63,68]. Women with a history of skin allergy or exfoliative dermatologic disorders may not be good candidates for the patch. Approximately 86% of breast symptoms are reported to be mild or moderate [68]. Breakthrough bleeding or spotting may be more prevalent in cycles 1 and 2 than noted with OCPs. The incidence of nausea, emotional lability, and headaches are similar to that noted with OCPs. The mean gain in weight is reported to be 0.3 kg [68]. The risk of thromboembolism is not known but is estimated to be the same as with the OCPs [58]. The patch produces a similar lipid profile as noted with other OCPs containing EE and norgestimate [69].

Using the contraceptive patch does not require direct genital contact or daily compliance, which makes this contraceptive method popular with many students [70]. Some may find that using the patch is more convenient than daily pill dosing and more user controlled and more readily reversible than Depo-Provera [29]. In addition, for students who have difficulty swallowing pills or gastrointestinal disturbances with OCPs, the patch may be a good alternative. There are no hormonal peaks and troughs as noted with OCPs, and cycle control and ovulation suppression is similar to Ortho-Cyclen [29,56]. Taking oral antibiotics, such as tetracycline, does not disturb the contraceptive hormone levels [65,66].

Progestin-only pills

Contraceptive mechanisms of POPs include thickening of the cervical mucus and endometrial involution. Ovulation is not reliably inhibited and pregnancy rates can be 1 to 3 pregnancies per 100,000 [1]. POPs are recommended by some clinicians when estrogen is contraindicated (eg, patients who have severe hypertension or coronary heart disease). Common side effects of POPs include irregular uterine bleeding and amenorrhea. POPs should not be used by women who have a history of ectopic pregnancy and women taking medications such as anticonvulsants, griseofulvin, and rifampin. Progestins used in POPs include 0.35 mg of norethindrone (Micronor, Nor-Q.D) and 0.075 mg of norgestrel (Ovrette).

Emergency contraceptives

Emergency contraceptives (ECs) are among the most controversial and under-prescribed contraceptive methods. The following ECs are currently available:

Ovral: 2 tablets followed by 2 tablets in 12 hours
Lo/Ovral, Nordette, or Levlen: 4 tablets and 4 more in 12 hours
TriPhasil or Tri-Levlen (yellow tablets only): 4 tablets, and 4 more in 12 hours
Ovrette: 20 tablets and 20 more in 12 hours
Preven EC kit (off the market)
Plan B: levonorgestrel, 0.75 mg followed by 0.75 mg in 12 hours

Various OCPs can be taken after coital activity to prevent pregnancy, including Ovral (2 pills followed in 12 h by 2 more pills) and the following various brands, which require 4 pills followed by 4 pills in 12 hours: Lo-Ovral, Levlen, and Nordette. In 1998, the FDA approved the Preven emergency kit as an EC, and in 1999, the FDA approved Plan B, a progestin-only EC method that consists of 2 tablets of 0.75 mg of levonorgestrel [32]. The first tablet of Plan B is taken immediately and the second tablet is taken 12 hours later; more recent studies have shown that Plan B is equally effective when both pills are taken at the same time as soon as possible after unprotected intercourse [32,71]. Because Plan B contains no estrogen, nausea and vomiting are uncommon and there is no need to obtain a pregnancy test before administration. Thus, Plan B may be better tolerated than other ECs that contain estrogen [71]. Although initially approved for use within 3 days of coitus, more recent studies have shown that Plan B may be effective in pregnancy prevention if taken up to 5 days after unprotected coitus.

The expected pregnancy rate of 8% from an episode of unprotected coitus in the second or third week of the menstrual cycle is reduced to less than 1% with Plan B use [64,72]. If ECs were more widely available, they could prevent

1.7 million unintended pregnancies and reduce abortions by 50%. Whenever college students seek ECs, they should be counseled regarding effective contraceptive methods. Although ECs are an over-the-counter (OTC) product in Europe, the FDA has not yet approved Plan B for OTC use in the United States [73–75].

The misconception that Plan B can interrupt an established pregnancy has politicized the process of FDA approval for this effective and safe contraceptive method for OTC use.

ECs are very effective in preventing pregnancy, yet they are not well known among adolescents and college students [76]. College students should be clearly taught that ECs can be used in the following situations [77–80]:

- Having unplanned sex without protection
- Condom slipping/breaking
- Dislodgment of a diaphragm, cervical cap, IUD
- Missing more than 2 OCPs in a row
- Being more than 14 weeks from the last Depo-Provera injection

Without proper instruction, students do not use ECs effectively [81]. Providing the EC for the patient to take home before it is needed may improve efficacy [82]. Barriers to the use of ECs are as follows:

1. Religious/cultural pressures from the university, clinic providers, staff
2. Inability to pay for the services needed to obtain contraceptives
3. Fear of the absence of confidentiality
4. Fear of contraceptive side effects
5. Failure of health care providers to educate students about ECs
6. Failure of health care providers to prescribe ECs
7. Fear of liability
8. Fear it will undermine students' use of more efficacious contraception

A 2001 survey of college health centers noted that one third of centers did not provide EC services; 57% of these centers cited moral issues for not prescribing ECs [76]. Another study noted that 47.8% of college health centers did not prescribe ECs [83]. An EC hotline is available in the United States (1-888-668-2528 or 1-888-NOT-2-LATE); there is also Web site: http://opr.princeton.edu/ec/.

NuvaRing vaginal ring

NuvaRing is a soft, flexible, transparent vaginal ring made of an ethylene vinyl acetate copolymer. It has an outer diameter of 54 mm and a cross-section of 4 mm [54]. There are two steroid reservoir cores in the ring that provide a daily hormonal release of 15 µg of EE and 120 µg of etonogestrel (an active metabolite of desogestrel) [16,40,70]. Etonogestrel implants with depot testosterone is under study as a long-acting male contraceptive [84].

The NuvaRing provides hormone bioavailability comparable to an OCP such as Desogen or Ortho-Cept. It is inserted by the woman and removed after 3 weeks. After 1 week, a new ring is inserted for the next month. If the ring is expelled, it is washed and reinserted; if it is out for more than 3 hours, a back-up contraceptive method is recommended until the ring is back in place for 7 days in a row. This contraceptive method is popular with college students who are comfortable with their bodies and accept this form of contraceptive technology. Patients should be educated that the ring does not prevent STDs but provides contraceptive efficacy similar to combined OCPs [85,86].

The advantages of the ring are as follows [54,85–88]: (1) it provides good contraceptive efficacy, (2) it offers continuous hormone release, (3) gastrointestinal absorption is not required, (4) it is easily inserted and removed by the wearer, (5) wearer has rapid return to ovulation after stopping its use, and (6) it is a confidential method. Studies have shown that this contraceptive method is well accepted by women and their partners [89–91]. Side effects include prolonged menstrual bleeding lasting more than 7 days in 25% of cycles, vaginal discomfort, vaginitis, and foreign body sensation.

The other side effects noted in those using the NuvaRing are similar to OCP users. Because ovulation returns during the first cycle after stopping ring use, there is the possibility of pregnancy immediately after discontinuing use [92].

Vaginal barrier contraceptives

Barrier contraceptives are as follows: diaphragm, cervical cap (Prentif), vaginal contraceptive sponge, vaginal spermicides, female condom (Reality), and male condom. These are potentially good contraceptive methods for those individuals who are highly motivated to avoid pregnancy, are comfortable with their bodies, and can use these methods correctly with each act of coitus [1]. Many college students are well motivated and may choose these techniques over others discussed in this article.

Diaphragm and vaginal spermicides

Contraindications to diaphragm use are as follows:

- Allergy to rubber or spermicides
- Anteversion (severe, forward tilting of uterus)
- Complete uterine prolapse
- Perineal tears

- Retroversion (severe, backward tilting of uterus)
- Short anterior vaginal wall
- Vesicovaginal (or rectovaginal) fistulas
- Toxic shock syndrome

Health care clinicians can learn how to fit diaphragms, providing the female student with the correct size and instructions on how to successfully use this barrier method [93]. Box 6 outlines available types of diaphragms.

The diaphragm is used with vaginal cream or foam and can be used in conjunction with the condom for increased contraceptive efficacy and increased protection from STDs. Vaginal contraceptives or spermicides include foams, creams, jellies, suppositories, and a film; The advantages of vaginal contraceptives are as follows:

- The pair can share contraceptive responsibility when used with a condom
- Can reduce dyspareunia, if present (vaginal lubricant)
- Minimal cost
- No prescription needed
- Effective contraception is provided, especially if used in conjunction with condom or diaphragm
- Few side effects
- Useful for young women who have only occasional coitus

Side effects of these agents include vaginal odor and, rarely, allergic reactions. The diaphragm has been associated with an increased risk of urinary tract infections in some women, such as in those with diabetes mellitus. Rarely, toxic shock syndrome has occurred in women using a vaginal diaphragm, and this method is contraindicated in women who have a past history of toxic shock syndrome.

Cervical cap

The FDA approved the cervical cap (Prentif cavity-rim cervical cap) in 1988 because it has similar contraceptive efficacy as other barrier contraceptives [1,2]. This cervical cap is a small latex cap (with spermicide added inside) that is about half the size of a diaphragm; the cap fits around the cervix by suction. Four cervical cap sizes are available. Approximately 25% of women cannot be fitted, and some women find it difficult to insert the cap. Cervical cytology screening should be done before or at the time of fitting the cervical cap because cervical dysplasia has been noted in some women using a cap. Screening is also done 3 months after the fitting. Cervical laceration, cervical scarring, and a history of toxic shock syndrome are contraindications to using cervical caps.

Box 6. Diaphragm types

Coil-spring diaphragm (suited for general use)

A metal wire is inserted in the rim of the coil-spring diaphragm. The wire is round and spiral-coiled and folds in one plane.

Flat-spring diaphragm (Mensinga; suited for an anteverted uterus and/or a cervix that is long and posteriorly pointed)

This type is similar to the coil-spring type but firmer.

Matrisalus diaphragm (Bowbent; suited for those with a cystocele or vaginal-wall relaxation)

This diaphragm contains a steel band that is strong and flat; the band is curved and placed in the rim.

Arching-spring diaphragm (Findley; suited for those with poor muscle tone or who have a cervix that is pointed posteriorly)

This diaphragm has a double metal spring on its rim; an arc is formed when the rim is compressed.

Vaginal contraceptive sponge (Today)

The vaginal contraceptive sponge is an OTC, disposable, polyurethrane sponge with a concave shape; it can be inserted up to 2 days before coitus and left in 6 to 24 hours afterward [1]. Vaginal malodor, vulvar rash, pruritus, candidiasis, and increased risk for urinary tract infection and toxic shock syndrome may develop. Contraceptive efficacy is similar to other barrier contraceptives.

Female condom

The female condom is an OTC polyurethane bag or sheath that is placed in the vagina before coitus [1,94]. It is not used with a male condom. The female condom offers some STD protection and provides contraceptive efficacy similar to other barrier contraceptives.

Male condom

Male condoms are recommended to reduce the risk of STDs and to prevent pregnancy. They do not eliminate the risk of STDs and are less effective in preventing the transmission of human papillomavirus and possibly herpes virus infection than other STDs [38,39]. The contraceptive effectiveness of condoms is equivalent to other barrier contraceptives, if used correctly with each coital act. The advantages of condoms are as follows:

- They allow men to actively take part and share in the contraception of the pair.
- They are an effective contraceptive agent.
- Many types are available.
- They may decrease dyspareunia.
- There are minimal side effects.
- They are available without a prescription.
- There is decreased risk of STDs.

Reasons for not using condoms or inconsistent condom use are listed in Box 7 [9,10,95–98].

The latex condom is preferred because it is more effective at STD prevention (especially viral STDs) than the Kraton polyurethrane condom (eZ•on) and lamb cecum condoms. Many different kinds of condoms are available [39]. Latex condoms are associated with increased breakage rates when exposed to high temperatures or ultraviolet light; they are also weakened by oil-based lubricants. Latex sensitivities develop in up to 7% of the general population and 17% to 25% of health care workers [99]. Health care professionals should present the subject of condoms in a positive light. College students often do not use the condom and need physician encouragement in this regard [26,100].

Box 7. Reasons for not using condoms as contraceptives

Condom may rupture
Cost
Disrupts foreplay
Failure of clinicians to recommend condoms
Failure of pharmacists to make condoms easily available
Proper technique needed each time
Reduced penile sensation during coitus
Refusal of contraceptive responsibility
Religious beliefs
Stigma of using a method that is associated with promiscuity and STDs
Individual prefers other contraceptive method
Individual feels he is at low risk for STD acquisition
Criticism that condoms are not 100% effective in STD protection and thus should not be used

---

Injectable contraceptives

Medroxy-progesterone acetate (Depo-Provera) is the main injectable contraceptive available in the United States [51,70,101]. It inhibits ovulation and induces a thin endometrium and a thick cervical mucus. Depo-Provera is given as an intramuscular dose of 150 mg every 3 months, and has a pregnancy failure rate of only 0.3%. FDA approval was delayed until 1992 because of concern over possible increased risk of breast cancer and mutagenic properties, even though this contraceptive had been used for many years in other countries; none of these concerns have ever been substantiated. Because Depo-Provera does not contain estrogen, it can be used by women for whom estrogen is contraindicated. A partial list of adverse effects of Depo-Provera is shown in Box 8. Bone loss is noted in adolescents on this agent, and thus it should be avoided in those at risk for low bone density, such as adolescents who have chronic renal disease, anorexia nervosa, and possibly those who are wheelchair-bound [1]. Depo-Provera users often stop menstruating, especially with prolonged use.

Benefits of this contraceptive method include reduced incidence of dysmenorrhea and premenstrual tension syndrome. It may reduce seizure activity in some women who have epilepsy. Fertility can be delayed for 1 year of more after discontinuation because of the prolonged duration of contraceptive efficacy [51].

In 2000, the FDA approved another injectable contraceptive, Lunelle (5 mg of estradiol cypionate and 25 mg of medroxyprogesterone acetate); it is given intramuscularly every month (every 28–30 d) and has very high contraceptive efficacy. It is available as Cyclo-Provera and as Cyclofem in other countries. Because this injectable agent contains estrogen, amenorrhea and dysfunctional uterine bleeding (DUB) are less common than noted with Depo-Provera [51]. The mean cycle length is 28 days, and there is a predicable bleeding-free interval and less breakthrough bleeding than is noted with OCPs. There also is a rapid return

---

Box 8. Partial list of side effects of Depo-Provera

Acne
Amenorrhea
Behavioral changes (depression, anxiety, irritability)
Breast tenderness
Decreased bone density
Dizziness
Fatigue
Glucose intolerance
Hair loss
Irregular menstrual bleeding
Nausea
Weight gain

to fertility after discontinuation. One study noted that there was a weight gain of 0.9 to 1.8 kg if the woman weighed less than 68 kg versus a weight gain of 1.4 to 3.6 kg if the woman weighed more than 68 kg [70]. Another progestin-estrogen product that is injectable and available outside the United States is Mesigyna (with 50 mg of norethindrone and 5 mg of estradiol valerate) [102].

Finally, Norplant is a long-acting, levonorgestrel-containing contraceptive designed to be implanted subcutaneously in the upper arm [1]. Each of the six matchstick-sized capsules is 34 mm long and 2.4 mm in diameter and contains 36 mg of levonorgestrel. Contraindications to its use include the following: active thrombophlebitic or thromboembolic disorder, undiagnosed or abnormal genital bleeding, known or suspected pregnancy, acute liver disease (including benign or malignant liver tumors), and known or suspected carcinoma of the breast. It was withdrawn from the US market in 2000.

Intrauterine device

There are three IUDs that currently are used in the United States: Progestasert, the ParaGard (Copper T380A), and the Mirena [1,16,40]. Progestasert was first made available in 1976; it is replaced annually and has an expulsion rate of 2.7%. ParaGard was introduced in 1983 and has a lower failure rate than the Progestasert IUD; it is replaced every 8 to 10 years and has a reported expulsion rate of 5%. ParaGard may help protect women against endometrial carcinoma. There are various other copper IUDs in the world market but only ParaGard is available in the United States. The IUD has been linked in the past with inducing increased rates of PID, even though careful analysis noted that the risk is minimal [16,30]. Most clinicians will not insert an IUD in a college student, however, unless she is in a mutually monogamous relationship, has no history of PID or ectopic pregnancy, and has demonstrated her fertility. The IUD is used by 12% of adult women using contraception in the world versus 1% in the United States [103].

The Mirena IUD (levonorgestrel-containing IUD) is a second generation of steroid-releasing IUDs and is called the levonorgestrel intrauterine system. It has a 32 mm × 32 mm Nova T-shaped polyethylene-barium sulfate frame (1.25" tall and wide, made of plastic), with a reservoir around the vertical stem that contains silicone and 52 mg of levonorgestrel. Two threads for removal are attached to the end of the stem [104]. It is packaged in a sterile state inside a disposable insertion device.

This IUD releases 20 µg of levonorgestrel per 24 hours over the first 5 years of use; the levonorgestrel that is released decreases to 10 µg per day after 5 years. Concentrations in the plasma stabilize to 150 to 200 pg/mL, which is less than noted with OCPs or Norplant. Mirena has been available in Europe for more than 10 years and has been used by more than 2 million women worldwide. The Mirena IUD was approved by the FDA in 2001 for 5 years' use in the United States, although it is used in Europe for 7 to 10 years before replacement is recommended. It is a highly effective contraceptive, with a failure rate of 0.2% in the first year and 0.7% at 5 years [94,104–106].

The Mirena IUD is inserted before day 7 of the cycle and is not effective if inserted postcoitally. A newer insertion device allows easy insertion with minimal uterine perforation risks. It exerts a local effect on the endometrium and the cervical mucus and can initially lead to systemic effects [70,107]. The contraceptive mechanisms of IUDs are as follows:

1. They prevent fertilization.
2. They interfere with ovum development.
3. They interfere with sperm movement and ability to penetrate ovum.
4. They inhibit sperm survival.
5. They help prevent egg release.
6. They thicken cervical mucus.

This IUD has been used to reduce heavy menstrual bleeding in women because, eventually, menstrual blood loss may be decreased by up to 90% [108–110]. Ovulation can continue and amenorrhea may develop because of endometrial thinning [101]. Box 9 lists the side effects of the Mirena IUD [70,104,111]. The most common side effect is menstrual bleeding; there is increased bleeding and spotting during the first 3 to 6 months after insertion but this usually decreases

---

Box 9. Mirena intrauterine device side effects

Common

  Initial increased menstrual bleeding
  Abdominal pain

Uncommon

  Acne/other skin problems
  Back pain
  Breast tenderness
  Headache
  Nausea
  Mood changes

Rare

  Hypersensitivity reaction
  IUD becomes embedded in myometrium
  Perforation of uterus or cervix

thereafter [70].The benefits of the Mirena IUD include the following [112,113]: (1) effective contraception, (2) eventual reduction in menstrual flow, (3) frequent amenorrhea, (4) decreased dysmenorrheal, (5) decreased premenstrual syndrome, and (6) very low rates of infectious complications. Contraindications to Mirena use include active pelvic inflammatory disease, prosthetic heart valves, history of subacute bacterial endocarditis, and distorted uterine cavity.

Summary

Contraception is an important concept for the more than 80% of college students who are sexually active, usually without a desire for pregnancy to develop from their coital behavior. This article has reviewed important, effective, and safe contraceptive methods that can be used by college students. The promotion of sexual responsibility should be the charge of all health professionals caring for high school and college students [114,115]. The framework of sexual responsibility includes prevention of pregnancy, STDs, and premature child-bearing [116]. The integration of effective contraceptive methods with the desire and maturational state of the student often is difficult. The potential of contraceptive failure should be noted by the student and alternatives to this failure must be understood [20]. (See addendum for a list of Internet sites on contraception.)

Abstinence is a highly recommended method of contraception; however, coitus interruptus is not recommended because of its high failure rate, 19% per year [117]. Care must be used in prescribing an IUD for the college student because of the concern for PID [20]. Finally, sterilization is a method of contraception normally not recommended for the college student.

Addendum

Useful Internet sites on contraception

American College of Obstetrics and Gynecology: http://www.acog.org
Alan Guttmacher Institute: http://www.agi-usa.org/index.html
Association of Reproductive Health Specialists: http://www.arhp.org
Cochrane Library: http://hiru.mcmaster.ca/cochrane/cochrane/cdsr.htm, or http://www.update-software.com
Journal of the American Medical Association (JAMA): http://www.ama-assn.org/special/contra.html (JAMA Contraception Information Center)
CONRAD: http://www.conrad.org
European Journal of Contraception and Reproductive Health: http://www.tandf.co.uk/journals
Family Health International: http://www.fhi.org
Health People 2010: http://www.health.gov/healthypeople/

Reproductive Health Online: http://www.reproline.jhu.edu/
WHO medical eligibility criteria: http://www.who.int/reproductivehealth/
publications/RHR_00_2_medical_eligibility_second_edition/index.ht
Emergency Contraception info: http://www.not-2-late.org
Managing Contraception: www.managingcontraception.com
Center for Young Women's Health: http://www.youngwomenshealth.org

References

[1] Greydanus DE, Patel DR, Rimsza ME. Contraception in the adolescent: an update. Pediatrics 2001;107(3):562–73.
[2] Greydanus DE, Patel D. Contraception in the adolescent: preparation for the 1990's. Med Clin North Am 1990;74(5):1205–24.
[3] Matytsina LA. Contraception and sexual activity among teenagers in Ukraine. Fourth Congress of the European Society of Contraception, Barcelona. Eur J Contracept Reprod Health Care 1996;2:121.
[4] Zite NB, Shulman LP. New options in contraception for teenagers. Curr Opin Obstet Gynecol 2003;15:385–9.
[5] Rimsza ME. Contraception in adolescents. In: Greydanus DE, Patel DR, Pratt HD, editors. Essentials of adolescent medicine. New York: McGraw-Hill; 2005. p. 27.
[6] Greydanus DE, Pratt HD, Dannison LL. Sexuality education programs for youth: current state of affairs and strategies for the future. J Sex Educ Ther 1995;21(4):238–54.
[7] Reinisch J, Hill C, Sanders S, et al. High-risk sexual behavior at a Midwestern university: a confirmatory survey. Fam Plann Perspect 1995;27:79–82.
[8] Institute of Medicine. College students fail the grade in condom use. CDC, college groups target behavior. Contracept Technol Update 1998;19:63–5.
[9] Prince A, Bernard AL. Sexual behaviors and safer sex practices of college students on a commuter campus. J Am Coll Health 1998;47(1):11–21.
[10] Sawyer RG, Pinciaro PJ, Anderson-Sawyer A. Pregnancy testing and counseling: a university health center's 5-year experience. J Am Coll Health 1998;46:221–5.
[11] Siegel DM, Klein DI, Roghmann KJ. Sexual behavior, contraception, and risk among college students. J Adolesc Health 1999;25(5):336–43.
[12] Patrick K, Covin JR, Fulop M, et al. Health risk behaviors among California college students. J Am Coll Health 1997;45:265–73.
[13] Douglas K, Collins J, Warren C, et al. Results from the 1995 National College Health Risk Survey. J Am Coll Health 1997;46:55–67.
[14] Simon DA, Roach JP, Dimitrievich E. Assessment of knowledge and practice of high risk sexual behavior at a private Midwestern university. S D J Med 2003;56:265–9.
[15] Linn ES. Progress in contraception: new technology. Int J Fertil Womens Med 2003;48:182–91.
[16] Herndon EJ, Zieman M. New contraceptive options. Am Fam Phys 2004;69:853–60.
[17] Hillard PJA, Deitch HR. Menstrual disorders in the college age female. Ped Clin North Am 2005;52(1).
[18] Olenick I. US teenagers' birthrate and pregnancy rate fall during the mid-1990s. Fam Plann Perspect 1998;30:292.
[19] Warren CW, Santelli JS, Everett SA, et al. Sexual behavior among US high school students, 1990–1995. Fam Plann Perspect 1998;30:170–2.
[20] Rome ES. Adolescent sexuality. In: Greydanus DE, Patel DR, Pratt HD, editors. Essentials of adolescent medicine. New York: McGraw-Hill Medical Publishers; 2005. p. 500–20.
[21] Katz A, Davis P, Findlay SS. Ask and ye shall plan. A health needs assessment of a university population. Can J Public Health 2002;93:63–6.

[22] Zabin LS. Teenage pregnancy. In: Wallace HM, Patrick K, Parcel GS, Igoe JBPrinciples and practices of student health, vol. 1. Oakland, CA: Third Party Publishing; 1992. p. 135–45.

[23] Swinford P. Pregnancy, contraception, and issues of sexuality for college students. In: Wallace HM, Patrick K, Parcel GS, Igoe JB, editors. Principles and practices of student health, vol. 3. Oakland, CA: Third Party Publishing; 1992. p. 660–70.

[24] Baxter TL. College health. In: Hofmann AD, Greydanus DE, editors. Adolescent medicine. 3rd edition. Stamford, CT: Appleton & Lange; 1997. p. 755–9.

[25] Dale T, Woodrum P. Women's health issues and contraception in college and university health services. In: Turner HS, Hurley JL, editors. The history and practice of college health. Lexington KY: University Press of Kentucky; 2002. p. 118–40.

[26] Yarnall KS, McBride CM, Lyna P, et al. Factors associated with condom use among at-risk women students and nonstudents seen in managed care. Prev Med 2003;37(2):163–70.

[27] Hewitt G, Cromer B. Update on adolescent contraception. Obstet Gynecol Clin North Am 2000;27:143–62.

[28] Black A, Rowe T. 2004 contraceptive guidelines. J Obstet Gynaecol Can 2004;26:197–8.

[29] Archer DF, Bigrigg A, Smallwood GH, et al. Assessment of compliance with a weekly contraceptive patch (Ortho Evra/Evra) among North American women. Fertil Steril 2002; 77(Suppl 2):S27–31.

[30] Grimes DA. Intrauterine device and upper-genital tract infection. Lancet 2000;356:1013–9.

[31] Forinash AB, Evans SL. New hormonal contraceptives: a comprehensive review of the literature. Pharmacotherapy 2003;23:1573–91.

[32] Plourd DM, Rayburn WF. New contraceptive methods. J Reprod Med 2003;48:665–71.

[33] Murphy PA. New methods of hormonal contraception. Nurse Pract 2003;28:11–21.

[34] Zieman M, Guillebaud J, Weisberg E, et al. Contraceptive efficacy and cycle control with the Ortho Evra/Evra transdermal system: the analysis of pooled data. Fertil Steril 2002; 77(Suppl 2):S13–8.

[35] Skouby SO. Contraceptive use and behavior in the 21st century: a comprehensive study across five European countries. Eur J Contracept Reprod Health Care 2004;9:57–68.

[36] Anonymous. Yasmin. An oral contraceptive with a new progestin. Med Lett Drugs Ther 2002; 44:55–7.

[37] Rudolf PM, Bernstein IBG. Counterfeit drugs. N Engl J Med 2004;350:1384–6.

[38] National Institute of Allergy and Infectious Diseases. Workshop summary: scientific evidence on condom effectiveness for sexually transmitted diseases (STD) prevention. Available at: http://www.niaid.nih.gov/dmid/stds/condomreport.pdf. Accessed 2001.

[39] Kulig J. Condoms: the basics and beyond. Adolesc Med 2003;14:633–45.

[40] Petitti DB. Combination estrogen-progestin contraceptives. N Engl J Med 2003;349:1443–4.

[41] Sheldon T. Venous thromboembolism and oral contraceptives. BMJ 2002;324:869.

[42] Anonymous. Seasonale. Med Lett 2004;46:9.

[43] Burkman RT, Miller L. Extended and continuous use of hormonal contraceptives. Dialogues Contracept 2004;8:1–4.

[44] World Health Organization. Improving access to quality care in family planning—medical eligibility criteria for contraceptive use. Geneva, Switzerland: World Health Organization; 1996.

[45] World Health Organization. Medical eligibility criteria for contraceptive use. Geneva, Switzerland: Reproductive Health and Research, World Health Organization; 2000 [Publication #WHO/RHR/00.02].

[46] Greydanus DE. Contraception. In: Greydanus DE, Patel DR, Pratt H, Bhave S, editors. Course manual for adolescent health. New Delhi, India: Cambridge Press; 2002. p. 309–24.

[47] Vandenbrouke JP, Rosing J, Bloemenkamp KWM, et al. Oral contraceptives and the risk of venous thrombosis. N Engl J Med 2001;344:1527–35.

[48] Anonymous. Mottram Hall guidelines. Evidence-guided prescribing of the pill. Carnforth, UK: Parthenon; 1996.

[49] Davidson NE, Helzlsouer KJ. Good news about oral contraceptives. N Engl J Med 2002;346: 2078–9.

[50] Glasier A. Drug interactions and combination oral contraceptives. Dialogues Contracept 2000;6(5):1–4.

[51] Freeman S. Contraceptive efficacy and patient acceptance of Lunelle. J Am Acad Nurse Pract 2002;14:241–6.

[52] Rosenberg M, Waugh MS. Causes and consequences of oral contraceptive noncompliance. Am J Obstet Gynecol 1999;180:S276–9.

[53] Rosenberg M, Waugh MS. Oral contraceptive discontinuation: a prospective evaluation of frequency and reasons. Am J Obstet Gynecol 1998;179:577–82.

[54] Bjarnadottir RI, Tuppurainen M, Killick SR. Comparison of cycle control with a combined contraceptive vaginal ring and oral levonoregestrel/ethinyl estradiol. Am J Obstet Gynecol 2002;186:389–95.

[55] Williams JK. Rationale for new oral contraceptive dosing. Int J Fertil Womens Med 2004; 49:30–5.

[56] Dittrich R, Parker L, Rosen JB, et al. Transdermal contraception: evaluation of three transdermal norelgestromin/ethinyl estradiol doses in a randomized, multicenter, dose-response study. Am J Obstet Gynecol 2002;186:15–20.

[57] Audet MC, Moreau M, Koltun WD, et al. Evaluation of contraceptive efficacy and cycle control of a transdermal contraceptive patch vs. an oral contraceptive. A randomized controlled trial. JAMA 2001;285:2347–54.

[58] Anonymous. Ortho Evra—a contraceptive patch. Med Lett 2002;44:8.

[59] Sicat BL. Ortho Evra, a new contraceptive patch. Pharmacotherapy 2003;23:472–80.

[60] Burkman RT, Mishell Jr DR, Shulman LP. Transdermal contraceptive system. Dialogues Contracept 2001;7(3):1–4.

[61] Burkman RT. The transdermal contraceptive patch: a new approach to hormonal contraception. Int J Fertil Womens Med 2002;47(2):69–76.

[62] Smallwood GH, Meador ML, Lenihan JP, et al. Efficacy and safety of a transdermal contraceptive system. Obstet Gynecol 2001;98:799.

[63] Rubinstein ML, Halpern-Felsher BL, Irwin CE. An evaluation of the use of the transdermal contraceptive patch in adolescents. J Adolesc Health 2004;34:395–401.

[64] Faculty of Family Planning and Reproductive Health Care Clinical Effectiveness Unit. New product review: norelgestromin/ethinyl oestradiol transdermal contraceptive system (Evra). J Fam Plann Reprod Health Care 2004;30:43–5.

[65] Abrams LS, Skee DM, Natarajan J, et al. Pharmacokinetics of a contraceptive patch (Evra/Ortho Evra) containing norelgestromin and ethinyl estradiol at four application sites. Br J Clin Pharmacol 2002;53(2):141–6.

[66] Abrams LS, Skee DM, Natarajan J, et al. Pharmacokinetic overview of Ortho Evra/Evra. Fertil Steril 2002;77(Suppl 2):S3–12.

[67] Zacor HA, Hedon B, Mansour D, et al. Integrated summary of Ortho Evra/Evra contraceptive patch adhesion in varied climates and conditions. Fertil Steril 2002;77(Suppl 2):S32–5.

[68] Sibai BM, Odlind C, Meador ML, et al. A comparative and pooled analysis of the safety and tolerability of the contraceptive patch (Ortho Evra/Evra). Fertil Steril 2002;77(Suppl 2): S19–26.

[69] Creasy GW, Fisher AC, Hall N, et al. Transdermal contraceptive patch delivering norelgestromin and ethinyl estradiol. Effects on lipid profile. J Reprod Med 2003;48:179–86.

[70] Keder LM. Tips for clinicians: new developments in contraception. J Pediatr Adolesc Gynecol 2002;15:179–81.

[71] Anonymous. Emergency contraception OTC. Med Lett 2004;46:10–1.

[72] Trussel J, Kowal D. The essentials of contraception. Efficacy, safety and personal considerations. In: Hatcher RA, Trussel J, Stewart F, et al, editors. Contraceptive technology. New York: Ardent Media; 1998. p. 211–47.

[73] Drazen JM, Greene MF, Wood AJJ. The FDA, politics, and plan B. N Engl J Med 2004;350: 1561–2.

[74] Steinbrook R. Waiting for plan B—The FDA and nonprescription use of emergency contraception. N Engl J Med 2004;350:2327–9.

[75] Vastag B. Plan B for "plan B"? FDA denies OTC sales of emergency contraceptive. JAMA 2004;291:2805–6.

[76] Brening RK, Dalve-Endres AM, Patrick K. Emergency contraception pills (ECPs): current trends in United States college health centers. Contraception 2003;67:449.

[77] Trussell J, Ellertson C, Steward F, et al. The role of emergency contraception. Am J Obstet Gynecol 2004;190(Suppl 4):S30–8.

[78] Gold MA, Sucato GS, Conrad LAE, Hillard PJA. Provision of emergency contraception to adolescents. Position paper of the Society for Adolescent Medicine. J Adolesc Health 2004; 35:66–70.

[79] Virjo I, Virtala A. Why do university students use hormonal emergency contraception? Eur J Contracept Reprod Health Care 2003;8(3):139–44.

[80] Porter JH. Use of hormonal emergency contraception at a university health centre over a 6 year period. J Fam Plann Reprod Health Care 2001;27(1):47–8.

[81] Free C, Ogden J. Contraceptive risk and compensatory behaviour in young people in education post-16 years: a cross-sectional study. J Fam Plann Reprod Health Care 2004;30(2):91–4.

[82] Raine T, Harper C, Leon K, Darney P. Emergency contraception: advance provision in a young, high-risk clinic population. Obstet Gynecol 2000;96:1–7.

[83] McCarthy SK. Availability of emergency contraceptive pills at university and college student health centers. J Am Coll Health 2002;51(1):15–22.

[84] Anderson RA, Kinniburgh D, Baird DT. Suppression of spermatogenesis by etonogestrel implants with depot testosterone: potential for long-acting male contraception. J Clin Endocrinol Metab 2002;87(8):3640–9.

[85] Mulders TMT, Dieben TOM. Use of the novel combined contraceptive vaginal ring NuvaRing for ovulation inhibition. Fertil Steril 2001;75:865–70.

[86] Mulders TM, Dieben TO, Bennick HJ. Ovarian function with a novel combined contraceptive vaginal ring. Hum Reprod 2002;17:2594–9.

[87] Killick S. Complete and robust ovulation inhibition with NuvaRing. Eur J Contracept Reprod Health Care 2002;7(Suppl 2):13–8.

[88] Vree M. Lower hormone dosage with improved cycle control. Eur J Contracept Reprod Health Care 2002;7(Suppl 2):25–30.

[89] Dieben TOM, Roumen FJME, Apter D. Efficacy, cycle control, and user acceptability of a novel combined contraceptive vaginal ring. Obstet Gynecol 2002;100:585–93.

[90] Novak A, de la Loge C, Abetz L, et al. The combined contraceptive vaginal ring, NuvaRing: an international study of user acceptability. Contraception 2003;67:187–94.

[91] Szarewski A. High acceptability and satisfaction with NuvaRing use. Eur J Contracept Reprod Health Care 2002;7(Suppl 2):31–6.

[92] Roumen F. Contraceptive efficacy and tolerability with a novel combined contraceptive vaginal ring, NuvaRing. Eur J Contracept Reprod Health Care 2002;7(Suppl 2):19–24.

[93] Harvey SM, Bird ST, Branch MR. A new look at an old method: the diaphragm. Perspect Sex Reprod Health 2003;35:270–3.

[94] Foran TM. New contraceptive choices across reproductive life. Med J Aust 2003;178:616–20.

[95] Civic D. College students' reasons for nonuse of condoms within dating relationships. J Sex Marital Ther 2000;26(1):95–105.

[96] Parsons JT, Halkitis PN, Bimbi D, Borkowski T. Perceptions of the benefits and costs associated with condom use and unprotected sex among late adolescent college students. J Adolesc 2000;23:377–91.

[97] Zaleski EH, Schiaffino KM. Religiosity and sexual risk-taking behavior during the transition to college. J Adolesc 2000;23(2):223–7.

[98] Tulloch HE, McCaul KD, Miltenberger RG, et al. Partner communication skills and condom use among college students. J Am Coll Health 2004;52(6):263–7.

[99] Steiner MJ, Dominik R, Rountree RW, et al. Contraceptive effectiveness of a polyurethane condom and a latex condom: a randomized controlled trial. Am J Obstet Gynecol 2003; 101(3):539–47.

[100] McDermott RJ, Noland VJ. Condom use history as a determinant of university students' condom evaluative index. Psychol Rep 2004;94(3 Pt 1):889–93.

[101] Power J, Guillebaud J. Long-acting progestogen contraceptives. Practitioner 2002;246:332–9.

[102] Affandi B. Long-acting progestogens. Best Pract Res Clin Obstet Gynecol 2002;16(2):169–79.

[103] Arias RD. Compelling reasons for recommending IUDs to any woman of reproductive age. Int J Fertil 2002;47(2):87–95.

[104] Anonymous. A progestin-releasing intrauterine device for long-term contraception. Med Lett 2001;43:7–8.

[105] Baldaszti E, Wimmer-Puchinger B, Loschke K. Acceptability of the long-term contraceptive levonorgestrel-releasing intrauterine system (Mirena): a 3-year follow-up study. Contraception 2003;67:87–91.

[106] Grimes D, editor. FDA approves levonorgestrel-releasing intrauterine system (Mirena). Contracept Rep 2001;12:9–14.

[107] Phillips V, Graham CT, Manek S, et al. The effects of levonorgestrel intrauterine system (Mirena coil) on endometrial morphology. J Clin Pathol 2003;56:305–7.

[108] Henshaw R, Coyle C, Low S, et al. A retrospective cohort study comparing microwave endometrial ablation with levonorgestrel-releasing intrauterine device (Mirena) in the management of heavy menstrual bleeding. Aust N Z J Obstet Gynaecol 2002;42(2):205–9.

[109] Hidalgo M, Bahamondes L, Perrotti M, et al. Bleeding patterns and clinical performance of the levonorgestrel-releasing intrauterine system (Mirena) up to two years. Contraception 2002;65(2):129–32.

[110] Monteiro I, Bahamondes L, Diaz J, et al. Therapeutic use of levonorgestrel- releasing intrauterine device in women with menorrhagia: a pilot study. Contraception 2002;65(5):325–8.

[111] Pereira A, Coker A. Hypersensitivity to Mirena—a rare complication. J Obstet Gynaecol 2003; 23:81.

[112] Bounds W. Use of Mirena in epilepsy. Br J Fam Plann 1997;23:12.

[113] Bounds W, Guillebaud J. Observational series on women using the contraceptive Mirena concurrently with anti-epileptic and other enzyme-inducing drugs. J Fam Plann Reprod Health Care 2002;28(2):78–80.

[114] Brooks RL, Shrier LA. An update on contraception for adolescents. Adolesc Med 1999; 10(2):211–9.

[115] Riain A. Increasing the effectiveness of contraceptive usage in university students. Eur J Contracept Reprod Health Care 1998;3:124–8.

[116] Alan Guttmacher Institute. Into a new world: young women's sexual and reproductive lives. New York: Alan Guttmacher Institute; 1998.

[117] Hatcher R, Trussell J, Stewart Jr FH, et al, editors. Contraceptive technology. 17th edition. New York: Irvington; 1998.

Human Papilloma Virus, Papanicolaou Smears, and the College Female

Anna-Barbara Moscicki, MD

Department of Pediatrics, Division of Adolescent Medicine, University of California, San Francisco, 3333 California Street, Suite 245, San Francisco, CA 94118, USA

Although human papilloma virus (HPV) for decades was predominantly referred to as the "wart" virus, its strong association with invasive cervical cancer has draw, recent public attention [1]. Worldwide, more than 650,000 cases of invasive cancer are diagnosed per year. The largest burden of cervical cancer, however, lies in developing countries where cervical cancer remains the leading cause of cancer mortality [2]. In contrast, cervical cancer is the seventh leading cancer in industrialized countries. This discrepancy is predominantly associated with cervical cancer screening programs that are well entrenched in industrialized countries compared with the virtual lack of any programs in developing countries. With the introduction of the Papanicolaou smear, rates of invasive cancer have plummeted in the United States over the last four decades [3]. There has been a slight increase observed in younger women over the last two decades [2]. In the United States, cervical cancer screening is bit of a misnomer. That is, cervical cancer screening is expected to detect "precancer" lesions, and failure is often referred to as the detection of invasive cancer, even when found in early treatable stages. Precancer lesions in the past have included the group termed cervical intra-epithelial neoplasia (CIN) I, II, and III. These terms in the United States have been reclassified using the terminology referred to as the Bethesda System for Rating Cytology outlined in Table 1 [4]. The ratings 1 through 3 (and terms low and high) are based on their progression potential (see later in Natural History). It is worth mentioning that in the United States, the Bethesda system for cytology combines CIN 2 and 3, which many believe have different potential

This study received funding support from the National Cancer Institute grants #CA051323 and CA87905.

E-mail address: annam@itsa.ucsf.edu

Table 1
Clinical classification

Bethesda classification	WHO classification

ASCUS (ASC)
  Undetermined significance (ASC-US)
  Cannot exclude HSIL (ASC-H)
	Atypia

LSIL (low-grade squamous intraepithelial lesions)	Condyloma, Cervical intraepithelial neoplasia (CIN)-1
HSIL (high-grade squamous intraepithelial lesions)	CIN-2, CIN-3, Carcinoma in situ

for progression [5]. However, because inter-rater reliability for separating CIN 2 and 3 is quite poor, these have been combined clinically so that clinicians are aware that these lesions have higher potential of progression as compared with a CIN 1 or low-grade squamous intraepithelial lesions (LSIL).

Unfortunately, the Pap smears have several limitations, which include a lack of sensitivity unless used repeatedly and a lack of specificity. Most high-grade squamous intraepithelial lesions (HSIL) lesions defined by histology are identified by the referral of LSIL and atypical squamous cells of undetermined significance (ASCUS) diagnosis on cytology [6]. On the other hand, most cytologic LSIL and ASCUS are LSIL and not HSIL. These limitations have resulted in screening practices, which are set up to miss few to no cases of invasive cancer. Consequently, large numbers of women without true precancer disease are also referred. Recent efforts have been made to decrease this over-referral of young women and new guidelines are reviewed later.

Unique to cervical cancer screening is that a precancer screening test became available before the cause was recognized. The recent association between HPV persistence and invasive cancer has introduced HPV testing into the clinical market [7,8]. This time of transition has created quite a bit of confusion for both clinicians and consumers. The next few paragraphs explain the rationale for using HPV testing in clinical diagnosis.

Viral pathogenesis

Studies have shown that more than 99.5% of invasive cervical cancers are associated with one of 18 different HPV types with HPV 16 responsible for almost 60% [1]. For comparison, high-risk HPV types, specifically HPV 16, are the most common HPV seen in young women with normal cytology [1,9]. Consequently, HPV type alone does not explain ultimate risk. Clearly, cervical carcinogenesis is a multi-step process with numerous host and viral factors involved. Although HPV is considered necessary but not sufficient for cancer development, laboratory studies have demonstrated the presence of several HPV proteins that have oncogenic properties. The functions of these HPV gene products and their role in the pathogenesis of SIL and squamous cell cancer have been increasingly well defined.

HPV is thought to require access to basal epithelial cells through a wound or abrasion. The virus may remain dormant for a period of time before expression of these oncogenes. The early (E) region contains the open reading frames (ORF) capable of encoding proteins that function as transactivating factors that regulate cellular transformation (the E6 and E7 ORF) [10–16]. Studies of HPV 16-infected cervical tissues have demonstrated that the transformation proteins, E6 and E7, are found to be expressed in all grades of lesions with levels of expression increasing from LSIL to HSIL [17–19]. Expression of E4 is known to interact with the cytoskeleton structure of squamous cells resulting in the perinuclear halo described for HPV. Consequently, expression of HPV E6, E7, and E4 induce histologic changes including basal cell proliferation, abnormal mitotic figures, enlarged nucleus, and a perinuclear halo. These changes define SIL. Consequently, SIL is the histologic manifestation of an active viral infection. LSIL is considered a benign and reversible change. The morphologic changes of HSIL (aneuploidy, altered chromatin texture, increased nuclear volume) suggest that HSIL changes are due in part to the expression of these viral genes in the epithelial stem cells which have lost the capacity to differentiate or at least in the nondifferentiated, replicating basal and parabasal cells [15]. The epithelial stem cells experience mutagenic consequences resulting in viral integration [20]. How this expression suddenly occurs in nonterminally differentiated cells is unknown, but E6 and E7 are abundantly expressed in these cells as well as the terminally differentiated cells. HSIL and carcinomas are found to have a higher number of HPV genomes integrated into the host genome than LSIL [21,22]. Through loss of the regulatory protein E2, integration of E6 and E7 promotes expression of itself. Questions remain on what are the final steps to carcinogenesis.

Natural history

With the advent of molecular techniques to detect HPV, several epidemiologic and virologic studies of HPV have shed light on the natural history of this virus. The early studies begun in the 1980s showed that HPV was extremely common with at least a 70% chance of exposure over a women's sexual life. Moscicki et al [9] showed that 50% of sexually active women will acquire a cervical HPV infection within 5 to 7 years after initiating vaginal intercourse. Initially, most believed that HPV was similar to other viral infections such as cytomegalovirus or Epstein Barr Virus, when these infections are lifelong. However, the striking difference in prevalence rates for HPV among young women as compared with older women suggested otherwise. Rates of HPV in women under 25 years of age are four times that of women over 35 years [23]. Notably, HPV rates are highest in young populations with multiple sexual partners and cervical cancer rates are highest in the older population with the lowest rates of HPV. This dichotomy suggests two things: as there are no antiviral therapies for HPV, the decline in HPV prevalence reflects a true spontaneous "loss" of HPV and second, time is an important component of the development of invasive cancer. What happens during this "time" is clearly key to our understanding of HPV's onco-viral potential.

With the high rates of HPV in young women, it would be expected that LSIL, a cellular manifestation of HPV, would also be highest in this young population. Although some believe that all HPV results in LSIL, the prevalence rates of HPV usually outnumber LSIL rates. A recent study in young women showed that risks for the acquisition of HPV and those for LSIL development were different [9]. Cigarette smoking was associated with LSIL development, whereas new sexual partners and herpes simplex infections were associated with HPV. These data suggest that changes associated with LSIL are uniquely influenced. The reason for this high rate of HPV acquisition and LSIL in young women is thought to be in part due to the inherent vulnerability of the "immature" cervix [24]. The cervix of an adolescent, in contrast to a woman 10 to 20 years older, is covered predominantly by columnar and metaplastic epithelium whereas squamous epi-thelium predominates in the older women (Fig. 1). The thinly layered columnar epithelium allows for easy access to the basal cell layer for infection. The meta-plastic epithelium is reflective of a transitional state referred to as squamous meta-plasia. This epithelium reflects rapid replication and differentiation as columnar epithelium transitions to squamous epithelium, a process most commonly found during the period of adolescents. This epithelial type with its rapid replication and differentiation is a perfect host for HPV replication since HPV replication and patterns of transcription depend on the differentiation program of keratinocytes [25]. This process and high rates of new sexual partners explains the high rate of HPV and LSIL in young women [9,26]. However, it must be underscored that these high rates do not reflect risk for invasive cancer. The explanation for the difference in prevalence among ages is that the majority of HPV infections result in regression; 50% to 90% of infections in young women regress within 1 to 3 years of observations [27–29]. As LSIL is a manifestation of HPV, it might be expected that the rates of LSIL regression should parallel those for HPV. Studies

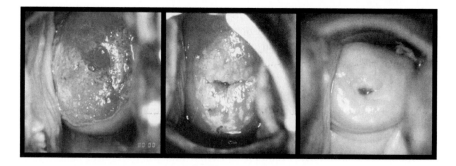

Fig. 1. Colpophotographs of cervices after the application of 3% acetic acid. (*Left panel*) ado-lescent cervix largely covered by columnar epithelium. (*Middle panel*) adolescent cervix largely covered by transitional squamous metaplastic epithelium. (*Right panel*) adult cervix covered by ma-ture squamous epithelium.

in adult women (ie, mean ages over 30 years) show that 50% to 70% of LSIL will spontaneously regress [5,30,31]. Recent data show that regression in younger women is even more striking with 91% of young women showing LSIL regression within 3 years of detection [32]. The higher rate of regression in young women compared with older women may reflect a more benign natural history for HPV infection in these young women. On the other hand, the natural history of HPV suggests that HPV or LSIL detection in older women reflects a persistent infection that was acquired many years before detection. Thus LSIL in many adult women reflects a "failed" immune response to HPV rather than an acute acquisition [33].

In the natural history of HPV, it is important to return to the significance of the "lack" of regression of HPV infections. Persistence of HPV is strongly linked to the development of HSIL and invasive cancers. With persistent HPV, the expression of E6 and E7 are expected to increase with increasing cellular abnormalities causing the development of HSIL. Whether LSIL is a necessary precursor to HSIL remains controversial; however, it is well accepted that HPV persistence (with or without the detection of a LSIL) is a risk for the appearance of HSIL and invasive cancer [7,8,27,28]. However, not all studies suggest persistence is necessary for HSIL development. Woodman et al [34] noted that 3% of HPV-negative and 7% of HPV-positive adolescents developed HSIL shortly after HPV detection. How long HPV persistence is "necessary" is not known and most likely relies on other genetic and environmental factors (eg, smoking cigarettes, p53 mutations, *C. trachomatis* infections) [35–39].

In the natural history of lesions, all lesions that do not regress do not necessarily progress. In fact, the vast majority of LSIL and HSIL do not "progress." In adolescents and young women, progression from LSIL to HSIL is quite low (3%) [9]. Studies performed in adult women show higher rates of progression with 20% to 30% of LSIL progressing to HSIL/invasive cancer [5,30,31]. Again this discrepancy may be that many of the LSIL in adult women reflect a failed-to-clear LSIL. Schlecht et al [40] reported that in women who had LSIL persistence, 20% progressed to HSIL/invasive cancer during follow-up.

Studies of HSIL progression are confusing as some studies depended on biopsy confirmation whereas other depend on cytology increasing the possibility of misclassification. In addition, WHO categories CIN 2 and 3, which are combined in the United States as HSIL, may behave quite differently [5]. Some believe that the only true precancer is CIN 3 or carcinoma in situ. The importance of these differences is that CIN 2 lesions make up the majority of HSIL in adolescents and young women whereas CIN 3 is quite rare [24,41]. Studies suggest that CIN 2 lesions in young women reflect a "bad case of HPV" with regression rates closer to CIN 1 than CIN 3. Syrjanen et al [5] reported 56% of CIN 1, 53% of CIN 2, and 14% of the CIN 3 lesions regressed. Progression rates had similar patterns where 14% and 21% of the CIN 1 and CIN 2 groups, respectively, progressed compared with 69% of the CIN-3 group. Nasiell et al [30] found similar rates of regression for CIN-2 lesions but with slightly higher progression rates overall (30%).

Time frames for progression are also vague. Nasiell et al [30] observed that the time of progression for women with CIN-2 to a carcinoma in situ or cancer over age 51 was 70 to 80 months, 41 to 42 months for women aged 26 to 50 years, and 54 to 60 months for women under 25 years of age. Schlecht [40] showed that women over 30 year of age with LSIL progressed more rapidly than younger women (16 to 30 years) with a mean of 77.9 month and 88.4 months, respectively. No data were available for progression of CIN 2 in this study.

Although no recent studies of CIN 2 have been performed, the low prevalence rates of invasive cancer in women support the notion that HSIL rarely progresses in today's young women. A relatively recent large review of cytology showed that 0.7% of adolescent women aged 15 to 19 years of age have HSIL and 0.8% of women aged 20 to 24 years [24] with no cases of invasive cancer in the adolescent age group. Other large studies have shown that invasive cancer is rare to almost nonexistent in the adolescent group with low rates in the 20- to 24-year-old group [24,41]. SEER data statistics [3] underscore these observations. Between 1995 and 1999, the incidence of invasive cancer of the cervix was 0 per 100,000 for ages 10 to 14 years; 0 per 100,000 for ages 15 to19 years, and 1.7 per 100,000 for ages 20 to 24. Thus the cost of missing HSIL in 15 to 19 year olds by not screening or treating these lesions is 1.7 cases of cervical cancer per 100,000 (the incidence for 20 to 24 year olds). It is not known, however, whether certain factors are associated with these 1.7 per 100,000 cases—for example, how many of them were for found in women who were immunosuppressed or HIV positive and what stage the cancers were. HIV remains an important risk for the development of HSIL and invasive cancer [42].

Rates of abnormal cytology in college-aged women

Although the younger women predominates in many colleges, it is not uncommon for older women to enroll into colleges and universities. Unfortunately, few studies have included college women. Moscicki et al [9] performed a prospective study that included approximately 300 women aged 17 to 22 from a University Clinic setting. In this study, University Clinic students had similar rates of acquisition and regression of HPV and LSIL as the younger adolescents when the analysis corrected for years sexually active. Bauer et al [43] showed that although 46% of college women were found to have a genital HPV infection, less than 3% had abnormal cytology which was predominantly ASCUS and LSIL. It is expected that older women in colleges have similar natural histories of HPV to studies involving adolescent and adult women. Many older women attending colleges have their own health insurance and therefore do contribute to general statistics in the student health clinics. In general, there is no reason to suggest that college-bound women are at higher risk than other women their age. In some settings, they may be at lower risk than urban high-risk populations since they generally have higher socioeconomic status and greater access to heath care. On the other hand, rampant alcohol and substance use at most colleges often leads to increased risk sexual behavior [44–46].

New guidelines for cytology screening

Cytology screening has clearly made a significant impact on decreasing cervical cancer rates in industrialized countries [47]. Traditionally, screening guidelines recommended that cervical cancer screening begin at age 25 years. With the advent of HPV molecular studies, it became clear that HPV and abnormal cytology was highly prevalent in young women. These observations quickly transformed into guidelines that resulted in aggressive screening of young women and not unexpectedly an explosion of referrals for adolescents and young women for colposcopy and treatment. American Medical Association, US Preventive Services, American College of Obstetrics and Gynecolgoy, and the National Cancer Institute recommend that screening begin with the onset of sexual activity or at 18 years of age, whichever occurs first or if the sexual history is unreliable [48–50]. Once screening is initiated, a woman is recommended to have three consecutive annual Pap smears. If all three are normal, then recommended screening frequencies vary from every 1 to 3 years; specifically "high-risk" women, which includes women who initiate intercourse early, should have annual screening. Recent review of the data now informs us that: (1) adolescents and young women have high prevalence and incidence of HPV and LSIL; (2) the majority of HPV and LSIL regresses spontaneously; and (3) prevalence rates of CIN 3 and invasive cancer are extremely low in this group. Because of these observations, the risk for overtreatment of lesions is greater for younger women than older. These observations led the American Cancer Society to review current guidelines and make new recommendations on when to initiate screening based on these current data [51]:

- Can be delayed until 3 years after the onset of sexual activity.
- No later than 21 years of age.
- Does not include immunocompromised women.
- Women need reproductive health care including pregnancy prevention and STD screening with the onset of sexual activity.

The new recommendation supports screening within 3 years of the onset of vaginal intercourse but no later than 21 years of age. It should be noted that these recommendations are still considered by other industrial countries to be unnecessarily aggressive. Most European nations recommend that cytology screening begin no earlier than 24 years of age [52–55].

In contrast to most recommendations, these guidelines are based on a more important risk criterion than chronological age: the age of onset of a behavior. Many college women have delayed sexual activity until they arrive at college. Twenty to thirty percent of college women report they have not yet experienced vaginal intercourse [56,57]. The risk associated with the development of significant HPV-associated disease is associated with persistence of HPV, which in turn depends on the time from possible exposure (ie, the age of onset of sexual activity). The limit of 21 years of age is based on the premise that some women may not reveal accurate information regarding sexual activity and some health care providers may be remiss in their screening for risk behaviors.

New guidelines for triage of abnormal cytology

Unfortunately, new infections are also quite common with new sexual partners, resulting in high incident rates of HPV in young women [9]. The cycle of frequent acquisition and regression results in overall high prevalence rates of LSIL in adolescent and young women, making triage imperative. ASCUS diagnosis remains one of the more common cytologic diagnoses in women. ASCUS is a nonspecific diagnosis, so any triage is welcomed. HPV reflex testing has been shown to have a higher sensitivity to detect HSIL than repeating cytology 4 to 6 months later [58]. Triage can either be done by asking the patient to return for HPV testing, by obtaining a second swab for storage, or by obtaining the initial cytology in a liquid-based cytology medium. The liquid-based cytology medium can be directly used for HPV testing. Although liquid-based cytology is becoming routine at many institutions, the cost for cytology is higher. Returning for a second visit is less cost effective than either of the other two. However, space for storage of the sample for HPV testing is a problem at many laboratories. HPV triage for ASCUS is approved by the US Food & Drug Administration for all ages. Fig. 2 summarizes current recommended strategies.

With studies showing the high rate of regression of LSIL in young women, the new guidelines now allow for cytologic follow-up of LSIL in adolescent populations [58]. The current guidelines for older women continue to recommend colposcopic referral for LSIL on cytology. This recommendation is probably too aggressive for young women who recently began sexual activity. In contrast to LSIL in adult women, adolescents may be managed with a repeat smear in 6 months; if the smear remains abnormal (ASCUS or greater), guidelines recommend referral to colposcopy. Alternatively, an HPV test may be performed one year after the index LSIL cytology. If positive for high-risk HPV types, referral to colposcopy is recommended. The increased sensitivity of HPV testing to detect HSIL allows for the greater interval between testing [6,58]. The guidelines are summarized in Fig. 3.

The guidelines for management of histologically confirmed LSIL have also changed [59]. Preferred management for LSIL with satisfactory colposcopic examinations includes follow-up with repeat cytology at 6 and 12 months or HPV testing at 12 months. Referral to colposcopy is recommended if the repeat smear is ASCUS or worse or if the HPV test is positive for high-risk types. Decision to treat remains a decision between provider and patient; however, observations up to 24 months are quite acceptable. Guidelines for referral of HSIL have not

Management of Women with Atypical Squamous Cells of Undetermined Significance (ASC-US)

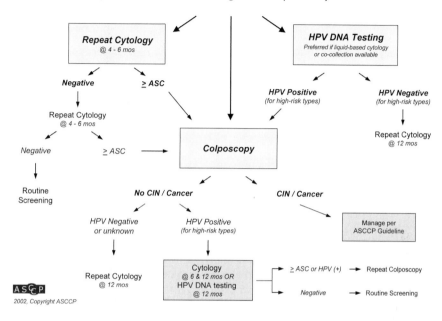

Fig. 2. Guidelines for the triage of atypical squamous cells of undetermined significance. (*From* The American Society for Colposcopy and Cervical Pathology. ASCCP algorithm for the management of women with atypical squamous cells of undetermined significance (ASC-US). The Journal of Lower Genital Tract Disease 2002;6(2); with permission.)

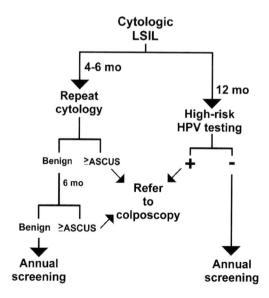

Fig. 3. Preferred management of LSIL in adolescents.

changed and all HSIL on cytology should be referred. Biopsy-confirmed HSIL is generally referred for treatment. There is a clause in the new guidelines that reflects expert opinion only in that adolescents with CIN 2 may be observed if patient is reliable for follow-up [59]. It is believed (although the evidence is not adequate) that many HSIL in young women under age of 25 years will undergo spontaneous regression [59]. These guidelines can be reviewed in the 2001 Consensus Guidelines for the Management of Women with Cervical Cytological Abnormalities and the 2001 Guidelines for Management of Women with Cervical Intraepithelial Neoplasia (www.asccp.org).

Human papilloma virus education

With the advent of HPV testing coming into the clinical market, there have been large debates on how best to handle telling a women she has a positive test for "HPV." The discussion directed toward a Pap smear diagnosis was different since many referred to the dysplastic changes as "precancer" changes. Now SIL is referred to as changed due to "a sexually transmitted infection (STI)". Clearly, the stigma of having an STI is often greater than having a nondescriptive "pre-cancer." In a study, college women were asked hypothetically how they would feel if told they had HPV [60]. The predominant answers were scared, angry, guilty, anxious, confined, dirty, regretful, and panicky. Another problem is the inconsistent stories given by health care providers. HPV in young women most likely reflects recent acquisition and transient infections. In older women, HPV most likely reflects a "failed clearance." Unfortunately, most women immediately want to know where they got it. The explanation must be carefully worded and should underscore the possibility that it was acquired years ago. On the other hand, the HPV test may reflect a more recent acquisition and a measure of infidelity of the partner or the patient. Several groups have now begun newsletters and websites to help inform patient populations. *HPV News*, supported by the American Social Health Association, is informative and consumer friendly (www.ashastd.org).

Education regarding initiation of Pap smear screening

The recommendations to delay screening until after 3 years of sexual activity or age 21 years also require efforts to educate women as well as health care providers. Traditionally, the pelvic examination has been equated with the "Pap smear." With these new guidelines, the need for gynecologic health care that includes pregnancy and sexually transmitted disease prevention and screening must be underscored. The cost of overscreening does not support the public continuing to equate their entire gynecologic health with "Pap smear" screening. A current history of STI infection or hormonal contraceptive use in a young woman does not make her an immediate risk for HSIL. Consequently, history of either of these is not an indication to initiate cervical cancer screening. In addition, these recommendations and arguments do not apply to immunocompromised women [42]. Immunocompromised women have higher rates of HSIL and invasive cancer. Unfortunately, immunocompromised women also have more recurrences making this a difficult population to treat. All ASCUS and LSIL in HIV infected women, regardless of age, should be referred for colposcopy and biopsy. LSIL, however, should be managed conservatively with follow-up since the high rate of recurrences result in repeated aggressive treatment often resulting in scarring and distortion [58].

Human papilloma virus testing as an adjunct to cytology

As described in the natural history, persistence of HPV is uncommon and reflects a risk for developing HSIL and invasive cancer. The frequent cycle of acquisition and regression in young women make clinical interpretation of HPV detection confusing in these women. On the other hand, HPV detection in women over 30 years when monogamy is more common appears to reflect "persistence." These infections most likely reflect acquisition that occurred years before and clearance never occurred. Observation of the natural history led to studies that examined the utility of HPV testing to detect HSIL in older women. A recent review by Wright et al [6] highlighted the enhanced sensitivity by combing cytology and HPV testing. Reviewing seven studies, the sensitivity of the Pap smear to detect HSIL or cancer ranged from 33.8% to 94%. HPV fared better with sensitivities ranging from 84.9% to 100%. In combination, sensitivities ranged from 87% to 100%. The specificity of HPV testing in general is less than that of a Pap smear alone; thereby combination of the two lowers the specificities of a Pap smear alone to range between 69.5% and 95.8%. The negative predictive value for the combination is in the range of 99.9% to 100%. Consequently, using the combination increases the sensitivity and the high negative predictive value allows for a greater interval between testing. Based on these data, HPV testing is now FDA approved in the United States as an adjunct to cervical cytology for primary screening in women aged 30 years or older. If negative for both, a woman can be screened at 3-year intervals.

Summary

New guidelines for cancer screening in women are less conservative and more cost-effective, saving many women from unnecessary procedures. The new recommendations to initiate screening within 3 years of the onset of sexual activity is in the right step in preventing over-referral and overtreatment of adolescents and young women. Additionally, young women with LSIL on cytology do not require immediate referral to colposcopy. Rather these women can be observed safely with HPV testing or cytology. In women of all ages, biopsy-confirmed LSIL can also be safely followed with HPV testing or cytology.

New guidelines for screening and management of adolescent and young women for cytologic abnormalities are important in delivering better health care to this group. Screening can be delayed up to 3 years after the initiation of vaginal intercourse but no later than 21 years of age, and LSIL can be followed by repeat cytology or HPV testing instead of immediate referral to colposcopy.

Acknowledgments

I would like to acknowledge Anthony Kung for his assistance in preparing the manuscript.

References

[1] Munoz N, Bosch FX, de Sanjose S, et al. Epidemiologic classification of human papillomavirus types associated with cervical cancer. N Engl J Med 2003;348(6):518–27.

[2] Franco ELF. Epidemiology of anogenital warts and cancer. Obstet Gynecol Clin N Am 1996;23(3):597–623.

[3] Ries LAG, Eisner MP, Kosary CL. SEER cancer statistics review, 1973–1999. Bethesda, MD: National Cancer Institute; 2002.

[4] Solomon D, Davey D, Kurman R, et al. The 2001 Bethesda System: terminology for reporting results of cervical cytology. JAMA 2002;287(16):2114–9.

[5] Syrjanen K, Kataja V, Yliskoski M, et al. Natural history of cervical human papillomavirus lesions does not substantiate the biologic relevance of the Bethesda System. Obstet Gynecol 1992;79:675–82.

[6] Wright TCJ, Schiffman M, Solomon D, et al. Interim guidance for the use of human papillomavirus DNA testing as an adjunct to cervical cytology for screening. Obstet Gynecol 2004;103(2):304–9.

[7] Wallin KL, Wiklund F, Angstrom T, et al. Type-specific persistence of human papillomavirus DNA before the development of invasive cervical cancer. N Engl J Med 1999;341(22):1633–8.

[8] Konno R, Sato S, Yajima A. Progression of squamous cell carcinoma of the uterine cervix from cervical intraepithelial neoplasia infected with human papillomavirus: a retrospective follow-up study by in situ hybridization and polymerase chain reaction. Int J Gynecol Pth 1992;11:105–12.

[9] Moscicki AB, Hills N, Shiboski S, et al. Risks for incident human papillomavirus infection and low-grade squamous intraepithelial lesion development in young females. JAMA 2001; 285(23):2995–3002.

[10] Werness BA, Levine AJ, Howley PM. Association of human papillomavirus types 16 and 18 E6 proteins with p53. Science 1990;248:76–9.

[11] Scheffner M, Werness BA, Huibregste JM, et al. The E6 oncoprotein encoded by human papillomavirus types 16 and 18 promotes the degradation of p53. Cell 1990;63:1129–36.

[12] Halbert CL, Demers GW, Galloway DA. The E7 gene of human papillomavirus type 16 is sufficient for immortalization of human epithelial cells. J Virol 1991;65:473–8.

[13] Dyson N, Howley PM, Munger K, Harlow E. The human papillomavirus-16 E7 oncoprotein is able to bind to the retinoblastoma gene product. Science 1989;243:934–7.

[14] Barbosa MS, Edmonds C, Fisher C, et al. The region of the HPV E7 oncoprotein homologous to adenovirus E1a and SV40 large T antigen contains separate domains for the Rb binding and casein kinase II phosphorylation. EMBO J 1990;9:153–60.

[15] Munger K, Werness BA, Dyson N, et al. Complex formation of human papillomavirus E7 proteins with the retinoblastoma tumor suppressor gene product. EMBO J 1989;8:4099–105.

[16] Nevins JR. E2F; A link between the Rb tumor supression protein and viral oncoproteins. Science 1992;258:424–9.

[17] Durst M, Glitz D, Schneider A, Zur HH. Human papillomavirus type 16 (HPV 16) gene expression and DNA replication in cervical neoplasia: analysis by in situ hybridization. Virology 1992;189:132–40.

[18] Broker TR, Chow LT, Chin MT, et al. A molecular portrait of human papillomavirus carcinogenesis. Cancer Cells 1989;7:197–208.

[19] Firzlaff JM, Kiviat NB, Beckmann AM. Detection of human papillomavirus capsid antigens in various squamous epithelial lesions using antibodies directed against the L1 and L2 open reading frames. Virology 1988;164:467–77.

[20] Duensing S, Duensing A, Flores ER, et al. Centrosome abnormalities and genomic instability by episomal expression of human papillomavirus type 16 in raft cultures of human keratinocytes. J Virol 2001;75(16):7712–6.

[21] Durst M, Kleinheinz A, Hotz M, Gissman L. The physical state of human papillomavirus type 16 DNA in benign and malignant genital tumours. J Gen Virol 1985;66(7):1515–22.

[22] Schwarz E, Freese UK, Gissmann L, et al. Structure and transcription of human papillomavirus sequences in cervical carcinoma cells. Nature 1985;314(6006):111–4.

[23] Herrero R, Hildesheim A, Bratti C, et al. Population-based study of human papillomavirus infection and cervical neoplasia in rural Costa Rica. J Natl Cancer Inst 2000;92(6):464–74.

[24] Mount SL, Papillo JL. A study of 10,296 pediatric and adolescent Papanicolaou smear diagnoses in northern New England. Pediatrics 1999;103(3):539–46.

[25] Taichmain LB, LaPorta RF. The expression of papillomaviruses in epithelial cells. In: Salzman NP, editor. The papovaviridae. New York: Plenum; 1986. p. 109–30.

[26] Moscicki AB, Grubbs-Burt V, Kanowitz S, et al. The significance of squamous metaplasia in the development of low grade squamous intra-epithelial lesions in young women. Cancer 1999; 85:1139–44.

[27] Moscicki AB, Shiboski S, Broering J, et al. The natural history of human papillomavirus infection as measured by repeated DNA testing in adolescent and young women. J Pediatr 1998;132:277–84.

[28] Ho GY, Bierman R, Beardsley L, et al. Natural history of cervicovaginal papillomavirus infection in young women. N Engl J Med 1998;338(7):423–8.

[29] Evander M, Edlund K, Gustaffson A, et al. Human papillomavirus infection is transient in young women: a population-based cohort study. J Infect Dis 1995;171:1026–30.

[30] Nasiell K, Nasiell M, Vaclavinkova V. Behavior of moderate cervical dysplasia during long term follow-up. Obstet Gynecol 1983;61:609–14.

[31] Nash JD, Burke TW, Hoskins WJ. Biologic course of cervical human papillomavirus infection. Obstet Gynecol 1987;69:160–2.

[32] Moscicki AB, Shiboski S, Hills NK, et al. High rate of regression of low-grade squamous intra-epithelial lesions (LSIL) among adolescents and young women. Lancet 2004;364:1678–83.

[33] Scott M, Stites DP, Moscicki AB. Th1 cytokine patterns in cervical human papillomavirus infection. Clin Diagn Lab Immunol 1999;6(5):751–5.

[34] Woodman CB, Collins S, Winter H, et al. Natural history of cervical human papillomavirus infection in young women: a longitudinal cohort study. Lancet 2001;357(9271):1831–6.

[35] Schachter J, Hill EC, King EB. Chlamydial infection in women with cervical dysplasia. Am J Obstet Gynecol 1975;123(7):753–7.

[36] Munoz N, Bosch FX, de Sanjose S, et al. Risk factors for cervical intraepithelial neoplasia grade III/carcinoma in situ in Spain and Colombia. Cancer Epidemiol Biomarkers Prev 1993;2: 31–43.

[37] Hakama M, Lehtinen M, Knekt P, et al. Serum antibodies and subsequent cervical neoplasms: a prospective study with 12 years of follow-up. Am J Epidemiol 1993;137(2): 166–70.

[38] Munoz N, Kato I, Bosch FX, et al. Cervical cancer and herpes simplex virus type 2: case-control studies in Spain and Colombia, with special reference to immunoglobulin-G sub-classes. Int J Cancer 1995;60(4):438–42.

[39] Koyamatsu Y, Yokoyama M, Nakao Y, et al. A comparative analysis of human papillomavirus types 16 and 18 and expression of p53 gene and Ki-67 in cervical, vaginal, and vulvar carcinomas. Gynecol Oncol 2003;90(3):547–51.

[40] Schlecht NF, Platt RW, Duarte-Franco E, et al. Human papillomavirus infection and time to progression and regression of cervical intraepithelial neoplasia. J Natl Cancer Inst 2003;95(17):1336–43.

[41] Sadeghi SB, Hsieh EW, Gunn SW. Prevalence of cervical intraepithelial neoplasia in sexually active teenagers and young adults. Am J Obstet Gynecol 1984;148:726–9.

[42] Centers For Disease Control. USPHS/IDSA Guidelines for the prevention of opportunistic infections in persons infected with human immunodeficiency virus: A summary. Morb Mortal Wkly Rep 1995;44:1–34.

[43] Bauer HM, Ting Y, Greer CE, Chambers JC, Tashiro CJ, Chimera J, et al. Genital human papillomavirus infection in female university students as determined by a PCR-based method. JAMA 1991;265:472–7.

[44] Hingson R, Heeren T, Winter MR, Wechsler H. Early age of first drunkenness as a factor in college students' unplanned and unprotected sex attributable to drinking. Pediatrics 2003; 111(1):34–41.

[45] Hingson RW, Heeren T, Zakocs RC, Kopstein A, Wechsler H. Magnitude of alcohol-related mortality and morbidity among US college students ages 18–24. J Stud Alcohol 2002;63(2): 136–44.

[46] Sax LJ. Health trends among college freshmen. J Am Coll Health 1997;45(6):252–62.

[47] American Cancer Society. Cancer Facts and Figures. Atlanta: American Cancer Society, Inc.; 2002.

[48] American College of Obstetricians and Gynecologists. Recommendations on Frequency of Pap Test Screening 1995;152.

[49] NIH. NIH Consensus Statement 1996; April 13, 1996. p. 1–38.

[50] American Medical Association. Guidelines for adolescent preventive services. Chicago, IL: American Medical Association; 1992.

[51] Saslow D, Runowicz CD, Solomon D, Moscicki AB, Smith RA, Eyre HJ, et al. American Cancer Society guideline for the early detection of cervical neoplasia and cancer. CA Cancer J Clin 2002;52(6):342–62.

[52] Working IARC. Group on Evaluation of Cervical Cancer Screening Programmes. Screening for squamous cervical cancer: duration of low risk after negative results of cervcal cytology and its implication for screening policies. BMJ 1986;293:659–64.

[53] Laara E, Day NE, Hakama M. Trends in mortality from cervical cancer in the Nordic countries: association with organised screening programmes. Lancet 1987;1(8544):1247–9.

[54] Sasieni PD, Cuzick J, Lynch-Farmery E. Estimating the efficacy of screening by auditing smear histories of women with and without cervical cancer. The National Co-ordinating Network for Cervical Screening Working Group. Br J Cancer 1996;73(8):1001–5.

[55] Bos AB, van Ballegooijen M, van Gessel-Dabekaussen AA, Habbema JDF. Organised cervical-cancer screening still leads to higher coverage than spontaneous screening in The Netherlands. Eur J Cancer 1998;34:1598–601.

[56] Shapiro J, Radecki S, Charchian AS, Josephson V. Sexual behavior and AIDS-related knowledge among community college students in Orange County, California. J Community Health 1999; 24(1):29–43.

[57] Wiley DC, James G, Furney S, Jordan-Belver C. Using the Youth Risk Behavior Survey to compare risk behaviors of Texas High School and college students. J Sch Health 1997;67(2): 45–9.

[58] Wright TCJ, Cox JT, Massad LS, Twiggs LB, Wilkinson EJ. 2001 Consensus Guidelines for the management of women with cervical cytological abnormalities. JAMA 2002;287(16): 2120–9.

[59] Wright TCJ, Cox JH, Massad LS, Carlson J, Twiggs LB, Wilkinson EJ. 2001 Consensus Guidelines for the Management of Women with Cervical Intraepithelial Neoplasia. Am J Obstet Gynecol 2003;189(1):295–304.

[60] Ramirez JE, Ramos DM, Clayton L, Kanowitz S, Moscicki AB. Genital human papillomavirus infections: knowledge, perception of risk, and actual risk in a nonclinic population of young women. J Women's Health 1997;6:113–21.

PEDIATRIC CLINICS

OF NORTH AMERICA

ELSEVIER
SAUNDERS

Pediatr Clin N Am 52 (2005) 179–197

Menstrual Disorders in the College Age Female

Paula J. Adams Hillard, MD[a],*, Helen R. Deitch, MD[b]

[a]*Division of Adolescent Medicine, Cincinnati Children's Hospital Medical Center,
3333 Burnet Avenue, ML 4000, Cincinnati, OH 45229-3039, USA*
[b]*Centre Medical and Surgical Associates, Obstetrics and Gynecology, 1850 East Park Avenue,
Suite 103, State College, PA 16870, USA*

Obstetric and gynecologic issues are the most common reason for 18- to 21-year-old women to visit a health care provider, and 75% of older adolescents will perceive a problem with menstruation [1]. Common complaints include dysmenorrhea, menorrhagia, and delayed or irregular menses.

Approximately 50% of 17 year olds have had intercourse [2], and unintended pregnancy rates are the highest in the 18- to 24-year-old age group [3]. Adolescents have been shown to wait typically a year or more after first intercourse before they seek medical advice for contraception [4]. Because many adolescents are unable or unwilling to divulge their current or planned sexual debut, particularly if they are not aware that they can do so confidentially, any young woman presenting for evaluation of abnormal bleeding (either infrequent or excessive bleeding) should have a pregnancy test performed, regardless of her stated sexual history. The consequences of missing a pregnancy-related complication are simply too great to omit this testing.

This article addresses normal menstrual function, excessive bleeding, infrequent or absent menses, pain with menses, menstrual-related mood disorders, and recommendations about routine gynecologic examinations and evaluation.

Normal menstruation

The average age of menarche in the United States is 12.88 years for white girls, and 12.16 years for black girls [5]. Initially, anovulatory cycles are the

---

* Corresponding author.
E-mail address: paula.hillard@cchmc.org (P.J.A. Hillard).

norm, as seen in a Hungarian study that documented that the frequency of ovulatory cycles was 10% to 13% after the first 7 to 10 menstruations and rose to 50% ovulatory cycles after 20 menstruations [6].

The expected series of events in an ovulatory cycle begins with the sloughing of the endometrium from the previous cycle. The follicular phase lasts from

A

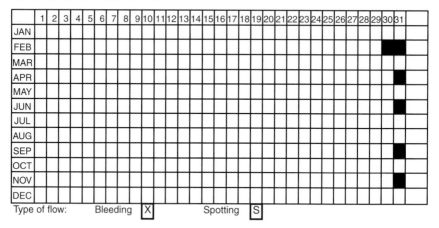

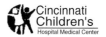

MENSTRUAL FLOW CHART

	1	2	3	4	5	6	7	8	9	10	11	12	13	14	15	16	17	18	19	20	21	22	23	24	25	26	27	28	29	30	31
JAN																															
FEB																													■		
MAR																															
APR																													■		
MAY																															
JUN																													■		
JUL																															
AUG																															
SEP																													■		
OCT																															
NOV																													■		
DEC																															

Type of flow: Bleeding |X| Spotting |S|

Please have this chart with you when you call or visit your health care provider

B

WHAT IS A NORMAL PERIOD?

Normal Periods:
- ❖ Start before age 16
- ❖ Last one week or less
- ❖ Are between 21 and 42 days from the first day of one period to the first day of the next period
- ❖ When you bleed, you fill less than one pad per hour

If your periods are <u>NOT</u> "normal," talk with your clinician.

WRITE YOUR PERIODS DOWN ON A CALENDAR

**This information is provided to you as a courtesy through:
Cincinnati Children's Hospital Medical Center
Teen Health Center, Adolescent & Pediatric Gynecology
If you need an appointment, please call (513)636-4681**

Fig. 1. (*A,B*) Menstrual calendar (a two-sided card 4 1/4 × 5 1/2 inches).

the first day of menses until ovulation. The follicular phase is marked by the elevation of follicle stimulating hormone (FSH) from the anterior pituitary, resulting in the recruitment of a dominant ovarian follicle. The dominant follicle matures under FSH stimulation and produces estrogen that stimulates growth of the endometrial lining. Ovulation generally occurs around day 14 of the cycle and is triggered by a surge in luteinizing hormone (LH) production. The second half of the menstrual cycle, or luteal phase, is marked by progesterone production from the corpus luteum that replaces the follicle under the stimulus of LH. Progesterone acts to slow the growth of the estrogen stimulated endometrium and to induce changes that make it a supportive environment for implantation should conception occur. In the absence of implantation of an embryo, the progesterone production declines, resulting in endometrial shedding and menstruation.

Despite the frequent lack of ovulation, most cycles during adolescence will fall within a cycle length of 21 to 42 days with 2 to 8 days of flow [7]. In adults and older teens, regular, ovulatory menstrual cycles occur every 21 to 35 days and last up to 7 days with an average blood loss of 25 to 69 mL [8]. Cycles shorter or longer than these norms, prolonged bleeding, or excessive menstrual flow may be evidence of underlying pathophysiology and deserve further evaluation. It is not unusual for young women to complain of abnormal menses when their cycles fall within normal variation. Whereas most college women understand the basics of menstrual physiology and understand that an average 28-day cycle is counted from day 1 of one period until day 1 of the subsequent cycle, some women will complain that they have "2- to 3-week cycles" when they are counting from the end of one menstrual period until the beginning of the next, failing to add 5 to 7 days of menstrual flow to the count. Other patients complain of "two periods a month," failing to realize that this is not abnormal if the number of cycle days falls within the range of norms noted earlier with a minimum of 21 days. Some girls complain of "skipping a month" when they have a period at the end of 1 month, miss a month, and then a period at the beginning of the subsequent month; again, this is not abnormal if the range is not greater than approximately 35 to 42 days. Charting of menstrual flow on a menstrual calendar can be helpful in documenting menstrual cycle normalcy or irregularities (see Fig. 1).

Excessive bleeding

Excessive menstrual bleeding can be described as menses more frequently than every 21 days, lasting for more than 7 days, or greater than 80 mL of blood loss per cycle. A menstrual calendar is helpful in documenting the frequency and duration of menses. Subjectively, a patient's complaint of heavy menstrual bleeding may not correlate with the definition of more than 80 mL of blood loss, which is the volume of flow that will result in anemia if it occurs on an ongoing basis. In a study from Glasgow, Scotland, only 34% of women reporting menorrhagia had documented blood loss of more than 80 mL. Clinical features associated with blood loss in excess of 80 mL include the rate of changing sanitary protection during full flow, passage of clots >1.1 in, low ferritin, and the need to change protection during the night [9]. However, difficulties with containment of periods, compromised iron status, and pathologic findings were similar between women with blood loss of 50 to 119 mL [10].

Menstrual disorders resulting in excessive menstrual bleeding can be divided into those due to anovulatory bleeding and other causes. Anovulatory bleeding is common in the years after menarche as the hypothalamic-pituitary-ovarian-axis matures to provide regular ovulatory cycles, although as noted previously, even anovulatory cycles typically occur every 21 to 42 days, with bleeding lasting for less than 7 days.

Numerous disorders can disrupt the intricate interplay of hormonal signals necessary for ovulation to occur. In the absence of ovulation, the endometrium continues to proliferate under the stimulation of estrogen. This results in overgrowth of the endometrium that then sheds irregularly, causing unpredictable and sometimes heavy or prolonged uterine bleeding.

Coagulation disorders

Coagulation disorders are often first recognized at menarche with the onset of menorrhagia, occasionally severe enough to warrant hospitalization. Menorrhagia with menarche, or a history of heavy menses with the patient complaining of soaking through double protection or soiling the sheets at night, should be an indication for further evaluation. Personal or family history may reveal prolonged nosebleeds, easy bruising, excessive bleeding with procedures, or a family history of menorrhagia and hysterectomy. Studies of adolescents presenting to the emergency department with acute menorrhagia have found an incidence of an underlying bleeding disorder ranging from 3% to 33% [11–13]. Common diagnoses include platelet dysfunction, acute idiopathic thrombocytopenic purpura (ITP), and von Willebrand disease (VWD) [14]. Laboratory testing for these conditions should be performed before the initiation of any hormonal therapy, as estrogens impact clotting studies.

Laboratory evaluation for bleeding disorders in an older adolescent with menorrhagia will depend on the history and severity of bleeding. After excluding pregnancy, a complete blood count with differential and platelets, prothrombin time, and partial thromboplastin time is essential for the initial evaluation [15]. Further laboratory evaluation is warranted if bleeding is excessive, the initial evaluation is abnormal, the patient is anemic, symptoms have occurred since menarche, or there is a strong personal or family history of other bleeding events or hysterectomy for menorrhagia. Consultation with a hematologist may be helpful.

Von Willebrand disease has a prevalence of approximately 1% [16]. Screening for von Willebrand disease may include von Willebrand factor antigen, factor VIII activity, or Ristocetin co-factor. The bleeding time has been found to be inconsistent and insensitive in detecting mild to moderate von Willebrand disease or platelet function defects, and was found to be normal in five of eight patients given a diagnosis of an inherited bleeding disorder in one study [14]. Platelet function screening tests using the Platelet Function Analyzer (PFA-100; Dade-Behring, Inc., Deerfield, Illinois) are now being used more frequently as a screen for acquired or inherited platelet function abnormalities, including von Willebrand disease, and have been found to be more sensitive than the bleeding time for detecting VWD. Experts still caution that when clinical suspicion is strong, testing should be supplemented with assays of von Willebrand factor (VWF) and platelet aggregometry [17]. Desmopressin is a synthetic analog of antidiuretic hormone secreted by the posterior pituitary gland, which may be therapeutically useful in the treatment of VWD [18]. The mechanism of action includes the stimulation of endogenous release of VWF, the release of Factor VIII from storage sites, and increased platelet adhesion to vessel walls [19]. Patients with von Willebrand disease and other coagulopathies may benefit from the use of combined oral contraceptives or hormonally induced therapeutic amenorrhea [20].

Treatment of acute menorrhagia depends on the patient presentation. Any patient who is bleeding profusely or who is hypovolemic needs inpatient treatment with volume replacement. After stabilization and assessment of the need for transfusion, hormonal therapy with high dose estrogens followed by combination oral contraceptives are the most commonly used therapies. However, testing for bleeding disorders should be performed before the use of hormonal therapy, as coagulation parameters are impacted by estrogen use.

The goals of medical treatment are to alleviate acute bleeding, prevent future episodes of noncyclic bleeding, decrease the patient's risk of long-term complications from anovulation, and improve the patient's overall quality of life [21].

Infrequent menses

Oligomenorrhea refers to irregular menses, often described as occurring less frequently than every 35 days in adult women. Secondary amenorrhea has been variably defined as absence of menses for 6 months, although the evidence supporting this definition is not well established [22]. A more statistically based guideline would suggest evaluation of menses occurring less frequently than 90 days, as this value represents the 95% for menstrual cycle length in the first gynecologic years after menarche; by the fourth year after menarche, the 95th percentile for cycle length has declined from 90 days to approximately 50 days;. by 7 years after menarche, the 95th percentile is 38 days [23]. Women with menses occurring less frequently than every 90 days most definitely deserve an evaluation with a careful history, physical examination, and consideration of laboratory testing; depending on the number of years since menarche, evaluation for menses that are irregular and infrequent, but which occur less frequently than every 38 to 50 days, may be appropriate.

Polycystic ovary syndrome

Polycystic ovary syndrome (PCOS) is likely the most common endocrinologic problem of women and thus the most common cause of irregular and infrequent menses and anovulation. PCOS has been found to affect approximately 3.4% of black women and 4.7% of white women in the southeastern United States, 6.5% in Spain, and 6.77% in the Greek Island of Lesbos [24–26]. Other studies have suggested an even higher incidence. Stein and Leventhal [27] originally described this heterogeneous disorder in 1935, and today the basic pathophysiology of PCOS is still unknown. Diagnostic criteria have differed over the years, but a 2003 Rotterdam consensus workshop concluded that PCOS is a syndrome of ovarian dysfunction along with the cardinal features of hyperandrogenism and polycystic ovary (PCO) morphology [28]. The diagnosis requires two of the following three criteria: (1) oligo or anovulation; (2) clinical and or biochemical signs of hyperandrogenism; (3) polycystic ovaries as demonstrated on ultrasound. The workshop also recognized the variety in presentation of PCOS; some women with PCOS may have irregular cycles without clinical evidence of hyperandrogenism, whereas others may have hyperandrogenism with monthly cycles [28].

The hallmark symptoms of PCOS include irregular menses, infertility, and hyperandrogenism. In the college age population, PCOS patients may present to the gynecologist with a variety of complaints, including primary or secondary amenorrhea, unpredictable bleeding patterns, acne, hirsutism, acanthosis nigricans, obesity, and infertility. Menstrual irregularities may be difficult to document without the benefit of menstrual charting, and acne and excess terminal hair growth may be perceived as normal instead of reported as a problem in some young women, particularly if others in the family are hirsute. Other young women take great efforts to remove all evidence of body hair, given cultural expectations of air-brushed models. Therefore, evaluation of a patient with any of the findings of hyperandrogenism or any complaints of menstrual irregularities should trigger careful questioning and examination for evidence of androgen excess, and laboratory evaluation.

Physical examination for androgen excess requires careful inspection of the patient unclothed. In addition, sensitive questioning may reveal the practice and frequency of hair removal measures or efforts to hide hair growth, including waxing, shaving, plucking, use of depilatories, or bleaching. Pertinent physical findings include oily skin, acne on the face, chest, or back, and terminal hair growth on the face, back, upper arms, between the breasts, upper and lower abdomen, and inner thighs. Clitoromegaly, male pattern baldness, and severe, recent onset, or rapidly progressive hirsutism may be evidence of an androgen-secreting tumor. Additional helpful physical findings include acanthosis nigricans, most commonly occurring on the back of the neck, but also in the axilla, the groin, or other areas of the body, as evidence of insulin resistance. Hypertension, violaceous abdominal striae larger than 1 cm, and the "buffalo hump" cervical fat pad suggest Cushing's disease.

Often college-aged women have been treated for irregular cycles with oral contraceptives before an appropriate endocrinologic evaluation or a diagnosis. Acne and excess terminal hair growth may not be obvious on examination due to treatment of acne with topical or oral acne medications, or use of temporary or permanent hair removal techniques; alternatively, the patient simply may not have been examined completely disrobed. The diagnosis of PCOS may not have been considered, confirmed with labs, or discussed with the patient, thus missing an opportunity to provide health guidance and recommendations that may mitigate the potential long-term health risks associated with the condition.

The health risks of PCOS can range from the annoyance and embarrassment of unpredictable menses to infertility to the long-term risks of increased morbidity and mortality due to the development of type 2 diabetes, dyslipidemia, and the increased risk of endometrial cancer. The disorder also predisposes young women to low self esteem [29].

The underlying defect in PCOS has yet to be determined, and the presenting phenotypes can vary greatly. Although many women with PCOS are obese, the condition also occurs in women who are lean or of normal weight. The recommendations for testing vary widely, with most recommendations referring to the evaluation and treatment of adult women. Even in older adolescents, the findings associated with PCOS may be subtle, and measurement of free and total testosterone levels may reveal biochemical hyperandrogenism with minimal physical findings. An LH to FSH ratio of greater than 2:1 can be supportive of the diagnosis of PCOS, but the ratio may also be normal in PCOS, or elevated in a normal patient if drawn during the LH surge; thus, these measurements may not be clinically useful. Pelvic ultrasound is useful for excluding other causes of irregular menses such as fibroids, polyps, and ovarian cysts. The classic ultrasound finding of polycystic ovaries adds to the diagnosis, but they may also be found in 15% to 30% of regularly cycling women [30].

The ovulatory dysfunction, hyperandrogenism, and infertility associated with PCOS can also be evidence of other pathophysiologic states that must be excluded before the diagnosis of PCOS can be made. Primary and secondary amenorrhea may be seen in college age women for a variety of reasons. Hypothyroidism, hyperprolactinemia, and premature ovarian failure can be excluded by evaluation of TSH, prolactin, and FSH. Hypothalamic hypogonadotropic amenorrhea can be precipitated by chronic diseases such as diabetes and Crohn's disease, as can eating disorders and excessive exercise. New onset of hirsutism, suddenly worsening hirsutism, and virilization are all suggestive of androgen-secreting tumors that should be evaluated by dehydroepiandrosterone sulphate (DHEAS) and total testosterone levels, along with imaging of the ovaries and possibly adrenals. Other causes of hirsutism include late onset congenital adrenal hyperplasia and Cushing's syndrome.

Treatment of PCOS is aimed at regulating menses, decreasing circulating androgens, ovulation induction for patients desiring pregnancy, and reduction of long-term health risks. Oral contraceptives are an ideal treatment for young women with PCOS. The progestin component provides menstrual regulation and protection against endometrial hyperplasia and contraception in an age group with a high incidence of unintended pregnancy. Oral contraceptives also lower circulating androgen levels, which will improve acne and decrease hirsutism [31]. Patients with PCOS should be screened for dyslipidemia, type 2 diabetes, and insulin resistance, regardless of their weight.

Sexually transmitted infections

Abnormal uterine bleeding can be the only presenting symptom of sexually transmitted infections (STIs). Three million teenagers are infected with an STI each year, and women and adolescents are disproportionately affected by STIs and their sequelae. Among women in 2002, as in previous years, 15- to 24-year-olds had the highest rates of gonorrhea compared with women in all other age categories, and 20- to 29-year-old women had the highest rates of primary and secondary syphilis in 2002 [32]. These high rates in teens are due to early onset of sexual activity, low rates of condom use, increased health facilities for teenagers allowing better diagnosis and reporting, and the recognition of asymptomatic infections in males and females [33]. Oral contraceptives may promote the acquisition of STIs by contributing to the persistence of cervical ectopy, but they may also protect the cervix from STIs by thickening cervical mucus and reducing menstrual flow [34–36].

Cervicitis caused by *C trachomatis*, *N gonorrhoeae*, Trichomonas vaginalis can be associated with abnormal bleeding and post coital bleeding. The increased finding of cervical ectopy during adolescence is associated with increased rates of *C trachomatis* and *N gonorrhoeae* infection, most likely caused by exposure of the more vulnerable columnar cells of the endocervical canal to these pathogens [37]. The prevalence of *C trachomatis* among 16- to 24-year-old women entering the National Job Training Program was as high as 16.8%. Symptoms of chlamydial cervicitis may mimic a urinary tract infection. Clinical diagnosis is imprecise, suggesting that adolescent females with vaginal or urinary symptoms should be tested for both *C trachomatis* and urinary tract infections [38]. Anyone testing positive for one STI should be offered screening for other infections including HIV, syphilis, and Hepatitis B.

Pelvic inflammatory disease (PID) is a general term to imply inflammation of the upper genital tract. This includes inflammation of the endometrium (endometritis), uterine musculature (myometritis), ovaries (oophoritis), and uterine serosa and broad ligament (parametritis). *C trachomatis* and *N gonorrhoeae* are thought to be the primary causative agents of PID through an initial cervical infection that then ascends into the upper genital tract. The inflammatory response allows access of other vaginal flora into the upper genital tract, causing a polymicrobic infection. Studies by Sweet et al [39] revealed that *N gonorrhoeae* is more likely to be isolated in the first 24 to 48 hours of symptoms, but anaerobic bacteria are more common later in infection. Women presenting with a new onset of heavy, unusually painful, but regular menses may have a subclinical or low grade endometritis. Thus, this presentation should prompt STD testing.

Adolescents tend to delay seeking health care for PID symptoms when compared with adults [40]. Patients who present for treatment more than 3 days after the onset of symptoms are more likely to experience infertility and ectopic pregnancy than those who present earlier for care [41]. These patients may be more likely to have anaerobic organisms as a cause of their pelvic infections.

The PEACH (Pelvic Inflammatory Disease Evaluation and Clinical Health) Study was a randomized clinical trial evaluating the long-term outcomes of inpatient versus outpatient treatment of mild to moderate PID [42]. About 25% of the study participants were under 19, and 65% were under the age of 24. Long-term outcomes studied included the time to pregnancy, PID recurrence, chronic pelvic pain, and ectopic pregnancy. No difference in outcomes was found between the inpatient and outpatient arms of the study [42]. However, compliance may be an issue in younger patients that may warrant inpatient management of PID, even with minimal clinical findings.

The Centers for Disease Control published guidelines in 2002 for the treatment of STIs [32]. In this publication they recommend new minimal criteria for the diagnosis of PID to try to minimize the long-term complications that may be associated with missed or delayed diagnosis. In a woman with lower abdominal or pelvic pain, treatment for PID should be initiated if there is uterine/ adnexal tenderness or cervical motion tenderness on exam.

Thyroid disease

Thyroid disorders have been implicated in the cause of irregular menses, in both the cases of hyper- and hypothyroidism. Screening patients for thyroid disorders with a sensitive TSH assay is reasonable for women with irregular menses, as the testing is relatively inexpensive and simple.

Other

Other conditions including various chronic diseases can cause anovulation and irregular menstrual bleeding. College age women may be somewhat more likely than older women to experience irregular and infrequent bleeding that is unexplained by specific disease conditions. Unexplained, idiopathic, or the so-called "stress-induced" hypothalamic amenorrhea or oligomenorrhea may be a risk factor for the occurrence of osteopenia or osteoporosis, even with a normal hormonal profile. In one study, only six of 19 girls with "pure" dysfunction of the hypothalamic-pituitary-ovarian axis had normal bone density [43]. Thus, excessive delay in the evaluation and treatment of abnormal and infrequent menses may contribute to osteoporosis. Regular menstrual cyclicity is a sign of good health. Just as blood pressure and pulse are "vital signs," the menstrual cycle should be viewed as a vital sign that can lead to earlier detection and potentially prevention of osteoporosis [22].

Amenorrhea

Pregnancy-related complications

Pregnancy usually presents with missed menses, and in adults, the most common cause of secondary amenorrhea, defined as no bleeding for 3 to 6 months, is pregnancy. In a population such as college students in which unprotected sexual activity may be common, pregnancy should always be ruled out when a menstrual period is missed. Assessment of human chorionic gonadotropin (hCG) in the urine is simple, quick, and accurate, and this test should be available in all outpatient medical settings. In addition, as noted previously, bleeding irregularities can signal a pregnancy-related complication such as a spontaneous abortion or ectopic pregnancy.

Bleeding during pregnancy is a common occurrence, and an adolescent presenting for evaluation may not have considered pregnancy-related complications as a cause of her bleeding. In a stable patient, a positive pregnancy test accompanied by vaginal bleeding or pain requires evaluation and careful observation until the location and viability of the pregnancy can be determined. Pregnancy-related complications should be managed in consultation with an obstetrician-gynecologist.

First-trimester vaginal bleeding is a common complication that affects 16% to 25% of all pregnancies [44,45]. The incidence of spontaneous abortion after first-trimester bleeding is quoted to be 50% before sonographic evaluation for fetal viability [45,46]. If a viable fetus is noted at ultrasound examination after first-trimester vaginal bleeding, 95% to 98% of such pregnancies will still continue beyond 20 weeks of gestation [45,47].

In the absence of ultrasonographic confirmation of an intrauterine pregnancy, an ectopic pregnancy must be considered. In 1992, the Centers for Disease Control and Prevention reported an ectopic pregnancy rate of 19.7 per 1000 reported pregnancies, and in 1990 there were 64,000 hospital admissions for ectopic pregnancy [48]. Whereas more ectopic pregnancies are being diagnosed before rupture and acute presentation, ectopic pregnancies remain the most common cause of pregnancy-related death in the first trimester. African American women have an ectopic mortality ratio 18 times higher than white women [49]. Thus, the possibility of an ectopic pregnancy must always be considered in a patient presenting with bleeding or pain who has a positive pregnancy test.

Forty to 45% of ectopic pregnancies are thought to be secondary to a history of acute salpingitis, the most common cause of which is Chlamydia trachomatis. Thus, adolescents and college-age women must be considered to be at increased risk because of the frequency of Chlamydia and STDs in this age group. Contraception decreases the overall pregnancy rate, and therefore, the overall ectopic rate is decreased by about 90% in women using any method of contraception when compared with women not using contraception.

The classic symptoms of ectopic pregnancy are delayed menses, abdominal pain, and irregular vaginal bleeding. These symptoms are often difficult to differentiate from a threatened abortion, and in a stable, minimally symptomatic patient, it may take several days to make the correct diagnosis. Helpful tools in diagnosing ectopic pregnancy include the serum quantitative beta human chorionic gonadotropin (B-HCG) levels, serum progesterone, and pelvic ultrasonography. With a viable intrauterine pregnancy, B-HCG levels should increase by at least 66% in 48 hours. The production of B-HCG by an ectopic pregnancy is less than that of a normal pregnancy, and an increase of less than 66% should raise suspicion of an ectopic. However, 15% of normal intrauterine pregnancies will have abnormally rising B-hCG levels, and 17% of ectopic pregnancies will increase appropriately, giving false reassurance [50]. Because the management of women with suspected ectopic pregnancy can be challenging or may even become a surgical emergency, women with pregnancy-related bleeding should be referred for evaluation by an ob-gyn with surgical privileges.

Pelvic ultrasound can detect a normal intrauterine pregnancy using a transvaginal approach at 5 weeks gestation or with a B-hCG level of about 1500 mIU/mL. The absence of a gestational sac at this discriminatory level suggests an ectopic pregnancy but can also be seen with an abnormal intrauterine pregnancy or multiple gestations, and obesity and uterine fibroids can make the diagnosis difficult. Ultrasound findings suspicious for ectopic pregnancy have a good correlation with findings at the time of surgery, but absence of adnexal findings does not exclude an ectopic pregnancy.

Serum progesterone can be helpful in delineating between a normal intra-uterine pregnancy and a nonviable pregnancy or an ectopic pregnancy. Using a cutoff of <5ng/mL, 85% of those patients with lower levels will have a spontaneous abortion, 14% will have ectopic pregnancies, and 0.16% will have a normal intrauterine gestation [51]. Four percent of ectopic pregnancies have a progesterone level between 20 and 24.9 ng/mL, and 2% are > 25 ng/mL.

Uterine curettage with examination of the uterine contents for the presence of chorionic villi is an important diagnostic procedure in cases where the pregnancy is clearly abnormal but the location cannot be determined. The absence of products of conception gives the diagnosis of an ectopic pregnancy.

Eating disorders

Eating disorders, including anorexia and bulimia, have the highest incidence during the adolescent years. In the United State, the prevalence of anorexia nervosa is 1%; anorexia nervosa is found mainly in white adolescents of the middle and upper socioeconomic classes, although it can be observed in either sex and in individuals of any race, age, or social class [52]. It is not unusual for an adolescent with an eating disorder to present with the complaint of amenorrhea. The diagnosis of anorexia nervosa is based on specifically defined diagnostic criteria and includes the presence of amenorrhea (defined as the absence of three consecutive menstrual periods) among the required symptoms [53].

Amenorrhea can precede significant weight loss. Bulimia nervosa, characterized by purging behaviors, is associated with irregular and anovulatory cycles and can occur in individuals of normal weight or overweight. Individuals with disordered eating and binging/purging behaviors may be quite secretive or ashamed of these behaviors; sensitive questioning by astute clinicians is required. Subclinical eating disorders are common and may be associated with amenorrhea [54]. Eating disorders can be quite difficult to treat and often require a team approach or referral for specialized care [55,56]. Morbidity rates range from 10% to 20%, and only about half of patients recover completely [52]. Thus, intervention and management by clinicians skilled in the management are mandatory. The associated hypoestrogenism is of concern, leading to osteopenia or even frank osteoporosis that may not be entirely reversible. In the absence of weight recovery, estrogen replacement does not appear to be sufficient to reverse bone loss [57,58]. Amenorrhea persists at 6 months after appropriate weight gain in as many as 14% of young women [59].

The Female Athlete Triad is characterized by disordered eating, osteoporosis or osteopenia, and amenorrhea in the setting of excessive exercise. It was first described in the sports medicine literature, but its relationship to the psychiatric diagnoses of eating disorders is obvious [60]. Again, a multidisciplinary approach is indicated, and the involvement of sports medicine specialists, orthopedics specialists, and coaches may beneficial. Amenorrhea is only the symptom that may call medical attention to the serious underlying disorder.

Hypergonadotropic hypogonadism

In adolescents who present with amenorrhea, the possibility of an underlying ovarian failure or gonadal dysgenesis must be considered. Although premature ovarian failure is rare, affecting only 1 of 10,000 women by age 20 years, the occurrence of declining ovarian function (prodromal failure) may present with irregular menses [61]. This condition may be diagnosed with elevated gonadotropins. Young women presenting with loss of menstrual regularity or with oligomenorrhea (no menses for > 90 days) should be evaluated with laboratory testing that includes a pregnancy test, serum prolactin, FSH, LH, and estradiol. An elevated FSH (> 40 IU/L) is suggestive of premature ovarian failure and should prompt repeat testing. If persistent, a karyotype is required.

College-age women may occasionally present with primary amenorrhea. Between 10% and 15% of women with premature ovarian failure present in such a fashion. A chromosomal abnormality can be detected in nearly 40% of patients who present with primary amenorrhea in association with pubertal delay. Referral to a reproductive gynecologist or a pediatric and adolescent gynecologist can help in addressing these conditions that may be associated with autoimmunity. The hypoestrogenic state may prevent these women from achieving and maintaining adequate bone density, thus putting them at increased risk for osteoporosis and fractures later in life. The serious ramifications for future reproductive capabilities require a sensitive and knowledgeable clinician [62].

Ovarian failure may also occur as a consequence of previous radiation or chemotherapy for childhood or adolescent malignancies. Efforts to prevent ovarian failure from chemotherapy through the use of gonadotropin releasing hormone agonists are currently under investigation [63]. Clinicians may occasionally encounter a young woman who has received previous chemotherapy or radiation who has either not been compliant with previously prescribed hormone replacement therapy or who has not sought evaluation for oligomenorrhea or amenorrhea from this cause. Young women with elevated gonadotropins as a consequence of previous chemotherapy should be informed that while their likelihood of recovery of ovarian function, ovulation, and fertility is low, they should not consider it beyond the realm of possibility that a pregnancy could occur due to spontaneous recovery of ovarian function. Thus, those who are not desirous of an unplanned pregnancy (most college women) should use hormonal contraception that provides both adequate estrogen for bone growth and development in addition to adequate contraception.

Drug-induced amenorrhea

A number of prescription drugs can cause amenorrhea. Those drugs include, most notably and historically, antipsychotics; many of these drugs induce elevated levels of prolactin by their mechanism of action as dopamine receptor antagonists [22]. Drugs included in this category include risperidone, phenothiazine, haloperidol, butyrophenones, metoclopramide, sulpiride, and domperidone. Other drugs that elevate prolactin include the now uncommonly used antihypertensive drugs methyldopa and reserpine; neither of these drugs is likely to be in common use in a young adult college population. Verapamil, which may be used for migraine prophylaxis, may raise serum prolactin [64]. Psychotropic drugs used as mood stabilizers or anticonvulsants may be associated with menstrual irregularities. Divalproex has been associated with an increased risk of hyperandrogenism/PCOS and thus irregular menses are not uncommon on this drug.

Other drugs that may be more commonly used in a college-age population include contraceptive medications, which may induce amenorrhea when taken in the usually prescribed manner. These drugs include combination oral contraceptive pills, progestin-only contraceptive pills, depot medroxyprogesterone acetate, and the levonorgestrel-containing intrauterine system. In the absence of concerns about possible pregnancy (which may occur with missed pills and should be ruled out), such hormonally induced amenorrhea is not medically worrisome and in fact may be a desirable effect. The recent approval of an extended cycle oral contraceptive pills formulation, packaged in such a manner as to lead to a period only four times a year, capitalizes on some women's desires to have less frequent menstrual periods. However, clinicians need to be aware that unscheduled bleeding is common in the initial months of such extended pill use. Irregular bleeding may be due to missed or late oral contraceptive pills or possibly related to the substitution of generic pill formulations. Whether this is associated with lower contraceptive efficacy is unclear.

Pain

Dysmenorrhea

Primary dysmenorrhea is menstrual pain that is due to the excess production and action of prostaglandins, which cause uterine cramping and ischemia leading to pain. Menstrual molimina include such uncomfortable menstrual-related symptoms as dysmenorrhea, breast tenderness, bloating, and headaches and are typically associated with ovulatory cycles [65,66]. Primary dysmenorrhea should be treated with nonsteroidal anti-inflammatory drugs (NSAIDS) in appropriate doses and frequency as a first-line therapy, as they effectively decrease prostaglandin production and actions. Adolescents may be unaware of the differences between various over the counter analgesics containing acetaminophen or those that contain a mixture of drugs without proven benefit in relieving dysmenorrhea and those that contain the effective NSAIDS ibuprofen or naproxen. They also may not understand pharmacology of drugs—loading dose, half-life, duration of action, prophylactic treatment—that could result in more effective relief of primary dysmenorrhea. Although there is a paucity of high-quality evidence supporting the use of today's low-dose combination oral contraceptive drugs as therapy for primary dysmenorrhea, most clinicians base their practices on their clinical observations suggesting that these drugs are an excellent second-line therapy for dysmenorrhea that is ineffectively relieved by NSAIDS [67,68]. Adolescents with dysmenorrhea who do not respond to these treatments should be evaluated for secondary causes of dysmenorrhea. Other causes of secondary dysmenorrhea that may be common in older women, such as uterine leiomyomata, are very infrequent in college age women. Endometriosis is much more common among older women than among adolescents and young adults but is not rare. It should be suspected in adolescents with dysmenorrhea or noncyclic pelvic pain that is ineffectively relieved by NSAIDS and combination oral contraceptives. Referral for surgical confirmation of endometriosis should be considered in these patients.

Premenstrual syndrome

Premenstrual syndrome (PMS) has been defined as "the cyclic occurrence of symptoms that are of sufficient severity to interfere with some aspects of life and that appear with consistent and predictable relationship to the menses" [69]. The cause of PMS is not well understood, but circulating levels of progesterone, estrogen, and testosterone are normal. It has been suggested that there may be an underlying neurobiologic vulnerability to normal fluctuations of these hormones and that these fluctuations impact CNS neurotransmitters [70]. Among women of all ages, at least 85% report some premenstrual symptoms; however, only 5% to 10% report significant impairment of lifestyle as a result. Women over the age of 30 are most likely to seek treatment, although severe symptoms may occur at any age.

PMS encompasses both somatic and affective symptoms. Clinicians are frequently asked about management options which should be tailored to the specific symptoms involved. In addition, other conditions—both psychiatric and medical—should be considered and ruled out if appropriate. Depressive disorders are the most common condition that may be self-diagnosed as PMS, but individuals with depression report symptoms that are present virtually every day of the cycle. Major depression may be subject to menstrual magnification of the mood disorder. Depressive symptoms that occur only during the luteal phase may be given the diagnosis of premenstrual dysphoric disorder (PMDD). In addition, panic disorder and anxiety disorder should be considered as possible diagnoses. Common medical disorders that may involve menstrual magnification include migraine headaches and irritable bowel syndrome; thyroid disease should also be considered [70].

Oral contraceptives are helpful in alleviating the somatic symptoms of PMS including cramping and headaches, but are not as effective at treating the emotional symptoms. Selective serotonin reuptake inhibitors (SSRIs) such as sertraline, fluoxetine, and paroxetine (as an extended-release formulation), have been approved for the treatment of PMDD and are efficacious even when taken only during the luteal phase [71].

Preventive care

Annual visits for gynecologic care are recommended for adolescents of college age. The American College of Obstetricians and Gynecologists (ACOG) recommends that the first visit for gynecologic care should be around the ages of 13 to15; this visit should address preventive health guidance and assess risk-taking behaviors, including the risks of STDs and unplanned pregnancy [72]. Most young women currently in college will not have had the benefit of this preventive services visit and thus may present for an initial gynecologic visit or exam. Guidelines from the American Cancer Society suggest that the first cervical cytology (Pap smear) screening should be performed approximately 3 years after the initiation of vaginal sexual intercourse or by age 21 [73]. In addition, the US Centers for Disease Control STD Treatment Guidelines recommends screening for Chlamydia trachomatis at least annually in all asymptomatic sexually active adolescents and annual in individuals aged 20 to 25 [74]. Urine DNA-based testing makes such screening possible without a pelvic examination [75].

In spite of these very specific guidelines for preventive care and assessment, many college age women are not getting appropriate gynecologic health care screening. The ACS Guidelines for Pap screening are not widely known to the general public. Compliance with STD screening guidelines is well below practice guidelines [76,77]. Sixty percent of adolescents wait more than 1 year from the time of coitarche before seeking medical contraceptive advice [4].

Clearly, improvement is needed in providing appropriate screening and preventive reproductive health care to young women. Thus, college-age women who present to a clinician for menstrual-related concerns could and should receive preventive health care services as noted above. Quality of life for these women could be improved through appropriate evaluation and management of menstrual-related concerns, and future reproductive health could be preserved.

Summary

College-age young women frequently experience a variety of menstrual-related complaints, including dysmenorrheal, menorrhagia, irregular menses, and menstrual-related mood changes. These problems deserve careful evaluation; they may reflect normal ovulatory menstrual symptoms or be suggestive of significant pathology that can have a major impact on future reproductive and general health. The menstrual cycle is a vital sign whose normalcy suggests an overall good health and whose abnormality requires evaluation. Eating disorders and the female athlete triad increase the risk of osteoporosis; polycystic ovary syndrome is associated with future cardiovascular risks. Diagnosis and management of these problems will not only improve a young woman's current health, sense of well-being, and overall quality of life but may also lower her risks for future disease and ill-health.

References

[1] Ziv A, Boulet JR, Slap GB. Utilization of physician offices by adolescents in the United States. Pediatrics 1999;104(1 Pt 1):35–42.

[2] Singh S, Darroch JE. Trends in sexual activity among adolescent American women: 1982–1995. Fam Plann Perspect 1999;31(5):212–9.

[3] Henshaw SK. Unintended pregnancy in the United States. Fam Plann Perspect 1998;30(1): 24–9, 46.

[4] Guttmacher Institute. Sex and America's teenagers. New York and Washington: The Alan Guttmacher Institute; 1994.

[5] Herman-Giddens ME, Slora EJ, Wasserman RC, et al. Secondary sexual characteristics and menses in young girls seen in office practice: a study from the Pediatric Research in Office Settings network. Pediatrics 1997;99(4):505–12.

[6] Borsos A, Lampe L, Balogh A, et al. Ovarian function after the menarche and hormonal contraception. Int J Gynaecol Obstet 1988;27(2):249–53.

[7] World Health Organization. World Health Organization multicenter study on menstrual and ovulatory patterns in adolescent girls. II. Longitudinal study of menstrual patterns in the early postmenarcheal period, duration of bleeding episodes and menstrual cycles. World Health Organization Task Force on Adolescent Reproductive Health. J Adolesc Health Care 1986;7(4):236–44.

[8] Hallberg L, Hogdahl AM, Nilsson L, Rybo G. Menstrual blood loss—a population study. Variation at different ages and attempts to define normality. Acta Obstet Gynecol Scand 1966;45(3):320–51.

[9] Warner PE, Critchley HO, Lumsden MA, et al. Menorrhagia I: measured blood loss, clinical features, and outcome in women with heavy periods: a survey with follow-up data. Am J Obstet Gynecol 2004;190(5):1216–23.

[10] Warner PE, Critchley HO, Lumsden MA, et al. Menorrhagia II: is the 80-mL blood loss criterion useful in management of complaint of menorrhagia? Am J Obstet Gynecol 2004; 190(5):1224–9.

[11] Falcone T, Desjardins C, Bourque J, et al. Dysfunctional uterine bleeding in adolescents. J Reprod Med 1994;39(10):761–4.

[12] Claessens EA, Cowell CA. Acute adolescent menorrhagia. Am J Obstet Gynecol 1981; 139(3):277–80.

[13] Smith YR, Quint EH, Hertzberg RB. Menorrhagia in adolescents requiring hospitalization. J Pediatr Adolesc Gynecol 1998;11(1):13–5.

[14] Bevan JA, Maloney KW, Hillery CA, et al. Bleeding disorders: a common cause of menorrhagia in adolescents. J Pediatr 2001;138(6):856–61.

[15] Strickland JL, Wall JW. Abnormal uterine bleeding in adolescents. Obstet Gynecol Clin North Am 2003;30(2):321–35.

[16] Werner EJ. von Willebrand disease in children and adolescents. Pediatr Clin North Am 1996;43(3):683–707.

[17] Posan E, McBane RD, Grill DE, et al. Comparison of PFA-100 testing and bleeding time for detecting platelet hypofunction and von Willebrand disease in clinical practice. Thromb Haemost 2003;90(3):483–90.

[18] Mannucci PM. Treatment of von Willebrand's disease. N Engl J Med 2004;351(7):683–94.

[19] Camm JH, Murata SM. Emergency dental management of a patient with von Willebrand's disease. Endod Dent Traumatol 1992;8(4):176–81.

[20] ACOG Committee on Gynecologic Practice. von Willebrand disease in gynecologic practice. Washington, DC: American College of Obstetrics and Gynecology; 2001.

[21] ACOG Committee on Gynecologic Practice. Management of anovulary bleeding. Washington, DC: American College of Obstetrics and Gynecology; 2000.

[22] Nelson R, Bakalov V. Amenorrhea. eMedicine. Available at: www.emedicine.com/med/topic117.htm. Accessed June 17, 2004.

[23] Treloar AE, Boynton RE, Behn BG, Brown BW. Variation of the human menstrual cycle through reproductive life. Int J Fertil 1967;12(1 Pt 2):77–126.

[24] Knochenhauer ES, Key TJ, Kahsar-Miller M, et al. Prevalence of the polycystic ovary syndrome in unselected black and white women of the southeastern United States: a prospective study. J Clin Endocrinol Metab 1998;83(9):3078–82.

[25] Asuncion M, Calvo RM, San Millan JL, et al. A prospective study of the prevalence of the polycystic ovary syndrome in unselected Caucasian women from Spain. J Clin Endocrinol Metab 2000;85(7):2434–8.

[26] Diamanti-Kandarakis E, Kouli CR, Bergiele AT, et al. A survey of the polycystic ovary syndrome in the Greek island of Lesbos: hormonal and metabolic profile. J Clin Endocrinol Metab 1999;84(11):4006–11.

[27] Stein I, Leventhal M. Amenorrhea associated with bilateral polycystic ovaries. Am J Obstet Gynecol 1935;29:181–91.

[28] Rotterdam ESHRE/ASRM-Sponsored PCOS Consensus Workshop Group. Revised 2003 consensus on diagnostic criteria and long-term health risks related to polycystic ovary syndrome. Fertil Steril 2004;81(1):19–25.

[29] Dramusic V, Goh VH, Rajan U, et al. Clinical, endocrinologic, and ultrasonographic features of polycystic ovary syndrome in Singaporean adolescents. J Pediatr Adolesc Gynecol 1997;10(3):125–32.

[30] Guzick DS. Polycystic ovary syndrome. Obstet Gynecol 2004;103(1):181–93.

[31] Breitkopf DM, Rosen MP, Young SL, Nagamani M. Efficacy of second versus third generation oral contraceptives in the treatment of hirsutism. Contraception 2003;67(5):349–53.

[32] CDC. Sexually transmitted disease surveillance, 2002. Atlanta, GA: Centers for Disease Control and Prevention, US Department of Health and Human Services; 2003.

[33] American Academy of Pediatrics Committee on Adolescence. Sexually transmitted diseases. Pediatrics 1994;94(4 Pt 1):568–72.

[34] Banikarim C, Chacko M. Pelvic inflammatory disease in adolescents. Adolescent Med Clin 2004;15(2):273–85.

[35] Ness RB, Keder LM, Soper DE, et al. Oral contraception and the recognition of endometritis. Am J Obstet Gynecol 1997;176(3):580–5.

[36] Wolner-Hanssen P, Eschenbach DA, Paavonen J, et al. Decreased risk of symptomatic chlamydial pelvic inflammatory disease associated with oral contraceptive use. JAMA 1990;263(1):54–9.

[37] Chacko MR, Lovchik JC. Chlamydia trachomatis infection in sexually active adolescents: prevalence and risk factors. Pediatrics 1984;73(6):836–40.

[38] Huppert JS, Biro FM, Mehrabi J, Slap GB. Urinary tract infection and Chlamydia infection in adolescent females. J Pediatr Adolesc Gynecol 2003;16(3):133–7.

[39] Sweet RL, Draper DL, Hadley WK. Etiology of acute salpingitis: influence of episode number and duration of symptoms. Obstet Gynecol 1981;58(1):62–8.

[40] Spence MR, Adler J, McLellan R. Pelvic inflammatory disease in the adolescent. J Adolesc Health Care 1990;11(4):304–9.

[41] Hillis SD, Joesoef R, Marchbanks PA, et al. Delayed care of pelvic inflammatory disease as a risk factor for impaired fertility. Am J Obstet Gynecol 1993;168(5):1503–9.

[42] Ness RB, Soper DE, Holley RL, et al. Effectiveness of inpatient and outpatient treatment strategies for women with pelvic inflammatory disease: results from the Pelvic Inflammatory Disease Evaluation and Clinical Health (PEACH) Randomized Trial. Am J Obstet Gynecol 2002;186(5):929–37.

[43] Csermely T, Halvax L, Schmidt E, et al. Occurrence of osteopenia among adolescent girls with oligo/amenorrhea. Gynecol Endocrinol 2002;16(2):99–105.

[44] Bowe P, Murphy H. Complications of pregnancy following threatened abortion. Ir J Med Sci 1987;156(11):328–9.

[45] Farrell T, Owen P. The significance of extrachorionic membrane separation in threatened miscarriage. Br J Obstet Gynaecol 1996;103(9):926–8.

[46] Chung TK, Sahota DS, Lau TK, et al. Threatened abortion: prediction of viability based on signs and symptoms. Aust NZ J Obstet Gynaecol 1999;39(4):443–7.

[47] Uerpairojkit B, Charoenvidhya D, Tannirandorn Y, et al. Sonographic findings in clinically diagnosed threatened abortion. J Med Assoc Thai 2001;84(5):661–5.

[48] MMWR. Ectopic pregnancy–United States, 1990–1992. Morb Mortal Wkly Rep 1995;44(3): 46–8.

[49] Anderson FW, Hogan JG, Ansbacher R. Sudden death: ectopic pregnancy mortality. Obstet Gynecol 2004;103(6):1218–23.

[50] Kadar N, Caldwell BV, Romero R. A method of screening for ectopic pregnancy and its indications. Obstet Gynecol 1981;58(2):162–6.

[51] McCord ML, Muram D, Buster JE, et al. Single serum progesterone as a screen for ectopic pregnancy: exchanging specificity and sensitivity to obtain optimal test performance. Fertil Steril 1996;66(4):513–6.

[52] Liburd J. Eating disorder: anorexia. eMedicine. Available at: www.emedicine.com/ped/topic115.htm. Accessed June 17, 2004.

[53] American Psychiatric Association. Diagnostic and statistical manual of mental disorders: DSM-IV. 4th edition. Washington, DC: American Psychiatric Association; 1999.

[54] Selzer R, Caust J, Hibbert M, et al. The association between secondary amenorrhea and common eating disordered weight control practices in an adolescent population. J Adolesc Health 1996;19(1):56–61.

[55] Emans SJ. Eating disorders in adolescent girls. Pediatr Int 2000;42(1):1–7.

[56] Kreipe RE, Mou SM. Eating disorders in adolescents and young adults. Obstet Gynecol Clin North Am 2000;27(1):101–24.

[57] Munoz MT, Morande G, Garcia-Centenera JA, et al. The effects of estrogen administration on bone mineral density in adolescents with anorexia nervosa. Eur J Endocrinol 2002; 146(1):45–50.

[58] Golden NH, Lanzkowsky L, Schebendach J, et al. The effect of estrogen-progestin treatment on bone mineral density in anorexia nervosa. J Pediatr Adolesc Gynecol 2002;15(3): 135–43.

[59] Golden NH, Jacobson MS, Schebendach J, et al. Resumption of menses in anorexia nervosa. Arch Pediatr Adolesc Med 1997;151(1):16–21.

[60] Otis CL, Drinkwater B, Johnson M, et al. American College of Sports Medicine position stand. The Female Athlete Triad. Med Sci Sports Exerc 1997;29(5):i–ix.

[61] Nelson R, Bakalov V. Ovarian insufficiency eMedicine. Available at: www.emedicine.com/med/topic3374.htm. Accessed January 2, 2004.

[62] Bakalov V, Nelson L. Ovarian failure. Available at: www.emedicine.com/med/topic1700.htm. Accessed January 5, 2004.

[63] Blumenfeld Z. Ovarian rescue/protection from chemotherapeutic agents. J Soc Gynecol Investig 2001;8(1 Suppl Proceedings):S60–4.

[64] Abrahamson M, Snyder P. Causes of hyperprolactinemia. Up to Date Online. Available at: www.htdol.com/application/topic.asp?file=pituitar2850. Accessed March 24, 2004.

[65] Magyar DM, Boyers SP, Marshall JR, Abraham GE. Regular menstrual cycles and premenstrual molimina as indicators of ovulation. Obstet Gynecol 1979;53(4):411–4.

[66] Bates GW, Garza DE, Garza MM. Clinical manifestations of hormonal changes in the menstrual cycle. Obstet Gynecol Clin North Am 1990;17(2):299–310.

[67] Davis AR, Westhoff CL. Primary dysmenorrhea in adolescent girls and treatment with oral contraceptives. J Pediatr Adolesc Gynecol 2001;14(1):3–8.

[68] Proctor ML, Roberts H, Farquhar CM. Combined oral contraceptive pill (OCP) as treatment for primary dysmenorrhoea. [Systemic Review] Cochrane Menstrual Disorders and Subfertility Group, Cochrane Database of Systemic Reviews 2004;3.

[69] Gise L, Kase N, Berkowitz R, editors. Contemporary issues in obstetrics and gynecology, Vol. 2. The premenstrual syndromes. New York: Churchill Livingstone; 1988. p. 157.

[70] ACOG Committee on Gynecologic Practice. Premenstrual syndrome. Washington, DC: American College of Obstetrics and Gynecology; 2000.

[71] Freeman EW. Luteal phase administration of agents for the treatment of premenstrual dysphoric disorder. CNS Drugs 2004;18(7):453–68.

[72] ACOG. Guidelines for women's health care. Washington DC: American College of Obstetrics and Gynecology; 1996.

[73] Saslow D, Runowicz CD, Solomon D, et al. American Cancer Society guideline for the early detection of cervical neoplasia and cancer. CA Cancer J Clin 2002;52(6):342–62.

[74] CDC. Sexually transmitted diseases treatment guidelines 2002. Centers for Disease Control and Prevention. MMWR Recomm Rep 2002;51(RR-6):1–78.

[75] Kohl KS, Markowitz LE, Koumans EH. Developments in the screening for Chlamydia trachomatis: a review. Obstet Gynecol Clin North Am 2003;30(4):637–58.

[76] St. Lawrence JS, Montano DE, Kasprzyk D, et al. STD screening, testing, case reporting, and clinical and partner notification practices: a national survey of US physicians. Am J Public Health 2002;92(11):1784–8.

[77] Huppert JS, Adams Hillard PJ. Sexually transmitted disease screening in teens. Curr Womens Health Rep 2003;3(6):451–8.

ELSEVIER
SAUNDERS

Pediatr Clin N Am 52 (2005) 199–216

PEDIATRIC CLINICS

OF NORTH AMERICA

Genitourinary Issues in the Male College Student: A Case-Based Approach

William P. Adelman, MD[a], Alain Joffe, MD, MPH[b],*

[a]Department of Pediatrics and Adolescent Medicine, National Naval Medical Center,
Uniformed Services University of the Health Sciences, 8901 Wisconsin Avenue, Bethesda,
MD 20889, USA
[b]Student Health and Wellness Center, Johns Hopkins School of Medicine,
3400 North Charles Street, Baltimore, MD 21218, USA

There are few issues of greater concern to a male college student than those related to the health of his genitourinary system. In the United States, one sample of nearly 59,000 patient care interactions revealed that 5% of all ambulatory visits by men 18 years or older include genitourinary symptoms as a reason for the visit [1]. In this article, using typical, unusual, or otherwise instructive cases, the authors review a select group of genitourinary issues in the college male: warts (human papilloma virus), testicular cancer, varicoceles, urethritis, prostatitis, and sexual dysfunction. With understanding of these medical conditions, the practitioner should feel comfortable addressing the most challenging genitourinary health needs of this population.

Human papillomavirus (warts)

Case

A 20-year-old male is referred from the emergency department for evaluation and treatment of genital warts. He initially presented with severe crampy abdominal pain and bloody diarrhea and was treated for acute infectious diarrhea.

The views expressed in this article are those of the authors and do not reflect the official policy or position of the US Army, US Navy, US Department of Defense, or the US government.

* Corresponding author.
E-mail address: ajoffe@jhu.edu (A. Joffe).

He has noticed a few perianal bumps over the last 6 months and occasional blood on the toilet paper. He admits to multiple female sexual partners but denies anal receptive intercourse or sexual activity with men. He reports losing 22 pounds over the last 6 months in conjunction with increased physical activity, and has noted an increase in daily loose stools. Physical examination reveals a thin male in no distress. Genitourinary examination is noteworthy for fleshy, pedunculated growths in the gluteal fold extending along the midline from the dorsal side of the anus to the base of the scrotum. The growths are friable and moist. Rectal examination is noteworthy for slightly diminished tone with 1 cm lesions palpable in the rectal vault at 11 o'clock and 7 o'clock. His hemoglobin is 11gm/dL, and his erythrocyte sedimentation rate is 45 mm per hour. A colonoscopy with biopsy confirms the diagnosis of Crohn's disease with perianal cutaneous manifestations.

More than 5 million cases of HPV infection are estimated to occur in the United States annually, and anogenital HPV is the most common sexually transmitted infection [2,3]. It is therefore appropriate to consider HPV in the presence of perianal lesions in a sexually active male. Although HPV accounts for the greatest number of perianal cutaneous lesions in young adults, the case cited illustrates that understanding the breadth of the differential diagnosis of perianal lesions in college males is critical. Perhaps because HPV is so common an entity, other cutaneous diseases with similar presentation commonly are misdiagnosed as HPV [4,5]. HPV infects epithelial tissues and mucous membranes. Clinical manifestations of infection typically present as warts. More than 100 types of the DNA virus of the *Papillomaviridae* family have been identified. Because of known associations with cervical cancer, anogenital types have been dichotomized as low-risk types (eg, types 6 and 11) when they are associated with anogenital warts and mild dysplasias, and high-risk types (eg, types 16, 18, 31, 33, 35, and 45) when they are associated with anogenital cancers and high-grade dysplasias.

Anogenital warts most commonly are associated with HPV types 6 and 11 [6,7]. In both men and women, most anogenital HPV infections are asymptomatic. In men, the most common clinically apparent manifestation of genital HPV infection is anogenital warts, with squamous intraepithelial lesion (SIL) and carcinoma in situ on the anus, penis, or scrotum occurring less commonly, and penile, scrotal, or anal cancers occurring rarely [8].

Anogenital warts are flesh, brown, or gray colored; vary in size; and present as four distinct morphologic types: condylomata acuminatum, flat, papular, and keratotic. Condylomata acuminata have a characteristic cauliflower appearance and develop on moist, partially keratinized epithelium. They commonly present as single or multiple papules on the penis, perineum, or anal region. The penile shaft is the most common site for lesions in circumcised men, while the glans penis, coronal sulcus, frenulum, and inner aspect of the foreskin (preputial cavity) are infected most frequently in uncircumcised men [9]. Flat-topped warts appear macular or raised and are found on partially or fully keratinized epithelium. Papular warts are small, domed, flesh-colored lesions, and like keratotic warts, which are thick and crusty, they usually occur on fully keratinized epithelium

[10]. Most anogenital warts are asymptomatic, but complaints of itching, burning, friability, and tenderness are not uncommon [11,12].

The incubation period of HPV is unknown, but it is estimated to range from 3 months to several years [13]. Diagnosis of HPV infection usually can be made by direct visual inspection; the urinary meatus and fossa navicularis should not be overlooked if warts are suspected in the college-aged male, as in a patient who complains of bleeding from the meatus. Internal lesions often accompany external lesions, so some authors suggest anoscopy when perianal or perineal warts exist or if the patient has a history of receptive anal intercourse [14].

Histologic confirmation by means of biopsy occasionally may be necessary in cases of atypical appearance such as in bowenoid papulosis (pigmented red-brown verrucous papules that histologically demonstrate condylomatous architecture with squamous cell carcinoma in situ). Additionally, biopsy may be necessary if the diagnosis is uncertain; if neoplasia is suspected because of ulceration, induration, fixed nature of lesion or unusual pigment; in an immunocompromised host; or in those cases unresponsive to therapy. Although the use of dilute solutions of acetic acid (3% to 5%) occasionally may assist with identification of lesions, routine use is not indicated, because this technique has a low specificity and positive predictive value [15]. Because of the greater risk of malignant transformation among men who have sex with men (MSM), cytologic screening for anal HPV infection by means of Papanicolaou (Pap) smear has been recommended for homosexual men irrespective of HIV status [16].

The differential diagnosis for HPV anogenital lesions includes multiple wart types, the benign condition of pearly penile papules, molluscum contagiosum, skin tags, local infection, seborrhea, psoriasis, lichen planus, secondary syphilis (condyloma lata), perianal Crohn's disease, neurofibromatosis, Bowen disease, Reiter syndrome with associated skin changes (balanitis circinata), and neoplasm.

The main goal of treatment is to remove symptomatic or unsightly (to the patient) warts. Whether treatment alters the natural history of HPV is unclear. Patient-applied regimens include podofilox 0.5% solution or gel or imiquimod 5% cream. Provider-administered therapies include cryotherapy, podophyllin resin 10% to 25%, trichloroacetic acid (tca), bichloroacetic acid (bca) 80% to 90%, or surgical removal. Alternative regimens may include intralesional interferon or laser surgery. Management of sex partners is not necessary for management of genital warts, as no data indicate that reinfection plays a role in recurrences. It is reasonable, however, to refer sex partners for visual inspection for evaluation of possible symptomatic warts and for routine Pap smear screening.

Multiple studies have shown that the strongest risk factors for male HPV infection are number of lifetime partners and young age (18 to 35 years)[17–20]. HPV infection can result from nonpenetrating sexual activity [21], so the only certain way to prevent HPV infection is avoidance of genital contact. Therefore, promotion of abstinence, delayed sexual activity, and monogamy with an uninfected partner are viable primary preventive strategies for college-aged men.

There is surprisingly little evidence that condom use decreases risk for HPV infection [22]. Condoms have the obvious mechanical limitation of not covering the perineum or scrotum, where HPV is commonly found. Multiple lines of indirect evidence, however, appear to suggest that condom use may offer some protection against HPV. One meta-analysis summarizing individuals with consistent condom use show decreased risk for cervical cancer, cervical intraepithelial neoplasia, and anogenital warts [23]. Case-control studies have shown that males who always use condoms have less likelihood of having genital warts compared with those who occasionally or never use condoms [18,24].

Circumcision appears to play a protective role against HPV, although the role it might play in other than primary prevention is unknown. Circumcised men are less likely to have detectable penile HPV DNA than uncircumcised men, and warts are more common in uncircumcised men [17,25]. In addition, neonatal circumcision reduces the risk for penile cancer by at least 10-fold [26].

Testicular cancer

Case

A 19-year-old college sophomore presents with a complaint of a painful left testicle. He noted gradually worsening testicular pain over the past 2 to 3 days. His last sexual encounter was 8 weeks before the visit. He denies dysuria, penile discharge, back or flank pain, fever, chills or sweats, recent trauma, or any history of testicular problems. On physical examination, he has no gynecomastia, and his lung and heart exams are normal. He is Tanner stage 5 and circumcised. He has no skin lesions or appreciable lymphadenopathy. Examination of the right scrotal contents is completely normal. His left epididymis is palpable and nontender. The left spermatic cord is without visual or palpable varicosity. His left testicle is palpable and normal in size, lie, and shape, but is markedly tender to palpation at the inferior pole. Pain does not decrease with elevation of the testis. Ultrasound reveals a testicular tumor at the lower pole with bleeding into the tumor.

Perhaps the most serious disease to confront college health care providers is testicular cancer. It is projected that in 2004, 8980 new cases will be diagnosed, and 360 men will die of the disease in the United States [27]. Testicular cancer is predominantly of germ cell origin (95%), is the most common cancer of young men between the ages of 15 and 34 years, accounts for 3% of all cancer deaths in this age group, and uniquely affects young adults [28]. Forty per cent of germ cell tumors are seminoma, making it the most common testicular cancer of single cell type, but the incidence of seminoma peaks in the 25- to 45-year-old age group, while nonseminoma tumors (embryonal cell, choriocarcinoma, teratoma, yolk sac, and mixed forms) peak in the 15-30 year old group. Bilateral tumors occur in 2% to 4% of patients [29].

Testicular cancer is 4.5 times more common among white men than African-American men, with intermediate incidence rates for Hispanic, Native American, and Asian males. Males with cryptorchidism have 3 to 40 times the average risk of testicular cancer, and 12% of men with testicular cancer have a history of cryptorchidism. One percent to 5% of boys with a history of undescended testicle later develop germ cell tumors. There is also an increased risk for testicular cancer in males with gonadal dysgenesis and Klinefelter's syndrome. Men with a family history of testicular cancer may be at a higher risk of this disease. A history of testicular cancer is associated with a higher risk of a future contralateral tumor [30].

Testis tumor most commonly presents as a circumscribed, nontender area of induration within the testis that does not transilluminate. Most cases are felt to be asymptomatic and discovered by the patient. Many individuals with testicular anomalies will not seek care until prompted by other bothersome symptoms. Often there is a history of recent trauma, which draws attention to pre-existing pathology in the scrotum. It is not unusual for a patient to present with a painless mass in the traumatized testicle. Although symptoms may be lacking, signs of testicular pathology are often present (for example, swelling is noted by the provider in up to 73% of cases), so identifying and being familiar with normal and abnormal genital exams are crucial [31]. Patients may present with a sensation of fullness or heaviness of the scrotum. As in the case described, testicular pain is the presenting symptom in 18% to 46% of patients with germ cell tumors.

Acute pain may be associated with torsion of the neoplasm, infarction, or bleeding into the tumor. Signs and symptoms indistinguishable from acute epididymitis have been observed in up to 25% of patients with testicular neoplasms. Less common presentations may include gynecomastia secondary to human chorionic gonadotropin (HCG)-secreting tumors, or back or flank pain from metastatic disease.

In most cases of testicular tumor, the epididymis and cord feel normal. With more advanced tumors, the testis may be enlarged diffusely and rock hard. Secondary hydroceles may occur such that new onset of a hydrocele warrants careful evaluation for testicular cancer. If the testis cannot be palpated adequately, because of tenderness, hydrocele, or limitation in examination skills, ultrasonography is indicated to allow visualization of the testis sufficient to rule out a tumor. The presentation of seminoma may be unique in that the testis may be enlarged uniformly to 10 times its normal size without loss of normal shape [32]. Therefore, size comparison with the contralateral testis is important, or a seminoma may be missed on casual examination. Of particular note in sexually active adolescents, a swollen, tender testicle with fever and pyuria, thereby mimicking epididymitis, may characterize advanced testicular cancer. Also, epididymitis and testicular cancer can coexist. Significant delays in treatment have been observed in patients treated for presumed epididymitis. Thus, following an appropriate course of antibiotics for epididymitis, the patient should be re-examined to ensure that no residual mass is palpable. If the diagnosis is not clear-cut, ultrasonography is indicated.

The differential diagnosis includes: testicular torsion, hydrocele, varicocele, spermatocele, epididymitis, or other malignancies such as lymphoma. Rarely, genital tuberculosis, sarcoid, mumps, or inflammatory disease also can mimic cancer. Because 25% of patients with seminoma and 60% to 70% of those with a nonseminomatous germ cell tumor have metastatic disease at the time of presentation, any of the following symptoms should prompt examination of the testis: back or abdominal pain, unexplained weight loss, dyspnea (pulmonary metastases), gynecomastia, supraclavicular adenopathy, urinary obstruction, or a heavy or dragging sensation in the groin.

Ultrasonography can discriminate between a testicular neoplasm and the nonmalignant processes included in the differential diagnosis [33]. Even if an obvious mass is palpated on physical examination, an ultrasound should be performed on both testicles to rule out bilateral disease (2% to 4%). Once a tumor is suspected, tumor serum markers such as lactate dehydrogenase, beta HCG (elevated in choriocarcinoma and seminoma), and alpha fetoprotein (produced by yolk sac cells) are indicated. Further evaluation for staging, including additional laboratory studies, a computed tomography (CT) scan of the chest, abdomen, and pelvis, and other imaging as needed (eg, imaging of the brain in the case of a pure choriocarcinoma), should be performed in consultation with an oncologist. Treatment regimens vary by grade and stage of tumor. All patients undergo radical orchiectomy, followed by close surveillance for certain early stage tumors, or chemotherapy and radiation, with a usually positive prognosis. Overall, there is a 92% 5-year survival rate, and even among those with advanced disease at diagnosis, 5-year survival is almost 70% [34].

Because advances in treatment have afforded an overall excellent prognosis to those affected, it is unknown what impact screening and prevention measures may have on mortality. Testicular self-examination (TSE) is simple to teach, simple to perform, has negligible cost, and is more likely to be practiced if taught by a practitioner [35,36]. Therefore, many national organizations (the American Academy of Pediatrics, the American Medical Association, the American Urological Association, and the American Cancer Society) recommend teaching TSE or performing annual professional testicular examination for adolescent and young adult males.

It is unknown, however, whether screening by either a physician or by patients themselves actually affects the stage of cancer at detection, impacts morbidity, or reduces mortality. Therefore, organizations that rely on large controlled trials for evidence- based recommendations, like the US Preventive Services Task Force (USPSTF) and the Canadian Task Force on the Periodic Health Examination (CTFPHE), make no recommendations for or against routine screening of asymptomatic males for testicular cancer. The American Academy of Family Practice takes a selective approach, recommending clinical testicular examination for men aged 13 to 39 years who have the known risk factors of cryptorchidism, orchiopexy, or testicular atrophy.

Varicocele

Case

A 19-year-old scholarship football player presents with a chief complaint of a dull ache in his scrotum after prolonged standing on the sideline. This seems to get worse after long periods of being upright or vigorous exercise, and is usually relieved after lying down. He has noted a fullness above his left testicle but not his right one. He denies any difficulty with erections or ejaculation, and otherwise has no complaints. Physical examination reveals dilated veins above the left testicle evident on inspection. Both testes are palpable and are normal in size, lie, and shape. No testicular mass is noted. The patient's left testis is approximately 16 cc in volume, while the right testis appears to be 20 cc in volume. Semen analysis is normal. Following counseling, the patient opts to undergo unilateral varicocelectomy after the football season with satisfactory resolution of his symptoms.

Varicocele, or dilated scrotal veins, is the most common scrotal mass among teenagers and young adults. Varicoceles represent elongated, dilated, tortuous veins of the pampiniform plexus within the spermatic cord, secondary to incompetence and dilatation of the internal and external spermatic veins. Varicoceles are rare in preadolescents; multiple large studies show that the prevalence of varicocele in adolescents and adults is approximately 15% [37–40]. Varicoceles deserve careful evaluation and selective treatment during adolescence and young adulthood because of a possible link to infertility [41].

Unlike the case vignette, most varicoceles are asymptomatic and discovered incidentally on routine physical examination. Varicocele can be associated with a time-dependent decline in testicular function [42–44]. Prophylactic varicocelectomy may prevent future infertility [45,46], but only 15% to 20% of men with a varicocele seek treatment for infertility, suggesting most males with a varicocele are fertile or do not desire treatment [47]. Therefore, surgical correction of all varicoceles is not indicated. Among males 18 years of age or older, semen analysis is a simple and inexpensive test of fertility; in adolescent boys, this technique is less practical, and normal parameters are less clearly defined. For these younger males, impaired growth of the ipsilateral testis (hypotrophy) or an abnormality in the integrity of the hypothalamic-pituitary-testicular axis (as measured by luteinizing hormone [LH] and follicle-stimulating hormone [FSH]) suggests testicular damage. The absolute utility of these surrogate markers is a continuing area of research, and controversy remains regarding which adolescents to refer for varicocele surgery [48].

Anatomical reasons may explain why varicocele also is noted often on the left side, but they fail to explain why varicoceles are associated with infertility [49]. Certainly if a varicocele only had a pathophysiologic effect unilaterally, it would not be expected to be such a common cause of infertility in adults, as males with a single functioning testis are usually fertile. The presumption guiding research has been that although usually apparent only unilaterally, varicocele somehow transmits testicular damage bilaterally, perhaps by increased testicular temperature, increased thickness of the testicular lamina propria, impaired transformation of myofibroblasts to fibroblasts, or elevated nitric oxide levels in spermatic venous blood [50–52]. Recent reports, however, suggest that the incidence of bilateral varicocele may be underestimated [53,54]; one recent study provides support to the probability that varicocele is a bilateral disease [55].

Twenty-eight adolescents with varicocele underwent evaluation including contact scrotal thermography and bilateral venography. Using a reference gold standard of percutaneous retrograde venography, the authors found bilateral varicoceles in 85.7% of participants, even though physical exam suggested bilateral disease in only 10%.

Abnormal semen analysis is the most definitive indicator of testicular damage in adults. For males younger than 18 years of age, measurement of unstimulated LH and FSH and loss of testicular volume or failure of the testis to grow are used as surrogate markers for testicular damage [56]. In a recent study of fully mature (Tanner V) adolescents, testicular volumes were not predictive for testicular dysfunction, but LH and FSH levels with or without gonadotropin-releasing hormone (GnRH) stimulation were predictive of abnormal semen analysis [57]. This study supports prior work showing the utility of hormonal testing in predicting those who may benefit from varicocele repair, and casts doubt on the utility of testicular volume measurement as a marker of testicular dysfunction [58,59]. It is common practice to refer to urology adolescents with symptomatic, bilateral, or clinically evident varicoceles, and those with varicocele associated with one testis. Little evidence, however, exists to support or refute these practices.

Several surgical options are available for treatment of adolescent varicocele: traditional Ivanissevich inguinal and high inguinal Palomo procedures (which may spare the testicular artery), subinguinal microsurgical techniques, and laparascopic and sclerotherapy procedures. Among those with normal semen parameters who complain of intermittent dull discomfort, a conservative approach with use of an athletic supporter and intermittent monitoring is a reasonable alternative to surgery.

Urethritis

Case

A 21-year-old college senior presents with a complaint of dysuria and penile discharge. He had unprotected intercourse with a female classmate 3 days earlier. He awoke this morning with severe pain on urination. Physical examination is noteworthy for a purulent discharge from the meatus. There is no testicular or epididymal tenderness or abnormality. First-void urine shows numerous white blood cells, and a gram stain of the discharge demonstrates white blood cells and gram-negative intracellular diplococci. He is treated for gonococcal (and presumed chlamydial) urethritis and refers his sexual partners for treatment.

Urethritis is an infection of the urethra characterized by discharge of mucopurulent, purulent, or watery material, and it may be accompanied by dysuria or urethral pruritus. Most cases, however, are asymptomatic [60,61], or symptoms may be so transient or mild, they are overlooked [62,63]. In addition, spontaneous resolution of symptoms frequently occurs [64,65].

Urethritis in men traditionally is classified as gonococcal or nongonococcal. *Chlamydia trachomatis* is the most commonly identified cause of nongonococcal urethritis (NGU), accounting for 15% to 55% of cases [65–67]. The prevalence of *C. trachomatis* NGU is believed to be decreasing in the United States [68]. *Ureaplasma urealyticum*, *Mycoplasma genitalium*, and less commonly, *Trichomonas vaginalis*, have been implicated as additional causes of NGU [69–71].

Testing to determine the etiology of urethritis as gonococcal or chlamydial is recommended to identify and report infection to the state health department. Specific diagnostic tests for *U. urealyticum* and *M. genitalium* are not indicated, because they are difficult to detect, and knowledge of their presence does not alter therapy. Urethritis can be diagnosed if any of the following signs are present:

- Mucopurulent or purulent discharge
- Gram stain of urethral secretions demonstrating five or more white blood cells per oil immersion field
- Positive leukocyte esterase test on first-void urine
- Microscopic examination of first-void urine demonstrating 10 or more white blood cells per high power field

In the absence of any of these criteria, treatment should be deferred until the results of *C. trachomatis* and *Neisseria gonorrhoeae* tests are known, except among individuals at high risk for infection who are unlikely to return for follow-up. For these cases, empiric treatment is warranted. If definitive diagnosis is not immediately available (eg, unable to perform a gram stain to confirm gonorrhea, or results of nucleic acid amplification tests are not timely), but urethritis is present, empiric treatment for both infections is warranted.

For nongonococcal urethritis, the Centers for Disease Control and Prevention (CDC) recommend azithromycin 1 g orally in a single dose or doxycycline 100 mg orally twice a day for 7 days. For uncomplicated gonococcal urethritis, recommended regimens include cefixime 400 mg in a single dose, ceftriaxone 125 mg intramuscularly in a single dose, ciprofloxacin 500 mg in a single dose, ofloxacin 400 mg orally in a single dose, or levofloxacin 250 mg orally in a single dose. Treatment for chlamydia also is warranted if chlamydial infection has not been ruled out. Quinolones should not be used for infections acquired in Asia, the Pacific (including Hawaii), California, or in other areas with increased prevalence of quinolone resistance. Among MSM, quinolone therapy also is not recommended. The CDC recommends ceftriaxone 125 mg intramuscularly as first-line therapy for gonorrhea for MSM throughout the United States and for those whose infection was acquired in Asia, the Pacific Islands, Hawaii, California, or other high-prevalence areas [72].

Patients must avoid sexual activity for a minimum of 7 days after therapy is initiated and until they and their partners are treated, and all symptoms have resolved. Patients should return for re-evaluation only if symptoms persist or recur, and they should refer all sex partners of the past 60 days for treatment. Those with recurrent or persistent symptoms should be retreated with the initial regimen if they were noncompliant with therapy or were exposed to an un-treated sex partner. Otherwise an intraurethral swab for culture should be sent, and a first void urine specimen should be evaluated for *T. vaginalis*. If the patient was compliant with the initial regimen, and new exposure can be excluded, the CDC recommends treating with metronidazole 2 g orally in a single dose plus erythromycin base 500 mg orally four times a day for 7 days or erythromycin ethylsuccinate 800 mg orally four times a day for 7 days.

Prostatitis

Case

A 19-year-old male presents severely distraught with a complaint of bloody and painful ejaculate. He states that he has been feeling poorly for the past 5 days with intermittent fever, chills, and persistent malaise. He noted mild dysuria and hesitation one day before presentation, with cloudy urine, and he has had dull perineal and back discomfort that has not dissipated. Physical examination is significant for a temperature of 101° F and a normal genital examination; gentle rectal examination reveals an enlarged and tender prostate. He is treated presumptively for acute prostatitis and recovers without incident.

Prostatitis is an unusual condition in the adolescent and young adult. Acute prostatitis in the college-aged male is likely associated with an infectious process that creates an inflammatory condition in the prostate gland. Organisms may reach the prostate by means of reflux of infected urine, or by lymphogenous or hematogenic spread. Risk factors for acute prostatitis may include trauma (eg, bicycle or horseback riding), dehydration, and sexual abstinence, but well-controlled studies are lacking. Prostatitis also can occur in patients with chronic indwelling bladder catheters and even in those who perform intermittent catheterization [73]. Although often assumed to be a sexually transmitted infection, only minimal evidence links its etiology to *C. trachomatis* or *N. gonorrhoeae;* it is more likely caused by *U. urealyticum*, coliform bacteria such as *Escherichia coli, Staphylococcus saprophyticus, T. vaginalis*, and *M. hominis* [74,75].

Characteristic signs of acute bacterial prostatitis may include pain in the groin, penis, scrotum, suprapubic area, perineum, or back. Pain exacerbated by ejaculation is consistent with this condition. Bladder symptoms such as hesitation, dribbling, increased frequency, dysuria, or even anuria may point to prostate inflammation, as may hematuria, cloudy urine, or hematospermia. Acute prostatitis often causes systemic symptoms such as fever, chills, and malaise. Although the clinical features of prostate infection can mimic urinary tract infection (UTI), isolated acute cystitis does not occur commonly in adult men, in whom virtually all lower UTIs are caused by prostatitis or urinary instrumentation [76,77].

Patients with bacterial prostatitis may be acutely ill and need hospitalization for parenteral antibiotic therapy. In these cases, broad antibiotic coverage should be administered empirically pending the culture results.

Optimal testing for acute bacterial prostatitis is laborious and invasive and is performed using the segmental culture technique. This involves collection of four specimens: a first-void 10 mL sample, a midstream urine, prostatic secretions during prostatic massage, and a first-void 10 mL urine after prostatic massage. To confirm bacterial prostatitis, the third and fourth samples will grow more colonies of bacteria than the first two. If the first specimen contains the most leukocytes, this suggests urethritis, and if the second specimen contains the most growth then cystitis is most likely. Because this test is time consuming, expensive, and invasive, it is not recommended as a routine diagnostic test.

A typical clinical history combined with the finding of an edematous and tender prostate on physical examination should lead to a presumptive diagnosis of acute prostatitis. Empiric treatment is often successful, as the antibiotic penetration of the acutely inflamed prostate gland is excellent [78]. A urine culture should be obtained in all men suspected of having acute prostatitis. Gram stain of the urine, if positive, can be used as a guide to initial therapy. Confirmatory laboratory findings include pyuria, positive urine and occasionally blood cultures, and leukocytosis.

Multiple outpatient antibiotic choices for acute prostatitis exist and can be chosen according to urine gram stain results if available. For example, gram-positive cocci in chains usually indicate enterococcal infection, which can be treated with ampicillin at a dose of 500 mg every 6 hours or amoxicillin 500 mg every 8 hours for 7 days. In contrast, patients with gram-negative rods should be treated with trimethoprim-sulfamethoxazole 160/800 mg (double strength) every 12 hours or a fluoroquinolone such as ofloxacin 300 mg every 12 hours or levofloxacin 400 mg daily by mouth.

In the case of recalcitrant or chronic symptoms, specific diagnostic samples are helpful, although the etiology for these conditions in the young adult are not well understood.

Sexual dysfunction

Case

A 20-year-old male presents with a complaint of difficulty with erections and sexual performance with his girlfriend since the time of their first encounter 4 months ago, which he described as "awkward and ended sooner than I wanted it to." He has had two prior sexual relationships without difficulty. He notes erections upon awakening and he is able to obtain an erection when alone. When with his current partner, he is able to achieve erection 90 percent of the time, but loses his erection, without ejaculation, upon penetration. Past medical history is significant for a prior diagnosis of anxiety disorder for which he was briefly placed on a selective serotonin reuptake inhibitor (SSRI). He is currently on no medications and denies tobacco or illicit drug use. He drinks alcohol at parties on the weekend, with an average of 10 drinks per week. Physical examination is normal. He is referred for psychological counseling, with eventual improvement in sexual function.

Sexual dysfunction causes great distress in the young adult, and in this age group, it is usually psychological in nature or related to medication or substance use. Understanding the four elements necessary for sexual competency can summarize a clinically useful approach to assessment of male sexual dysfunction. First of all, he must have desire for his sexual partner (libido). Secondly, he must achieve penile tumescence and rigidity (erection) adequate for penetration, through diversion of blood from the iliac artery into the corpora cavernosae. Thirdly, he must discharge sperm, prostatic and seminal vesicle fluid through the urethra (ejaculation). Finally, he should experience a sense of pleasure (orgasm) [79]. Failure in any of these areas may be the presenting concern in young men. Impotence is defined as the inability to develop or sustain erection 75 percent of the time. It may caused by psychological causes, medications, hormonal abnormalities, neurologic, or vascular problems.

Decreased libido is found in depression, androgen deficiency, alcoholism, recreational drug use, and as an adverse effect from prescription medications [80]. Erectile dysfunction may reflect either inadequate arterial blood flow into (failure to fill) or accelerated venous drainage out of (failure to store) the corpora cavernosae and may represent vascular deficiency as is seen in diabetes or as a result of aging. Testosterone deficiency also may be implicated in erectile dysfunction, as testosterone is necessary to maintain intrapenile nitric oxide synthase levels [81]. Disorders of ejaculation occur if the bladder neck sphincter is damaged, such as during prostate surgery, or if alpha adrenergic impulses responsible for clamping down the bladder neck sphincter to facilitate antegrade ejaculation fail, resulting in retrograde ejaculation. Failure to reach orgasm in men with adequate erectile function is also a common adverse effect of antidepressant medication or secondary to internal psychological conflict.

A sexual history is important and often can point the provider in the direction of the likely cause of dysfunction in the young adult. Prominent impotence risk factors that should be addressed include a history of cigarette smoking [82], diabetes mellitus, hypertension, heavy alcohol use, drug abuse, and depression. Increasing evidence also implicates cycling as a potential risk factor [83].

Radical prostatectomy and genital tract trauma cause a sudden loss of male sexual function [84]. Absent history of such trauma, a patient who presents with acute onset of sexual dysfunction (ie, normal function, then sudden lack of performance) invariably is suffering from psychogenic impotence. This problem may be caused by performance anxiety, discomfort with the current sexual partner, or some other emotional problem. In this setting, psychological counseling is the appropriate therapy.

In men presenting with a complaint of inability to develop erections, the presence or absence of spontaneous erections is an important clue to diagnosis. A history of morning or rapid eye movement sleep erections confirms the integrity of the neurovascular complex responsible for corpora cavernosa blood flow. In contrast, complete loss of nocturnal erections is present in men with neurologic or vascular disease. If a history of nocturnal or early morning erections cannot be elicited from the patient or his partner, nocturnal penile tumescence testing may be performed.

Nonsustained erection with detumescence after penetration, as was present in this case, is most commonly caused by anxiety or the vascular steal syndrome. With anxiety, conscious or subconscious concern about maintaining an erection activates an adrenergic hormone release, which is contrary to maintaining erectile turgor and rigidity. In the case cited, the patient's perceived poor performance during his first encounter is a likely cause of his anxiety. Sensate focus exercises are effective in restoring erectile confidence and competence in this setting. In the vascular steal syndrome, an uncommon finding in young adults, blood is diverted from the engorged corpora cavernosae to accommodate the oxygen requirements of the thrusting pelvis. Vascular surgery is necessary to correct this problem [85].

A thorough medication history is necessary in the evaluation of sexual dysfunction, as multiple medications may cause sexual adverse effects [86]. A partial list includes:

- Spironolactone, which inhibits testosterone
- Medications like clonidine or methyldopa that are sympathetic blockers
- Thiazide diuretics, which have twice the sexual dysfunction rate compared with placebo according to the treatment of mild hypertension study [87]
- Multiple antidepressants including SSRIs
- Ketoconazole
- Cimetidine
- Drugs of abuse such as alcohol, heroin, and cocaine [88]

Following a complete history, physical examination with specific attention to clues suggesting possible organic causes of dysfunction is important. Femoral and peripheral pulses should be evaluated, as abnormal pulses may suggest a vascular cause for impotence. The presence of a femoral bruit may be a clue to pelvic blood occlusion. A visual field examination should be performed to rule out defects that may be present in hypogonadal men with pituitary tumors. The presence of gynecomastia is a physical sign that suggests Klinefelter's syndrome; it also may be present with illicit drug use or testicular tumor. A thorough genital exam should search for penile strictures indicative of Peyronie's disease. The testicles should be examined looking for atrophy, asymmetry, or masses that may be a clue to testosterone abnormalities. Finally, a normal cremasteric reflex, elicited by stroking the inner thigh and observing for elevation of the ipsilateral testicle, assures integrity of the thoracolumbar erection center at T-11 to L-2. The thoracolumbar erection center serves as a spinal cord way station that transfers psychogenic impressions to the pelvic vascular bed, directing blood into the corpora cavernosae and leading to an erection [89].

If the history or physical suggests a possible organic cause for dysfunction, appropriate laboratory testing includes evaluation of hormonal function and nocturnal penile tumescence testing. Testing should include measurement of serum testosterone, LH, FSH, prolactin, and thyroid function tests, as series of adults with sexual dysfunction has found hormonal disorders in 29% to 34% of patients [90,91]. If a history of nocturnal or morning erections is not obtained, nocturnal penile tumescence testing (NPT) can be performed. Home medical devices quantify the number, tumescence, and rigidity of erectile episodes, and thus may classify erectile activity as normal or impaired. Impotent men with normal NPT are considered to have psychogenic impotence, whereas those with impaired NPT are considered to have organic impotence, usually caused by vascular or neurologic disease. Testosterone-deficient hypogonadal men are capable of exhibiting some erectile activity during nocturnal penile tumescence studies [92]. Additional studies such as duplex Doppler ultrasonography or angiography of the penile deep arteries are indicated in men with impaired NPT to identify areas of arterial obstruction or venous leak that might be amenable to surgical reconstruction.

Treatment for adult sexual dysfunction is tailored according to the cause of dysfunction. In the young adult, treatment most commonly entails psychological counseling and removal of environmental or behavioral causes. (eg, stopping illicit drug use or changing prescription medications). A possible course of therapy may include the widely advertised phosphodiesterase-5 (PDE-5) inhibitors: sildenafil, vardenafil, and tadalafil. These are usually not necessary to overcome organic causes of sexual dysfunction in the college-aged male but may be used as an adjunct to counseling to promote sexual confidence in the maintenance of erections. These medications should not be prescribed empirically to college-aged males, as primary neurovascular causes of erectile dysfunction are rare in this group.

Summary

Genitourinary issues are of critical concern to the college male and often are encountered by health care providers. This article reviewed several commonly encountered and potentially serious entities, using illustrative cases to clinically center the discussion. This article allows practitioners to fully address the young adult's genitourinary complaints relating to the diagnosis of genital warts, testicular tumor, varicocele, acute prostatitis, and sexual dysfunction.

References

[1] Collins MM, Stafford RS, O'Leary MP, et al. How common is prostatitis? A national survey of physician visits. J Urol 1998;159:1224–8.
[2] Cates Jr W. Estimates of the incidence and prevalence of sexually transmitted diseases in the United States. American Social Health Association Panel. Sex Transm Dis 1999;26(Suppl 4):7.
[3] Dunne EF, Burstein GR, Stone KM. Anogenital human papillomavirus infection in males. Adolesc Med 2003;14:613–32.

[4] Stratakis CA, Graham W, DiPalma J, et al. Misdiagnosis of perianal manifestations of Crohn's disease. Clin Pediatr 1994;33:631–4.

[5] Darmstadt GL. Perianal lymphangioma circumscriptum mistaken for genital warts. Pediatrics 1996;98:461–3.

[6] Law C, Merianos A, Thompson C, et al. manifestations of anogenital HPV infection in the male partners of women with anogenital warts and/or abnormal cervical smears. Int J STD AIDS 1991;2:188–94.

[7] Gissmann L, Zur HH. Partial characterization of viral DNA from human genital warts (condylomata acuminata). Int J Cancer 1980;25:605–9.

[8] Palefsky JM. Human papillomavirus-related tumors. AIDS 2000;14:95.

[9] von Krogh G, Lacey CJ, Gross G, et al. European course on HPV associated pathology: guidelines for primary care physicians for the diagnosis and management of anogenital warts. Sex Transm Infect 2000;76:162.

[10] Koutsky LA, Kiviat NB. Genital human papillomavirus. In: Holmes KK, Sparling PF, Mardh PA, et al, editors. Sexually transmitted diseases. New York: McGraw-Hill; 1999. p. 347–59.

[11] Bonnez W, Reichman R. Papillomaviruses. In: Mandell GL, Bennett JE, Dolin R, editors. Principles and practice of infectious diseases. 5th edition. Philadelphia: Churchill Livingstone; 2000. p. 1630.

[12] Beutner KR, Reitano MV, Richwald GA, et al. External genital warts: report of the American Medical Association Consensus Conference. AMA expert panel on External Genital Warts. Clin Infect Dis 1998;27:796–806.

[13] American Academy of Pediatrics. Human papillomavirus. In: Pickering LK, editor. Red book 2003 report of the Committee on Infectious Diseases. 26th edition. Elk Grove Village, IL: American Academy of Pediatrics; 2003. p. 449.

[14] Palefsky JM. Anal squamous intraepithelial lesions in human immunodeficiency virus-positive men and women. Semin Oncol 2000;27:471.

[15] Wiley DJ, Douglas J, Beutner K, et al. External genital warts: diagnosis, treatment and prevention. Clin Infect Dis 2002;35(Suppl 2):2–24.

[16] Palefsky JM. Anal squamous intraepithelial lesions: relation to HIV and human papillomavirus infection. J Acquir Immune Defic Syndr 1999;21(Suppl 1):S42.

[17] Castellsague X, Bosch FX, Nunoz N, et al. Male circumcision, penile human papillomavirus infection, and cervical cancer in female partners. N Engl J Med 2002;346:1105–12.

[18] Hippelainen MI, Syrjanen S, Hippelainen MJ, et al. Prevalence and risk factors of genital human papillomavirus infections in healthy males: a study on Finnish conscripts. Sex Transm Dis 1993;20:321–8.

[19] Svare EL, Kjaer SK, Worm AM, et al. Risk factors for genital HPV DNA in men resemble those found in women: a study of male attendees at a Danish STD clinic. Sex Transm Infect 2002; 78:215.

[20] Wikstrom A, Lidbrink P, Johansson B, et al. Penile human papillomavirus carriage among men attending Swedish STD clinics. Int J STD AIDS 1991;2:105–9.

[21] Winer RL, Shu-Kuang L, Hughes JP, et al. Genital human papillomavirus infection: Incidence and risk factors in a cohort of female university students. Am J Epidemiol 2003;157:218–26.

[22] Workshop summary. Scientific evidence of condom effectiveness for sexually transmitted disease transmission. NIAID, NIH, HHS, Herndon, VA. June 12–13, 2000.

[23] Manhart LE, Koutsky LA. Do condoms prevent genital HPV infection, external genital warts, or cervical neoplasia? A meta-analysis. Sex Transm Dis 2002;29:725–35.

[24] Wen LM, Estcourt CS, Simpson JM, et al. Risk factors for the acquisition of genital warts: are condoms protective? Sex Transm Dis 1999;75:312–6.

[25] Oriel D. Genital human papillomavirus infection. In: Holmes KK, Mardh PA, Sparling PF, editors. Sexually transmitted diseases. New York: McGraw-Hill; 1990. p. 433–41.

[26] Moses S, Bailey RC, Ronald AR. Male circumcision: assessment of health benefits and risks. Sex Transm Infect 1998;74:368–73.

[27] American Cancer Society. Cancer facts and figures 2004. Atlanta (GA): American Cancer Society; 2004.

[28] Richie JP, Steele GS. Neoplasms of the testis. In: Walsh PC, Retik AB, Vaughan ED, et al, editors. Campbell's Urology. 8th edition. Philadelphia: WB Saunders; 2002. p. 2876–910.
[29] Thomas R. Testicular tumors. Adolescent Medicine State of the Art Reviews 1996;7:149–55.
[30] Henderson BE, Benton B, Jing J, et al. Risk factors for cancer of the testis in young men. Int J Cancer 1979;23(5):598–603.
[31] Adelman WP, Joffe A. The adolescent male genital examination: what's normal and what's not. Contemp Pediatr 1999;16(7):76–92.
[32] Small EJ, Torti FM. Testes. In: Abeloff MD, Armitage JO, Lichter AS, et al, editors. Clinical oncology. New York: Churchill Livingstone; 1995. p. 1493–520.
[33] Chen DCP, Holder LE, Kaplan GN. Correlation of radionuclide imaging and diagnostic ultrasound in scrotal diseases. J Nucl Med 1986;27:1774.
[34] Ries LAG, Miller BA, Hankey BF, et al, editors. SEER cancer statistics review, 1973–1991: tables and graphs. Bethesda (MD): National Cancer Institute; 1994.
[35] Goldenring JM, Purtell E. Knowledge of testicular cancer risk and need for self-examination in college students: a call for equal time for men in teaching of early cancer detection techniques. Pediatrics 1984;74:1093–6.
[36] Singer AJ, Tichler T, Orvieto R, et al. Testicular carcinoma: a study of knowledge, awareness, and practice of testicular self-examination in male soldiers and military physicians. Mil Med 1993;158:640–3.
[37] Oster J. Varicocele in children and adolescents. An investigation of the incidence among Danish school children. Scan J Urol Nephrol 1971;5:27–32.
[38] Akbay E, Cayan S, Boruk E, et al. The prevalence of varicocele and the varicocele-related testicular atrophy in Turkish children and adolescents. BJU Int 2000;86:490–3.
[39] Vasavada S, Ross J, Nasrallah P, et al. Prepubertal varicoceles. Urology 1997;50:774.
[40] Nussinovitch M, Greenbaum E, Amir J, et al. Prevalence of adolescent varicocele. Arch Pediatr Adolesc Med 2001;155:855–6.
[41] Diamond DA. Adolescent varicocele: emerging understanding. BJU Int 2003;92(Suppl 1): 48–51.
[42] Chehval MJ, Purcell MH. Deteriorations of semen parameters over time in men with untreated varicocele: evidence of progressive testicular damage. Fertil Steril 1992;57:174–7.
[43] Witt MA, Lipschultz LI. Varicocele: a progressive or static lesion? Urology 1993;42:541–3.
[44] Gorelick JI, Goldstein M. Loss of fertility in men with varicocele. Fertil Steril 1993;59:613–6.
[45] Okuyama A, Nakamura M, Namiki M, et al. Surgical repair of varicocele at puberty: preventive treatment for infertility improvement. J Urol 1988;139:562–4.
[46] Paduch DA, Niedzielski J. Repair versus observation in adolescent varicocele: a prospective study. J Urol 1997;158:1128–32.
[47] World Health Organization. The influence of varicocele on parameters of fertility in a large group of men presenting to infertility clinic. Fertil Steril 1992;57:1289–93.
[48] Adelman WP, Joffe A. Controversies in male adolescent health: varicocele, circumcision, and testicular self-examination. Curr Opin Pediatr 2004;16:363–7.
[49] Skoog SJ, Roberts KP, Goldstein M, et al. The adolescent varicocele: what's new with an old problem in young patients? Pediatrics 1997;100:112–22.
[50] Santoro G, Romeo C, Impellizzeri P, et al. A morphometric and ultrastructural study of the changes in the lamina propria in adolescents with varicocele. BJU Int 1999;83:828–32.
[51] Barbieri ER, Hidelgo ME, Venegas A, et al. Varicocele-associated decrease in antioxidant defenses. J Androl 1999;20:713–7.
[52] Rome C, Santoro G, Impellizzeri P, et al. Myofibroblasts in adolescent varicocele. An ultrastructural and immunohistochemical study. Urol Res 2000;28:24–8.
[53] Dubin L, Amelar RD. Etiologic factors in 1294 consecutive cases of male infertility. Fertil Steril 1971;22:469–74.
[54] Kursh ED. What is the incidence of varicocele in a fertile population? Fertil Steril 1987;48:510–1.
[55] Gat Y, Zukerman Z, Bachar GN, et al. Adolescent varicocele: is it a unilateral disease? Urology 2003;62(4):742–6.

[56] Pinto K, Kroovand RL, Jarow JP. Varicocele related testicular atrophy and its predicted effect upon fertility. J Urol 1994;152:788–90.

[57] Guarino N, Tadini B, Bianchi M. The adolescent varicocele: the crucial role of hormonal tests in selecting patients with testicular dysfunction. J Pediatr Surg 2003;38(1):120–3.

[58] Haans LCF, Laven JSE, Mali WPTM, et al. Testis volumes, semen quality and hormonal patterns in adolescents with and without varicocele. Fertil Steril 1991;56:731–6.

[59] Takihara H, Cosentino MJ, Sakatoku J, et al. Significance of testicular size measurements in andrology: II. Correlation of testicular size with testicular function. J Urol 1987;137:416–9.

[60] Kahn RH, Moseley KE, Thilges JN, et al. Community-based screening and treatment for STDs: results from a mobile clinic initiative. Sex Transm Dis 2003;30:654–8.

[61] Oh MK, Cloud GA, Wallace LS, et al. Sexual behavior and sexually transmitted diseases among male adolescents in detention. Sex Transm Dis 1994;21:127–32.

[62] Oh M, Sturdevant M, Genuardi F, et al. Asymptomatic C trachomatis urethritis in adolescent males. J Adolesc Health 1994;15:56.

[63] Handsfield HH, Lipman TO, Harnisch JP, et al. Asymptomatic gonorrhea in man: diagnosis, natural course, prevalence and significance. N Engl J Med 1974;290:117–23.

[64] Simpson T, Oh K. Urethritis and cervicitis in adolescents. Adolesc Med 2004;15:253–71.

[65] Centers for Disease Control and Prevention. Sexually transmitted diseases treatment guidelines 2002. MMWR Morb Mortal Wkly Rep 2002;51:30–2.

[66] Stamm WE, Hicks CB, Martin DH, et al. Azithromycin for empirical treatment of the non-gonococcal urethritis syndrome in men. A randomized double-blind study. JAMA 1995;274:545.

[67] Romanowski B, Talbot H, Stadnyk M, et al. Minocycline compared with doxycycline in the treatment of nongonococcal urethritis and mucopurulent cervicitis. Ann Intern Med 1993; 119:16.

[68] Burstein GR, Zenilman JM. Nongonococcal urethritis—a new paradigm. Clin Infect Dis 1999; 28(Suppl 1):S66.

[69] Horner P, Thomas B, Gilroy CB, et al. Role of *Mycoplasma genitalium* and *Ureaplasma urealyticum* in acute and chronic nongonococcal urethritis. Clin Infect Dis 2001;32(7):995–1003.

[70] Deguchi T, Maeda S. *Mycoplasma genitalium*: another important pathogen of nongonococcal urethritis. J Urol 2002;167(3):1210–7.

[71] Krieger JN, Verdon M, Siegel N, et al. Risk assessment and laboratory diagnosis of trichomoniasis in men. J Infect Dis 1992;166:1362.

[72] Anonymous. Increases in fluoroquinolone-resistant *Neisseria gonorrhoeae* among men who have sex with men—United States, 2003, and revised recommendations for gonorrhea treatment. MMWR Morb Mortal Wkly Rep 2004;53:335.

[73] Wyndaele JJ. Complications of intermittent catheterization: their prevention and treatment. Spinal Cord 2002;40:536.

[74] Ostaszewska I, Zdrodowska-Stefanow B, Badyda J, et al. *Chlamydia trachomatis*: probable cause of prostatitis. Int J STD AIDS 1998;9:350.

[75] De la Rosette JJMCH, Hubregtse MR, Meuleman EJH, et al. Diagnosis and treatment of 409 patients with prostatitis syndromes. Urology 1993;41:301.

[76] Lipsky BA. Urinary tract infections in men. Ann Intern Med 1989;110:138.

[77] Pfau A. Prostatitis. A continuing enigma. Urol Clin North Am 1986;13:695.

[78] Aagaard J, Madsen PO. Bacterial prostatitis: new methods of treatment. Urology 1991; 37(Suppl 3):4.

[79] Spark RF. Evaluation of male sexual dysfunction. Available at: www.uptodate.com. Accessed November 30, 2004.

[80] Reynolds CF, Frank E, Thase ME, et al. Assessment of sexual function in depressed, impotent and healthy men. Psychiatry Res 1988;24:231.

[81] Mills TM, Wiedmeier VT, Stopper VS. Androgen maintenance of erectile function in the rat penis. Biol Reprod 1992;46:342.

[82] Mannino DH, Klevens RM, Flaanders WD. Cigarette smoking: an independent risk factor for impotence? Am J Epidemiol 1994;140:1003.

[83] Marceau L, Kleinman K, Goldstein I, et al. Does bicycling contribute to the risk of erectile dysfunction? Results from the Massachusetts Male Aging Study (MMAS). Int J Impot Res 2001;13:298.

[84] Bolt JW, Evans C, Marshal VR. Sexual dysfunction after prostatectomy. Br J Urol 1987;59:319.

[85] Virag R, Bouilly P, Frydman D. Is impotence an arterial disorder? A study of arterial risk factors in 440 impotent men. Lancet 1985;1:181.

[86] Wein AJ, Van Arsdalen K. Drug-induced male sexual dysfunction. Urol Clin North Am 1988; 15:23.

[87] Grimm Jr RH, Grandits GA, Prineas RJ, et al. Long-term effects on sexual function of five antihypertensive drugs and nutritional hygienic treatment in hypertensive men and women. Treatment of Mild Hypertension Study (TOMHS). Hypertension 1997;29:8.

[88] Smith DE, Wesson DR, Apter-Marsh M. Cocaine- and alcohol-induced sexual dysfunction in patients with addictive disorders. J Psychoactive Drugs 1984;16:359.

[89] Krane RJ, Goldstein I, Saenz D, et al. Impotence. N Engl J Med 1989;321:1648.

[90] Slag MF, Morley JE, Elson MK, et al. Impotence in medical clinic outpatients. JAMA 1983; 248:1736.

[91] Spark RF, White RA, Connolly PB. Impotence is not always psychogenic. JAMA 1980;243:750.

[92] Kwan M, Greenleaf WJ, Mann J, et al. The nature of androgen action on male sexuality: a combined laboratory self-report study on hypogonadal men. J Clin Endocrinol Metab 1983; 57:557.

ELSEVIER
SAUNDERS

PEDIATRIC CLINICS
OF NORTH AMERICA

Pediatr Clin N Am 52 (2005) 217–228

Sexually Transmitted Infections: New Guidelines for an Old Problem on the College Campus

Mary Ellen Rimsza, MD, FAAP[a,b,*]

a*School of Health Services Administration and Policy, W.P. Carey School of Business, Student Health and Wellness Center, Arizona State University, PO Box 872104, Tempe, AZ 85287-210, USA*
b*Mayo Clinic College of Medicine, Scottsdale, AZ, USA*

Approximately 80% of college-age adolescents are sexually active and at risk for sexually transmitted infections (STIs). Over 4 million STIs occur in teen-agers annually and young adults between the ages of 18 and 24, while adolescents 15 to 17 years of age have higher rates of STIs than any other age group in the United States [1]. Thus, the prevention, diagnosis, and treatment of STIs are a critical part of college health care. This article will discuss the epidemiology, diagnosis, and management of some of the most common STIs (Box 1) encountered in the college-age group, with an emphasis on new guidelines for treatment.

Chlamydia trachomatis infection

Chlamydia trachomatis is a gram-negative, obligate intracellular bacterium. The life cycle of *C trachomatis* includes an extracellular form (elementary body) and an intracellular form (reticulate body). The elementary body penetrates columnar epithelial cells, transforms into the reticulate body, and then reproduces more elementary bodies. *C trachomatis* is the most common sexually transmitted bacterial pathogen in the United States [2].

---

 * School of Health Services Management and Policy, W.P. Carey School of Business, Arizona State University, PO Box 874506, Tempe, AZ 85287-4506.
 E-mail address: mrimsza@asu.edu

Box 1. Common agents of sexually transmitted infections in college students

Chlamydia trachomatis
Neisseria gonorrhoeae
Herpes simplex virus
Treponema pallidum
Trichomonas vaginalis
Hepatitis B virus
Hepatitis C virus

A variety of diagnostic tests may be used to identify *C trachomatis* infection in addition to culture (Box 2). The direct fluorescent antibody test uses a fluorescent-labeled antibody; it is rarely used today because it requires extensive time and expertise, because the specimen needs to be examined using a fluorescent microscope. Enzyme immunoassay uses an antibody against the elementary body of the chlamydia organism. Nucleic acid amplification tests (NAATs) measure nucleic acids rather than viable organisms using a variety of amplification techniques, including polymerase chain reaction, transcription-mediated amplification, strand displacement assay, and ligase chain reaction. NAATs are the most commonly used tests today because of their high sensitivity and specificity, which allows testing of urine as well as cervical or urethral specimens. Urine tests using any of the NAATs may be slightly less sensitive than cervical testing, but they are satisfactory for screening in women who do note otherwise need a pelvic examination. Testing the initial first-void urine specimen is more sensitive than testing subsequent "midstream" urine specimens. It is important to remember that because NAATs measure nucleic acid, not viable organisms, NAATs may remain positive for up to 3 weeks after effective treatment of *C trachomatis* infection [3].

A recent cross-sectional study of 4086 students enrolled at California State University and three local community colleges revealed that 3.4% of the students were infected with *C trachomatis*. The incidence rates for males (3.03%) and

---

Box 2. Laboratory tests for Chlamydia trachomatis infection

Culture
Direct fluorescent antibody test
Enzyme immunoassay
Molecular-based testing (DNA probe)
Nucleic acid amplification test

---

females (3.78%) were similar. The risk for infection was greatest in students who were over 25 years of age, whose ethnicity was other than white, who had more than one sexual partner in the preceding year or a new partner in the preceding 2 months, and who had current symptoms [4]. A similar study done at the University of Pittsburgh revealed that 2.3% of female students were infected with *C trachomatis*; in this study, infection was more common in students who were over 21 years of age, had symptoms, reported prior chlamydial infection or gonorrhea, reported exposure to a sexually transmitted disease, were black, or had cervical signs during examination [5,6]. These rates are similar to the nationally reported rates from the Centers for Disease Control and Prevention (CDC) of 2619 cases per 100,000 individuals among 15- to 19-year-olds and 2570 per 100,000 for 20- to 24-year-old women [7].

A study of male college students enrolled in Reserve Officer Training revealed that the prevalence of *C trachomatis* infection was 2.48%. This is much higher than the Chlamydia infection rates reported by the CDC among young men between 20 and 24 years of age (692/100,000). [7] Almost 94% of these college men who were infected with *C trachomatis* were asymptomatic [6]. This rate of asymptomatic infection is similar to the rate of asymptomatic infection reported in other male populations in the United States of 90% to 92% [8].

Clinically symptomatic infection in men usually is characterized by dysuria and white or clear urethral discharge. Because these symptoms may be transient and mild, the patient may not seek medical attention. In addition, because spontaneous resolution of symptoms without treatment is common, infected symptomatic men who do not seek treatment early in the infection may never come to medical attention due to the resolution of symptoms.

C trachomatis is also the most common cause of epididymitis among sexually active young men. Inflammation of the epididymis is associated with painful swelling of the epididymis, unilateral scrotal/testicular pain and tenderness. Signs or symptoms of urethritis may precede or be associated with the epididimyitis. However, in some patients, the first symptom of infection is the acute onset of scrotal pain. Thus, the differential diagnosis of epididymitis includes testicular torsion. Examination of the urine may be helpful in distinguishing between these conditions, because epididymitis is often associated with pyuria and bacteruria, while these findings are rare in patients who have testicular torsion. Doppler ultrasound examination and radionuclide testicular scanning also may be helpful in distinguishing between epididymitis and testicular torsion. The differential diagnosis of epididymitis also includes testicular tumor, trauma, and inguinal hernia. Other conditions associated with *C trachomatis* infection in men include prostatitis, proctitis, and Reiter's syndrome [9].

Women who have *C trachomatis* infections also usually are asymptomatic. The most common site of infection is the transitional epithelium of the endocervix. Younger adolescents who have cervical ectopy are more susceptible to infection than older adolescents and adults. Cervicitis may present as vaginal discharge, postcoital bleeding, dyspaureunia, or irregular menstrual bleeding. On examination, mucopurulent cervical discharge, erythema, and cervical friability may be noted. Women may also have urethritis, salpingitis, bartholinitis, or endometritis due to *C trachomatis* infection [9].

Because most men who have urethral infection and most women who have cervical infection are asymptomatic, the best method of identifying chlamydial infection in the college population is by periodic screening. However, the value of the screening tests depends on the prevalence of *C trachomatis* infection in the population, cost of the screening tests, and cost of treatment [2]. A cost-effectiveness analysis of a universal screening program for women using NAATs showed that screening was advantageous when the prevalence of infection was 6% or greater [10]. For males, Genc and Mardh [10] reported that leukocyte esterase–enzyme immunoassay screening programs are cost-effective when the prevalence of *C trachomatis* infection exceeds 2%. Thus, universal screening is not likely to be cost-effective in a college population. Current recommendations from the CDC are for annual screening of sexually active adolescents and women 20 to 25 years of age [11]. More frequent screening may be indicated for some women.

Recommended treatment regimens for uncomplicated urethritis and cervicitis are displayed in Box 3 [11]. Patients do not need to be retested for *C trachomatis* after completing treatment with azithromycin or doxycycline unless symptoms persist or reinfection is suspected. Because erythromycin may be less effective in treating C trachomatis, a test of cure may be considered 3 weeks after completion of erythromycin therapy. It is important to remember that nonculture tests (eg. NAAT) may remain positive even after successful treatment for 3 weeks [11]. Some experts recommend rescreening women who have had *C trachomatis* infection at 3- to 4-month intervals, because this population has a high prevalence of repeat infection.

Current sex partners of women or men infected with *C trachomatis* should referred for evaluation, testing, and treatment, as should any previous partner

---

Box 3. Treatment for uncomplicated urethritis/cervicitis due to Chlamydia trachomatis

Recommended

Azithromycin 1 g orally as a single dose **OR** doxycycline 100 mg orally twice a day for 7 days

Alternative regimens

Ofloxacin 300 mg orally twice a day for 7 days **OR** levofloxacin 500 mg orally for 7 days **OR** erythromycin base 500 mg orally four times a day for 7 days

who had sexual contact with the infected patient during the 60 days before the onset of symptoms or diagnosis [11].

Neisseria gonorrhoeae infection

Neisseria gonorrhoeae is a gram-negative diplococcus. In the United States, approximately 6,000,000 new *N gonorrhoeae* infections occur each year. Most infections among men are symptomatic and are characterized by dysuria, pyuria, urethral discharge, or any combination of these symptoms. Complications of *N gonorrhoeae* infection in men include epididymitis, prostatitis, conjunctivitis, and disseminated disease. In contrast, most infected women are asymptomatic until complications such as salpingitis, perihepatitis, bartholinitis, conjunctivitis, or disseminated disease occur. Less commonly, women may present with signs or symptoms of uncomplicated infections such as urethritis or cervicitis (eg, dysuria, dysfunctional uterine bleeding, dyspareunia, postcoital bleeding, cervical discharge).

Uncomplicated gonococcal infection (urethritis, cervicitis) can be treated with the regimens listed in Box 4 [11]. Unless concomitant chlamydia infection has been ruled out, the patient should also be treated with either azithromycin 1000 mg orally in a single dose or doxycycline 100 mg orally twice a day for 7 days [11]. Because quinolone-resistant *N gonorrhoeae* is increasingly common, it is inadvisable to treat gonorrhea with quinolones.

Disseminated gonococcal infection (DGI) is caused by the hematogenous spread of gonococcus and may occur in 0.5% to 3% of untreated mucosal gonococcal infection. The classic triad of symptoms includes dermatitis, polyarthritis, and tenosynovitis. The dermatitis is usually on the extremities and is characterized by small erythematous nonblanching papules that become necrotic. The tenosynovitis usually occurs in the fingers, but larger joints also may be involved. The arthritis is migratory and may involve any joint, especially the knee, wrist, ankle, and phalanges. Women are more likely to develop DGI when they are pregnant or during the perimenstrual interval. Complement deficiencies also predispose patients to DGI; up to 13% of patients who have DGI are found to have complement deficiency. Gonococcus may be recovered from the blood,

---

Box 4. Treatment of uncomplicated N gonorrhoeae urethritis/cervicitis

Cefixime 400 mg orally as a single dose
Ceftriaxone 125 mg intramuscularly in a single dose
Ciprofloxacin 500 mg orally in a single dose
Ofloxacin 400 mg orally in a single dose
Levofloxacin 250 mg orally in a single dose

synovial fluid, or skin lesions in up to 50% of patients who have DGI [12]. Patients who have DGI should be hospitalized and treated initially with intravenous or intramuscular ceftriaxone 1 g every 24 hours. After initial management with parenteral antibiotics, patients can be switched to oral therapy (eg, cefixime 400 mg, ciprofloxacin 500 mg twice daily) to complete a 7-day course of therapy.

Herpes simplex infection

Genital herpes is caused by herpes simplex virus type 1 (HSV-1) or herpes simplex virus type 2 (HSV-2). The infection is usually acquired through sexual contact with an infected partner after an incubation period of 2 to 12 days. Although the risk of transmission of HSV from an infected sexual partner is more likely when lesions are present, most transmission occurs when lesions are not present as a result of asymptomatic viral shedding.

Approximately 20% of genital herpes in the United States is caused by HSV-1 that is usually spread through oral–genital contact. In contrast, HSV-2 is usually spread through genital–genital contact. Direct contact other than coitus can result in viral transmission if the virus comes into contact with the skin or mucous membranes. The classical clinical presentation after the initial acquisition of HSV begins with painful genital papules that progress to vesicles and ulcers. Tender inguinal lymphadenopathy is often noted on examination. Approximately 60% of women and 40% of men have constitutional symptoms including headache, fever, malaise, and myalgias with the first clinical episode [13]. Central nervous system complications of genital herpes include aseptic meningitis, sacral radiculopathy, and transverse myelitis. The local and systemic symptoms of primary HSV-1 infection are generally the same as for primary HSV-2 infection. First episodes of HSV-2 infections in patients who have antibody to HSV-1 (nonprimary infection) are less commonly associated with systemic symptoms than first episodes of HSV-2 in patients who do not have antibody to HSV-1 (primary infection).

After the initial acquisition of HSV, the virus resides in a latent state in neuronal bodies indefinitely. Recurrences of HSV-2 may be symptomatic or asymptomatic. For symptomatic recurrences, a prodrome may occur 30 minutes to 48 hours before genital lesions are noted. This prodrome ranges from a mild tingling sensation to severe shooting pain in the genital region extending to the buttock or hip [14]. Within 12 months of the initial HSV-2 episode, 90% of patients will have had at least one recurrence and approximately 40% will have had 6 or more recurrences. Fortunately, recurrences tend to decrease over time [15]. HSV-2 genital infection is twice as likely to reactivate as HSV-1 infection and recurs 8 to 10 times more often than HSV-1 infection [16].

Genital herpes can usually be diagnosed by way of viral culture of the lesions or serologic testing. The optimal test is viral culture, but this requires the presence of new genital lesions, and the sensitivity of culture decreases with advancing age of ulcers. About 95% of vesicular lesions will grow HSV, whereas only 70% of ulcerative lesions and 30% of crusted lesions will grow HSV. Unroofing the vesicle increases the sensitivity of culture [3,13]. The ability to culture the virus is greater with primary infections because the viral load is greater than with recurrent infection [13]. Polymerase chain reaction assays for HSV DNA are highly sensitive, but their role in the diagnosis of genital ulcer disease has not been well defined. However, it is the test of choice for identifying HSV in spinal fluid [11]. Both type-specific and nonspecific serologic tests for HSV are available. Unfortunately, serologic testing is of little clinical value because it cannot be used to distinguish between current, recent, and past infection. However, type-specific serologic testing for HSV may be useful for diagnosis in patients who have symptomatic disease in the healing stages or in recurrent infections when cultures of lesions are less likely to yield the virus. The CDC recommends glycoprotein G tests, which have a high sensitivity (80% to 98%) and specificity (>96%). The glycoprotein G tests, which have been approved by the US Food and Drug Administration, include POCkit HSV-2 (Diagnology, Research Triangle Park, North Carolina), HerpeSelect-1 and 2 ELISA (Focus Technologies, Cypress, California), and HerpeSelect 1 and 2 Immunoblot (Focus Technologies) [11]. The Tzanck prep, which requires microscopic analysis of scrapings from the ulcer base, is not sensitive or specific for HSV infection [3,11].

The differential diagnosis of genital ulcers includes infectious and non-infectious illnesses; infectious causes include primary syphilis and chancroid. One or more painless lesions characterize primary syphilis caused by *Treponema pallidum*. A dark field microscopic examination of scrapings from the base of the lesion for spirochetes is helpful in establishing the diagnosis. Chancroid ulcers, caused by *Haemophilus ducreyi*, are usually painful and have purulent exudates. Noninfectious causes of genital ulcers include Behçet's syndrome, Crohn's disease, Reiter's syndrome, and trauma.

Herpes simplex genital infection can be treated orally with acyclic nucleoside analogs (acyclovir, valacyclovir, famciclovir). All of these antiviral agents are effective in the treatment of an acute first episode of genital herpes and for episodic treatment of recurrent herpes. Acyclovir is the least expensive regimen but must be taken at least 3 times a day (400 mg orally 3 times a day for 7–10 days). Valacyclovir (1000 mg orally twice a day for 7–10 days) and famciclovir (250 mg orally three times daily for 7–10 days) are more expensive and no more effective in the treatment of first episode of infection than acyclovir [13]. Although lesions should be cultured before starting treatment, it should not be delayed pending culture results because treatment is more effective if started earlier in the course of the infection. Topical antiviral treatment is not recommended because it offers minimal clinical benefit.

For recurrent genital herpes infection, acyclovir (800 mg orally twice daily for 5 days) decreases the time to resolution of signs and symptoms by approximately 1 day. It also decreases the time to healing and duration of viral shedding by 1 to 2 days. Valacyclovir (1000 mg orally once daily for 5 days) or famciclovir

(125 mg orally twice daily for 5 days) are equally effective as acyclovir but are more expensive [11]. Episodic treatment should be started at the first sign of recurrence. If recurrences are associated with a prodrome, the therapy should be started during the prodrome rather than waiting for the development of lesions. Patients should be counseled on the typical signs and symptoms of recurrences and provided with a supply of antiviral medication to be used as needed for recurrences [11].

Suppressive antiviral therapy to reduce the frequency of recurrent episodes of genital herpes infection should be considered for patients who have more than 6 episodes per year. For these patients, suppressive therapy can reduce the frequency of recurrences by 70% to 80%. Treatment options include acyclovir (400 mg twice daily), valacyclovir (500–1000 mg once daily) or famciclovir (250 mg twice daily). Suppressive antiviral therapy also reduces the number of days of subclinical viral shedding [11]. Because the number of recurrences decreases over time, it is wise to discuss discontinuation of suppressive therapy annually with patients. For patients who are immunosuppressed (eg, HIV-infected patients), the HSV lesions may be larger, more painful, and slower to heal than for immunocompetent patients. Immunosuppressed patients also are likely to have more frequent recurrences. Episodic or suppressive antiviral therapy may be especially helpful for these patients. Suppressive therapy is safe and reduces the risk of viral transmission of HSV to uninfected partners, because it reduces viral shedding. Therapy with 500 mg of valacyclovir once daily for 8 months has been shown to reduce the likelihood of acquisition of HSV-2 genital infection in the seronegative partner by 48% [17].

Counseling is an important part of the management of genital herpes infection. Key points to make when counseling patients should include the potential for recurrences and the effectiveness of antiviral medication for the treatment of recurrences. Because HSV infection may initially be asymptomatic, a symptomatic episode does not necessarily mean that the patient's current partner is not monogamous. Patients should be counseled regarding the possibility of transmission during periods of asymptomatic viral shedding and the need to abstain from sexual activity with uninfected partners when lesions or prodromal symptoms are present; they should also be encouraged to use condoms. They should also be advised that the risk of HSV transmission to an uninfected partner is not completely eliminated by taking these precautions and that genital ulcer disease increases the risk of transmission of HIV. High titers of HIV are found in genital herpes ulcers of HIV-infected patients, and the viral load of HIV is increased when HSV-2 infection is reactivated [18].

The diagnosis of genital herpes is emotionally devastating to the young man or woman who is infected. Indeed, the psychologic effects are often more severe than the physical ones. Infected patients are embarrassed and feel stigmatized by the infection. They fear transmitting the infection to others and this fear often interferes with their sexual functioning. Although it is advisable for patients to inform future sexual partners about their infection, it is also understandable that discussing this with a future partner can be difficult. It is very important for the physician caring for these patients to provide appropriate psychologic as well as medical support.

Syphilis

Syphilis is caused by the spirochete *Treponema pallidum*. The infection can be transmitted through sexual contact or blood transfusion or through the placenta. There are three stages of the disease. The first or primary stage is clinically characterized by an ulcer (chancre) at the site of inoculation. The incubation period for primary syphilis that is acquired through sexual contact is approximately 3 weeks but may range from 10 to 90 days. The chancre begins as a small papule at the site of inoculation that progresses to an indurated ulcer. The chancre is usually painless but may be tender on palpation. There may be single or multiple chancres; the most common site is the external genitalia, but they may also occur in the mouth, vagina, cervix, and anal area. In approximately 80% of patients there is also painless regional lymphadenopathy. Without treatment, the chancre heals in 1 to 12 weeks in 60% of patients, though an atrophic scar may persist at the site.

The secondary stage of syphilis begins approximately 6 weeks after primary syphilis in untreated patients. This is the bacteremic phase when dissemination to other organs occurs. The signs and symptoms of secondary syphilis are protean and often nonspecific. Patients may present with a flulike illness and low-grade fever, malaise, myalgias, headache, and anorexia that can be difficult to distinguish from a variety of other infections. Skin lesions are common but also protean. The lesions may be localized or generalized and vary in appearance (eg, papules, macules, pustules). Some lesions are annular and may resemble pityriasis rosea. Psoriatic-like lesions also may occur. Lesions on the palms and soles are common and may help distinguish secondary syphilis from many other dermatologic disorders that typically do not occur on the palms and soles. Condyloma lata are wartlike lesions associated with secondary syphilis that occur in the perianal region, on the external genitalia, and in other intertriginous areas (eg, nasolabial folds, axillae, finger webs). Similar lesions (mucous patches) occur on the mucous membranes (eg, mouth, vulva, cervix, glans). Both condyloma lata and mucous patches are highly contagious, teeming with spirochetes. Secondary syphilis is also associated with alopecia.

The secondary stage of syphilis is followed by a subclinical phase (latent syphilis). During this phase, the only evidence of infection is serologic testing. In a small number of infected patients, latent syphilis is followed by a tertiary phase in which there is progressive involvement of the central nervous system (neurosyphilis) and cardiovascular complications. Neurosyphilis may be asymptomatic or characterized by signs and symptoms of meningitis, cranial nerve palsies, paresis, or tabes dosalis. Patients also may develop granulomatous lesions (gumma) in any organ.

Parenteral penicillin G is the preferred drug for the treatment of all stages of syphilis. For primary and secondary syphilis, the recommended treatment regimen is benzathine penicillin G 2.4 million U intramuscularly as a single dose. All patients who have syphilis should be tested for HIV infection and in geographic regions that have a high prevalence of HIV infection; patients who have primary syphilis should be retested for HIV 3 months later if the first HIV test is negative. If patients who have syphilis also have neurologic symptoms or signs, a cerebrospinal fluid analysis should be performed. Similarly, if symptoms of uveitis are present, and ophthalmologic evaluation including slit-lamp evaluation should be performed.

It is often difficult to assess response to treatment, because definitive criteria are not available for cure or failure. Follow-up clinical examination and serologic testing should be performed 6 months and 12 months following treatment. Failure of nontreponemal test titers to decrease fourfold within 6 months of treatment for primary or secondary syphilis is probably indicative of treatment failure. HIV-infected patients should be followed more frequently at 3-month intervals. Some experts recommend cerebrospinal fluid analysis whenever treatment failures occur because of increased risk of central nervous system infection. Most experts feel that retreatment should consist of benzathine penicillin G 2.4 million U intramuscularly weekly for 3 weeks [11].

Trichomoniasis

Trichomoniasis is an STI caused by the protozoan *Trichomoniasis vaginalis*. This infection may be asymptomatic, but many infected women have symptoms of vaginitis, including a malodorous, yellow discharge and vulvar irritation. In men, the infection is usually asymptomatic, although they may have symptoms of urethritis including dysuria and urethral discharge. Trichomoniasis is usually diagnosed through examination of the vaginal secretions microscopically, although culture is available. The sensitivity of microscopic evaluation is only 60% to 70%. The recommended treatment for *T vaginalis* infection is a single dose of metronidazole 2 g orally. Alternatively, 500 mg orally twice a day for 7 days can be prescribed. Either of these regimens can result in a 90% to 95% cure rate. Although a topical metronidazole gel is available, it is much less efficacious (cure rate <50%) and is therefore not recommended. Follow-up is not indicated after treatment unless symptoms remain.

If treatment failure occurs with the single-dose, 2-g regimen, repeat treatment with the 7-day regimen is recommended. Alternatively, if this fails, a 2-g dose of metronidazole daily for 3 to 5 days is recommended [11]. Sexual partners should be treated and patients should abstain from sex until both the patient and their partner have completed treatment and they are both asymptomatic. Although in the past physicians were advised to avoid using metronidazole in pregnant women, the CDC has stated that they may be treated with metronidazole 2 g orally in a single dose [11], because research has shown no association between prenatal use of metronidazole and birth defects [19,20]. Vaginal trichomoniasis has been associated with adverse pregnancy outcomes (eg, premature rupture of membranes, preterm delivery), but treating asymptomatic women does not seem to lessen this association [11,21].

Hepatitis B virus infection

Every person who seeks STI screening or is diagnosed with an STI should be advised to obtain hepatitis B vaccination. Hepatitis A vaccination can also be offered as a combined vaccine, because with increasing international travel by college students, many will benefit from the hepatitis A vaccine. Sexual transmission accounts for most hepatitis B infection in the United States. Prevaccination serologic testing is not cost-effective, so the vaccine also should be offered to all college students who are (or who plan to become) sexually active. Hepatitis B vaccine is safe and well tolerated. The most common symptoms are mild pain at the site of injection.

Hepatitis C virus infection

Hepatitis C virus (HCV) infection is most efficiently transmitted through exposure to infected blood, but sexual transmission is possible. The low prevalence (0%–4.4%) of HCV in long-term sexual partners of HCV-infected people raises doubts about the sexual transmissibility of HCV [22], but other studies suggest that approximately 20% of HCV infection is sexually transmitted [23].

References

[1] Shafii T, Burstein GR. An overview of sexually transmitted infections among adolescents. Adolesc Med 2004;15:201–14.

[2] Simpson T, Oh MK. Urethritis and cervicitis in adolescents. Adolesc Med Clinics 2004;15: 253–71.

[3] Spigarelli MG, Biro FM. Sexually transmitted disease testing: evaluation of diagnostic tests and methods. Adolesc Med 2004;15:287–99.

[4] Sipkin DL, Grady A, Grady LB. Risk factors for Chlamydia trachomatis infection in a California collegiate population. J Am Coll Health 2004;52:236–8.

[5] Cook RL, St. George K, Lassak M, et al. Screening for Chlamydia trachomatis infection in college women with a polymerase chain reaction assay. Am J Epidemiol 2003;157:858.

[6] Sutton TL, Martinko T, Hale S, et al. Prevalence and high rate of asymptomatic infection of Chlamydia trachomatis in male college Reserve Officer Training Corps cadets. Adolescence 2004;39:19–38.

[7] Centers for Disease Control and Prevention. Sexually transmitted disease surveillance, 2002. Atlanta: US Department of Health and Human Services; 2003.

[8] Oh M, Sturdevant M, Genuardi F, et al. Asymptomatic C trachomatis urethritis in adolescent males. J Adolesc Health 1994;15:56.

[9] Hammerschlag MR. Chlamydia trachomatis and Chlamydia pneumoniae infections in children and adolescents. Pediatr Rev 2004;25:43–51.

[10] Genc M, Mardh A. A cost-effectiveness analysis of screening and treatment for Chlamydia trachomatis infection in asymptomatic women. Ann Intern Med 1996;124:1–7.

[11] Centers for Disease Control and Prevention. Guidelines for the treatment of sexually transmitted diseases. MMWR Morb Mortal Wkly Rep 2002;51:1–80.

[12] Cucurull E, Espinoza LR. Gonococcal arthritis. Rheum Dis Clin North Am 1998;24:305–22.

[13] Kimberlin DW, Rouse DJ. Genital herpes. N Engl J Med 2004;350:1970–7.

[14] Corey L, Wald A. Genital herpes. In: Holmes KK, Mardh PA, Sperling PF, et al, editors. Sexually transmitted infections. New York: McGraw-Hill; 1999. p. 285–312.

[15] Benedetti J, Corey L, Ashley R. Recurrence rates in genital herpes after symptomatic first-episode infection. Ann Intern Med 1994;121:847–54.

[16] Trager JDK. Sexually transmitted diseases causing genital lesions in adolescents. Adolesc Med 2004;15:323–52.

[17] Corey L, Wald A, Patel R, et al. Once-daily valacyclovir to reduce the risk of transmission of genital herpes. N Engl J Med 2004;350:11–20.

[18] Corey L, Handfield HH. Genital herpes and public health: addressing a global problem. JAMA 2000;283:791–4.

[19] Piper JM, Mitchel EF, Ray WA. Prenatal use of metronidazole and birth defects: no association. Obstet Gynecol 1993;82:348–52.

[20] Burtin P, Taddio A, Airburnu O, et al. Safety of metronidazole in pregnancy: a meta-analysis. Am J Obstet Gynecol 1995;172:525–9.

[21] Klebanoff MA, Carey JC, Hauth JC, et al. Failure of metrondiazole to prevent preterm delivery among pregnant women with asymptomatic Trichomas vaginalis infection. N Engl J Med 2001;345:487–93.

[22] Thomas DL, Zenilman JM, Alter MJ, et al. Sexual transmission of hepatitis C virus among patients attending Baltimore sexually transmitted disease clinics: an analysis of 309 sex partnerships. J Infect Dis 1995;171:768–75.

[23] Centers for Disease Control and Prevention. Recommendations for prevention and control of hepatitis C virus (HCV) infection and HCV-related chronic disease. MMWR Morb Mortal Wkly Rep 1998;47:1–39.

ELSEVIER
SAUNDERS

PEDIATRIC CLINICS
OF NORTH AMERICA

Pediatr Clin N Am 52 (2005) 229–241

Immunizations for the College Student: a Campus Perspective of an Outbreak and National and International Considerations

Ashir Kumar, MD[a],*, Dennis L. Murray, MD[b],
Daniel H. Havlichek, MD[c]

[a]Department of Pediatrics and Human Development, College of Human Medicine,
Michigan State University, B-240 Life Sciences, East Lansing, MI 48824-1317, USA
[b]Department of Pediatrics, Medical College of Georgia, Children's Medical Center,
1446 Harper Street, BG-1107A, Augusta, GA 30912, USA
[c]Department of Medicine, College of Human Medicine, Michigan State University,
B-320 Life Sciences, East Lansing, MI 48824-1317, USA

Universities provide unique educational and social experiences to young adults. Many of these experiences put college students at high risk of acquiring a variety of infectious diseases. For example, while at college many students are housed in dormitories in crowded conditions; some of these students share eating and bathroom spaces with students from different regions of the United States, as well as students from different countries. During the academic year 2002–2003, more than half a million (586,323) international students were enrolled in the United States at colleges and universities. Approximately half of these students were enrolled in undergraduate courses.

Recent history of infectious diseases on college campuses

In recent years, the subject of recommended/required immunizations for college students has taken on increased importance. Following the resurgence of measles disease in 1989–1991, many colleges and universities in the United

---

* Corresponding author.
E-mail address: kumara@msu.edu (A. Kumar).

States began to pay more attention to immunization requirements because the costs of containing outbreaks of vaccine-preventable diseases (VPDs) on campus often created a tremendous outlay on school and public health resources. More recently, the occurrence of multiple cases of meningococcal disease across many college campuses (some cases ending tragically in death), coupled with an improved understanding of the risk factors involved in facilitating transmission of this bacterium among college students, have led several states and colleges to mandate meningococcal vaccine for college entry [1,2]. Although college entry immunization requirements vary considerably from state to state, as of July 2004 only 16 states in the United States reportedly have no college-entry requirements for any VPD (Greg Yoder, personal communication, Merck Vaccine Division, Merck & Co. Inc.).

In all 50 states, as a result of the success of prematriculation immunization requirements (PIRs) for grades K through 12, as well as an emphasis on increasing and maintaining high levels of immunizations in the population of children 0 to 2 years of age, most VPDs have declined to record-low levels. Depending on the age of the college student and the states in which the student attended school for grades K through 12, immunizations to prevent diseases caused by a varicella-zoster virus and hepatitis B virus may have not been required. Furthermore, on a college campus the immunization status of international students reflects the prevalence of immunization practices and diseases in their home country. Because each country has their own recommended childhood immunization schedule, and because in some countries vaccines similar to those used in the United States are not readily available, international students attending colleges and universities in the United States may pose additional risks because of a susceptibility to a variety of VPDs.

Part I of this two-part article discusses the impact of meningococceal disease when it occurs on a college campus. Part II reviews immunizations for several VPD's of particular significance for college students.

Part I: meningococceal disease at a college campus and the lessons learned

At Michigan State University (MSU), a pioneer land grant university, approximately 42,000 students are enrolled annually; more than 3000 students from approximately 125 countries also attend MSU yearly. All freshmen are required to live on campus, and the residence halls house over 17,000 students. Because the occurrence of invasive meningococcal disease ranges from 1 to 3 cases per 100,000 per year for on-campus students, with a student population of 40,000 one should expect one case every 1 to 2 years [3,4].

In December 1996, an MSU student who lived off campus died of complications of group B meningococcemia. Following this case, students defined as "close contacts" were contacted and recommended to receive ciprofloxacin as prophylaxis. In February 1997, a second off-campus student died after a 5-day hospitalization from complications of meningitis caused by *Neisseria meningitidis* group C. Both students knew each other well and were from the same hometown; they were reported to have attended some of the same parties, and had a few classes together. Education and prophylaxis measures were again undertaken, and over 500 students received antibiotic prophylaxis. Heightened media attention began the day the second student was admitted to the hospital. Within the next week, another student (student 3) died from a noninfectious central nervous system disease, and two additional students (students 4 and 5) were admitted with aseptic meningitis at a local hospital. The third student had known the first two students and had suffered bacterial meningitis 2 years earlier; the same student (student 3) had also written an editorial for the student newspaper concerning meningitis.

Within 72 hours of the last student's hospital admission, a task force to be advisory to the University President concerning the meningitis issue was established and a massive meningitis educational program was initiated. Health updates were produced and sent to all students and employees by way of the Internet. Printed flyers were sent to students living in residence halls, and a 24-hour hotline was established. Hotline staff ultimately spoke to 2555 callers. The Web page fact sheet was visited 2295 times. In mid-March, another student (student 6) was admitted to the hospital with group C meningococcemia. Ciprofloxacin was offered to all residents of that dormitory; a total of 891 students received the drug. Pulse field gel electrophoresis of the two group C isolates ultimately indicated that they were unrelated. In the week following occurrence of the fourth meningococcal case on campus, there were 1958 calls handled by hotline staff.

Following the diagnosis of the fourth meningococcal case, the task force recommended a mass vaccination program that was directed at undergraduate students but was open to all students, faculty, staff, and family members ages 3 to 30 years who lived on campus. Vaccination was offered for 5 days at one of the gymnasiums on campus; details of this program and characteristics of the students who chose to receive the vaccine have been previously published [5]. In those 5 days, 17,937 students and 1314 staff and dependents were vaccinated. The estimated cost for management of this problem was $400,000. Approximately 85% of the cost was for the meningococcal vaccine. No additional cases of *N meningitidis* infection occurred at MSU again until October 1999.

Following these events, MSU continued with educational programs aimed at both students and parents beginning at student orientation. A very successful vaccination program entitled "Take the shot!" that is endorsed by varsity athletes has also been part of the overall vaccination effort. With the initiation of a Web-based vaccination reporting system and other efforts, MSU now has information on vaccine preventable diseases for over 90% of its students.

Multiple issues come into play when discussing the importance and role of a mass vaccination program for meningococeal infections. The task force's recommendation to vaccinate was not based on the Centers for Disease Control and Prevention (CDC) criteria for an outbreak. The CDC defines a meningococcal outbreak only when there are three cases with group identical strains during a 3-month period [5]. The recommendation arose because multiple cases of confirmed meningococcal disease and other suspected cases had disrupted the functioning of the University to the point where the majority of task force members felt that the intervention was necessary.

The importance of maintaining good communication between parents and the university is obvious, particularly at a time of crisis. Parents have immeasurable emotional ties and are usually geographically distant from their loved ones. Student–parent communication is often less than what the parent would desire; therefore, the university must assume this role and work diligently to ensure open communication between parents and the university. This can be in the form of information distributed through the mass media, parent-specific mailings, Web pages, and using other means of communications. Parents of students who are ill or who have died need special support from individuals and the university as a whole. High-level administrators need to communicate regularly with these parents. Confidentiality of medical information is an important issue. When several students are involved and contact tracing becomes necessary, it is likely that the identity of the ill student might become known to the media and others. Parents need to be made aware of this issue and need to be supported. Nonetheless, during all discussions with the media, every attempt should be made to maintain confidentiality. Media-related issues are best handled in an honest and candid manner through press conferences in which issues are presented by a group of experts and administrators. Discussion of likely questions by the university representative or spokespersons before the press conference is crucial in determining how to present issues intelligently and preferably with one voice. Unexpected or difficult questions should be expected, and honest answers are required. Handouts are especially important, because few in the media have the medical background to understand subtle distinctions made in an oral presentation, but will work off the written handout for their newscasts and published items.

In the end, however, the decision about how to handle a potential campus outbreak, or multiple cases of disease, rests with the university. Decisions must be made with the best interest of the students. Students are part of the larger community; therefore, the city, state, and county health departments must be consulted in these situations along with the students' representatives. It should clearly be understood that at the juncture when important and timely decisions need to be made, only incomplete information might be available.

Part II: immunizations for college students

The American College Health Association publishes a brochure entitled "Immunizations: They're Not Just for Children" that explains to both parents and students those VPDs that are of particular importance to college students [6]. Included in this brochure are brief descriptions of tetanus/diphtheria vaccine; hepatitis A and B virus vaccines; measles, mumps, and rubella vaccines; and varicella vaccine and meningococcal vaccine, along with a description of the diseases each vaccine prevents. Another source of concise information regarding immunizations for those adolescents preparing for college and their parents is "The Healthy Student: A Parents Guide to Preparing Teens for the College Years" [7]. Before matriculation, most colleges request information concerning what immunizations the student has previously received and when they received them. At a minimum, colleges/universities should know whether or not a tetanus/diphtheria booster was received within the past 10 years. Additionally, students will likely need to show proof of immunity to measles, mumps, and rubella through documentation of at least one dose of both mumps and rubella vaccines and two doses for measles vaccine. Laboratory evidence of detectable antibodies for measles, mumps, and rubella or evidence of past disease through certification of physician-diagnosed measles or mumps is also acceptable.

Unimmunized persons are at greater risk of contracting and spreading VPDs. The use of prematriculation immunization requirements (PIRs) by college and universities has been recommended by several groups, including the Advisory Committee on Immunization Practices (CDC) and the National Coalition for

---

Box 1. Currently recommended prematriculation immunizations for colleges and universities[a]

- Tetanus and diphtheria: every 10 years after primary series in childhood[b]
- Measles, mumps, and rubella: all students born after 1956, unless contraindicated[b]
- Varicella: all students without history of the disease or with a negative antibody titer, unless contraindicated[b]
- Hepatitis B: all college students[b]
- Hepatitis A: in some states and regions with high incidences and for high-risk groups of students (see text)
- Meningococcal vaccine: college freshmen living in dormitories and other high-risk groups of students
- Influenza: annually for all students; priority in high-risk groups
- Pneumococcal vaccine: high-risk groups; may need revaccination[b,c]

[a] Based on the guidelines from the American College of Health Association.
[b] Recommended routine childhood immunizations in the United States.
[c] Pneumococcal vaccine used for infants or young children differs form the vaccine used in older children and adults with underlying medical conditions.

Adult Immunization [8]. The American College Health Association has published guidelines regarding PIRs as well [9]. College campuses in states with mandated PIRs have previously been shown to have a lower risk of VPD (measles) outbreaks [10]. Currently recommended prematriculation immunizations for college and university students are given in Box 1. Furthermore, there are several steps that colleges and universities can take to enhance campus-wide immunization rates. Box 2 lists factors that are known to contribute to increased use of vaccines. Many of these vaccines have been used for several years as part of the routine childhood immunizations in the United States and have an excellent safety profile. Vaccines of particular value to college students are discussed below.

Box 2. Factors likely to enhance immunization rates on college campuses

- Defined institutional policy regarding vaccine requirements
- Allocated budget for health promotion including vaccines
- Promotional materials identifying the institution's commitment to disease prevention and health promotion
- Providing vaccine information statements and consent documents to students and parents in a prematriculation information packet
- During orientation, have designated booths for vaccine- and health-related issues with available vaccine information statements, consent documents, and health care workers to immunize students needing vaccines
- Readily accessible database for immunization records
- Commitment of student health care providers toward immunization
- Regular promotional activities on campus regarding health
- Involving athletes/coaches for good health practices promotions
- Articles/columns in student newspaper regarding vaccines and disease prevention
- Computer-generated reminders to students needing immunizations
- Special clinics for mass immunizations when needed (eg, during the fall for influenza vaccine)
- A walk-in, no-appointment-necessary service for immunization
- Availability of immunization-related services during evenings and weekends
- Publicizing success rates of programs/health status of the campus

Meningococcal vaccine

Meningococcal vaccine is of special importance for the college student [1,2]. Although it is not part of the routinely recommended childhood and adolescent immunization schedule, as of August 2004 10 states required that a student must receive meningococcal vaccine for attendance at college or university in that state [11]. Several other states and many individual colleges/universities require accepted students and their parents to be informed about meningococcal disease and the availability of a vaccine for preventing this disease. Students—and in some cases parents—may then be required to choose to either have the student receive the vaccine or to sign a waiver stating that they decided not to obtain the meningococcal immunization. Although meningococcal meningitis is relatively uncommon in college-age individuals, certain groups of students, particularly first-year students living in dormitories or residence halls, are at a sixfold or greater risk of acquiring this disease [3,12]. Reimmunization 3 to 5 years after the initial dose is also strongly suggested for those college students who may be planning to study in countries known to have endemic or epidemic meningococcal disease. The current vaccine, a quadrivalent polysaccharide vaccine containing groups A, C, Y, and W-135, covers approximately 70% of the reported meningococcal disease cases in the 18- to 23-year age group [1]. *N meningitidis* group B, which is responsible for 20% to 30% of cases in this age group, is not included in the currently available vaccine. Although highly effective, the vaccine's efficacy is not 100% [10]. A new polysaccharide-protein conjugate quadrivalent (A, C, Y, W-135) vaccine is likely to be licensed by the US Food and Drug Administration before the end of 2004. This conjugate vaccine should provide immunologic memory along with a more prolonged high affinity antibody response to immunization compared with the current polysaccharide vaccine [13,14]. Experience with other polysaccharide-conjugate bacterial vaccines (*Haemophilus influenzae* type b and *Streptococcus pneumoniae*) in the United States has also demonstrated a reduction in nasopharyngeal carriage of vaccine-associated bacteria. Such a reduction in the carriage of vaccine strains of *N meningitidis* should result in improved "herd immunity" (ie, protection of unimmunized contacts), and ultimately, a further decrease in the numbers of cases with invasive disease than what could be normally expected from immunization alone.

Influenza vaccine

Any college student with an underlying chronic medical condition (ie, asthma, diabetes mellitus, sickle cell disease, others) should receive an influenza immunization annually. Influenza immunization of such "high risk" persons has been recommended since the early 1960s [15]. Although not routinely recommended for otherwise healthy college students, any student who wishes to decrease the risk of disruption of academic activities by influenza disease can receive the vaccine unless otherwise contraindicated (eg, allergy to eggs).

Hepatitis A and hepatitis B virus vaccines

Both hepatitis A and hepatitis B virus (HBV) infections can be prevented through immunization. HBV can be transmitted through sexual activity, contact with blood from infected individuals, and by use of contaminated needles (eg, drugs, tattoos, body piercing, others). Many states require evidence of hepatitis B immunization for children in grades K through 12; however, not all states currently have elementary or secondary school requirements for HBV vaccine. For hepatitis A, certain areas of the United States have infection rates that are significantly greater than the national average. Furthermore, students contemplating overseas study, those with chronic liver problems, and men who have sex with men should definitely consider receiving a vaccine to prevent hepatitis A virus infection [6]. A study that examined the cost-effectiveness of hepatitis A and B immunizations for United States college students concluded that, until infant/child/adolescent immunization can produce immune cohorts of adults, college-based hepatitis B immunization could cost-effectively reduce disease transmission [16]. Additionally, although combined hepatitis A and B vaccine would result in a higher initial cost, societal costs related to these two infections would decrease by 12% [16].

Varicella (chickenpox) vaccine

A vaccine to prevent chickenpox (varicella) was first licensed in the United States in 1995. This vaccine is now part of the routine recommended childhood immunization schedule. Varicella disease in adolescents and adults is associated with increased morbidity and mortality [17]. Furthermore, attack rates in close contact varicella susceptible individuals are quite high. Although most college students today would be expected to be immune, secondary to either having had disease as a child or secondary to immunization, some college/university students may have escaped natural infection or may not have been successfully immunized. International students, especially those from tropical countries, may have even higher rates of susceptibility than students born in the United States [18]. While a single immunization is sufficient to produce immunity in most children below 13 years of age, two doses of varicella vaccine 4 to 8 weeks apart are necessary in persons above 13 years of age. A history of disease is highly predictive of immunity.

Vaccines for college students traveling abroad

Immunization is one of the key elements of the health advice that should be offered to a student going abroad [19]. Several factors need to be considered before recommending vaccines to an individual, including destination, length of stay, climate, severity of the potential disease, and boarding facilities while abroad. Host-related issues (eg, any chronic illness, medications, and pregnancy) also need to be considered before immunizations are given. Immunization records and travel itinerary should be carefully reviewed. A person traveling abroad should be up-to-date on routinely recommended immunizations. If a student is traveling to an area of the world where polio remains endemic, a dose of inactivated polio vaccine should be offered to provide an additional boost to the existing immunity. For students traveling to one of the developing countries with high endemic rates for hepatitis A infection, hepatitis A vaccine is recommended. If hepatitis A vaccine cannot be administered, then intramuscular immunoglobulin should be used for immunoprophylaxis. If it cannot be ascertained whether a student has received two doses of the measles vaccine, then measles immunization should be recommended because measles is still endemic in several countries in the continents of Africa and Asia [19]. Yellow fever vaccine is required as a condition of entry for travelers arriving from endemic regions of the world, mostly located in sub-Saharan Africa and South America [20]. Yellow fever vaccine is an attenuated live virus vaccine and is only available through designated centers. The CDC travel health Web site (www.cdc.gov/travel) should be consulted to obtain further information. For students traveling to areas where frequent meningococcal epidemics occur (mostly sub-Saharan Africa), meningococcal polysaccharide vaccine (A, C, Y, and W 135) should be strongly recommended. Japanese encephalitis, a mosquito-borne, life-threatening viral encephalitis, is endemic in Southeast Asia, China, Eastern Russia, and the Indian subcontinent. For students who plan to stay abroad for a considerable period—particularly during the transmission season of this viral disease—or who are traveling to rural farming areas where outdoor exposure increases their likelihood of acquiring this infection, this vaccine is highly desirable. A three-dose vaccination schedule should be completed at least 10 days before arriving in the endemic area [19–21].

Typhoid vaccine is recommended for students traveling to developing countries where they may be exposed to contaminated water or poor sanitation. Two typhoid vaccines are available in the United States. For oral live attenuated *Salmonella typhi* (Ty21a strain vaccine), one capsule given on alternate days for a total of four doses is required. Antimicrobial agents and mefloquine should not be taken during this period, because those agents can inhibit the growth of these microbes. The only injectable typhoid vaccine available in the United States for general use is Vi capsular polysaccharide vaccine, which requires one intramuscular injection. Because none of the typhoid vaccines have a high efficacy, proper hygiene and careful selection of food items is essential. If it is anticipated that students may encounter rabid animals (eg, wildlife and dogs) or their excursions might include spelunking, then they should be advised to get a three-dose pre-exposure rabies vaccine series as well [19,21]. University officials counseling students who travel abroad should also obtain information from the CDC, the World Health Organization, and other published literature regarding preparing the traveler [19].

Vaccines on the horizon

There are several vaccines that are currently being evaluated and will likely be of value to college-age individuals in the future. It is well established that immunity to pertussis wanes within 10 years of the last booster, which is typically given at 4 to 6 years of age [22,23]. A reservoir of pertussis illness undoubtedly exists within the adolescent and young adult population in the United States. To further reduce and, ultimately, eliminate pertussis in the United States, improved immunity in the adolescent and young adult population is paramount. A TdaP, or an adult tetanus and diphtheria vaccine further combined with an acellular pertussis vaccine, will likely be licensed in the near future and initially targeted to be given to individuals between 11 and 64 years of age. If licensed, this vaccine would eventually replace the tetanus/diphtheria booster and would be given every 10 years.

Another vaccine that will be important to adolescents and young adults is the human papillomavirus (HPV) vaccine. HPV infection is common among sexually active men and women and is associated with both genital warts and cervical cancer. It is estimated that in the United States 10% to 20% of persons between 15 and 49 years of age have molecular evidence of infection [24]. A study conducted in the state of Washington among 603 female university students between 1990 and 2000 demonstrated that the acquisition of first-time HPV infection at 24 months was 32.3% (95% CI 28.0, 37.1) [25]. HPV infection, unlike other sexually transmitted diseases, may not be completely prevented by the use of condoms. Therefore, prevention of HPV infection through immunization, especially infection by those types specifically associated with cervical cancer, may be of significant value to adolescents and young adults. HPV vaccines could be licensed within the next 5 years. Vaccines to prevent other sexually transmitted diseases caused by herpes simplex virus and *Chlamydia trachomatis* are also in development.

Students with partial immunization

It is likely that a small number of students either received less than the recommended number of immunizations or received no immunizations at the time of entry into college. Although all 50 states have PIRs for grades K through 12, all states allow for medical exemption. All but two states allow for religious exemptions, and 20 states allow exemptions for philosophical reasons. Furthermore, a significant number of international students may fall into the category of partial or no immunization.

Infectious diseases and immunization-related issues in international students

Over the past two decades there has been a dramatic increase in international students on college campuses in the United States. Today more than half a million international students are enrolled in United States colleges and universities, approximately two thirds of whom are from developing countries. With the political turmoil that exists in several parts of the world, it is also likely that some students migrated to the United States as refugees [26]. University administrators and physicians should be aware of the prevalence of infectious diseases, especially VPDs, in the country of origin of these students [27–29]. Similarly, immunization requirements vary tremendously throughout the world [30,31]. In several developing countries, particularly those in Africa and Asia, mumps and rubella vaccines are not given with the measles vaccine. Therefore, it is likely that a significant number of nonimmunized students for rubella and mumps may be on the campus at any given time. Varicella vaccine is also not routinely used in several countries. Hepatitis B infection is endemic in several Southeast Asian countries and in Africa. Although hepatitis B vaccine has been added to the routine childhood immunizations in several countries where hepatitis B disease is endemic, it cannot be assumed that students originally from those countries have received that vaccine and are not carriers of hepatitis B virus.

Tuberculosis is widely prevalent in developing countries in the continents of Africa, Asia, and South America. Vaccination with Bacillus Calmette–Gŭerin (BCG) is commonly used in many countries in Africa, Asia, South America, and Eastern Europe. In the United States, basic screening for tuberculosis is done by performing a Mantoux skin test [32]. Even though there is the potential for the BCG vaccination to influence a Mantoux test, it is believed that a reaction of 15 mm or more to a Mantoux test should never be attributed to the BCG vaccination. All decisions regarding treatment should be made after carefully considering guidelines from the CDC and other authoritative resources [32,33].

Over the past two decades concern has also been raised about the potency of the vaccines used and the authenticity and reliability of the medical and immunization records from other countries. A healthy dose of skepticism is essential when reviewing medical records from sources not familiar to the physician.

Summary

Although VPDs have declined to record-low levels throughout the United States, immunizations continue to play an important role in the health and well-being of the college student population. Meningococcal disease, in particular, has been associated with certain risk factors at colleges and universities. College students lacking immunity to a VPD, such as measles or varicella, could, if infected, cause a campus-wide outbreak leading to significant morbidity and potential mortality. With outbreaks there is disruption of educational activities besides universities incurring additional expenses in controlling the problem. Although PIRs may vary from state to state and from institution to institution, they have been shown to reduce campus-wide outbreaks and are recommended by national organizations. Therefore, it is essential that by implementing effective policies, administrators encourage the use of these safe and effective vaccines on college campuses to further reduce the risk of students contracting a VPD.

Acknowledgments

The authors appreciate Erika Wilson's assistance in the preparation of this manuscript.

References

[1] Centers for Disease Control and Prevention. Meningococcal disease and college students. Recommendations of the Advisory Committee on Immunization Practices (ACIP). MMWR Morb Mortal Wkly Rep 2000;49:11–20.

[2] American Academy of Pediatrics Committee on Infectious Diseases. Meningococcal disease prevention and control strategies for practice based physicians. Pediatrics 2000;106:1500–4.

[3] Harrison CH, Dwyer DM, Maples CT, et al. Risk of meningococcal infection in college students. JAMA 1999;281:1906–10.

[4] Kelleher JA, Raebel MA. Meningococcal vaccine use in college students. Ann Pharmacother 2002;36:1776–84.

[5] Paneth N, Kort E, Jurczak D, et al. Predictors of vaccination rates during a mass meningococcal vaccination program on a college campus. J Am Coll Health 2000;49:7–11.

[6] American College Health Association. Immunizations: they're not just for children. Brochure #HS-32. Baltimore (MD): American College Health Association; 2003.

[7] Neinstein L. The healthy student. A parent's guide to preparing teens for the college years. 2003 Available at: www.adolescenthealth.org. Accessed September 7, 2004.

[8] National Foundation for Infectious Disease. Prematriculation immunization requirement (PIR). Available at: www.nfid.org/factsheets/pir.html. Accessed September 7, 2004.

[9] American College Health Association. ACHA Guidelines. Recommendations for institutional prematriculation immunizations. March 2003. Available at: www.acha.org. Accessed September 7, 2004.

[10] Baughman AL, Williams WW, Atkinson WL, et al. The impact of college prematriculation immunization requirements on risks for measles outbreaks. JAMA 1994;272:1127–32.

[11] Lazar K. State will mandate shots for collegians. Boston Herald: July 30, 2004. p. 2.

[12] Bruce MG, Rosenstein NE, Capparella JM, et al. Risk factors for meningococcal disease in college students. JAMA 2001;286:688–93.

[13] Granoff DM, Feavers IM, Borrow R. Meningococcal vaccines. In: Plotkin SA, Orenstein WO, editors. Vaccines. 4th edition. Philadelphia: WB Saunders; 2004. p. 959–87.

[14] Offit PA, Peter G. The meningococcal vaccine—public policy and individual choices. N Engl J Med 2003;349:2353–6.

[15] Fukuda K, Levandowski RA, Bridges CB, et al. Inactivated influenza vaccines. In: Plotkin SA, Orenstein WO, editors. Vaccines. 4th edition. Philadelphia: WB Saunders; 2004. p. 339–70.

[16] Jacobs RJ, Saab S, Meyerhoff AS. The cost effectiveness of hepatitis immunization for US college students. J Am Coll Health 2003;51:227–33.

[17] Meyer P, Seward JF, Jumaan AO, et al. Varicella mortality: trends before vaccine licensure in the United States, 1970–1994. J Infect Dis 2000;182:383–90.

[18] Seward J, Wharton M. Epidemiology of varicella. In: Arvin A, Gershon A, editors. Varicella-zoster virus. Cambridge (UK): Cambridge University Press; 2000. p. 187–205.

[19] Spira AM. Preparing the traveller. Lancet 2003;361:1368–81.

[20] Centers for Disease Control and Prevention. Yellow fever vaccine Recommendations of the Advisory Committee on Immunization Practices, 2002. MMWR Recomm Rep 2002; 51(RR-17):1–10.

[21] American Academy of Pediatrics. Immunizations in special clinical circumstances. In: Pickering LK, editor. Redbook: 2003 Report of the Committee of Infectious Diseases. 26th edition. Elk Grove Village (IL): American Academy of Pediatrics; 2003. p. 95–8.

[22] Fine PE, Clarkson JA. Reflection on the efficacy of pertussis vaccines. Rev Infect Dis 1987;9:866–83.

[23] Cattaneo LA, Reed GW, Haase DH, et al. The seroepidemiology of *Bordetella pertussis* infections: a study of persons 1–65 years. J Infect Dis 1996;173:1256–9.

[24] Koutsky L. Epidemiology of genital HPV infection. Am J Med 1997;102:3–8.

[25] Winer RL, Shu-Kuang L, Hughes JP, et al. Genital human papillomavirus infection: incidence and risk factors in a cohort of female university students. Am J Epidemiol 2003;157:218–26.

[26] Barnett ED. Infectious disease screening for refugees resettled in the United States. Clin Infect Dis 2004;39:833–41.

[27] Hersh BS, Tambini G, Nogueira AC, et al. Review of regional measles surveillance data in the Americas. Lancet 2000;355:1943–8.

[28] Staat MA. Infectious disease issues in internationally adopted children. Pediatr Infect Dis J 2002;21:257–8.

[29] Barnett ED, Holmes AH, Geltman P, et al. Immunity to hepatitis A in people born and raised in endemic areas. J Travel Med 2003;10:11–4.

[30] Irons B, Smith HC, Carrasco PA, et al. The immunisation programme in the Caribbean. Caribb Health 1999;3:9–11.

[31] Immunization Schedule in PAHO Member Countries. EPI Newsletter 1994;16:6.

[32] Mandalakas AM, Starke JR. Tuberculosis screening in immigrant children. Pediatr Infect Dis J 2004;23:71–2.

[33] Centers for Disease Control and Prevention. The role of the BCG vaccine in the prevention and control of tuberculosis in the United States: a joint state by the Advisory Council for the Elimination of Tuberculosis and the Advisory Committee on Immunization Practices. MMWR Recomm Rep 1996;45:1–18.

ELSEVIER
SAUNDERS

Pediatr Clin N Am 52 (2005) 243–278

PEDIATRIC CLINICS
OF NORTH AMERICA

Cardiovascular Disorders in the College Student

Eugene F. Luckstead, Sr, MD, FACC, FAAP

Department of Pediatrics, Texas Tech Medical School–Amarillo, 1500 Coulter Street, Amarillo,
TX 79106, USA

College students with possible congenital or acquired heart disease concerns often seek care from college health physicians. Information is provided in this article to help address such cardiac care needs in college students [1]. The major objective is to provide information enabling college physicians to diagnose and medically guide students. College student issues include severe chest pain, syncope, murmurs, possible dysrhythmias, hypertension, hyperlipidemia, mitral valve prolapse, and congenital and acquired heart anomalies. Those students with greater sudden cardiac death risk and surgically and interventionally treated congenital or acquired cardiac abnormalities merit special attention. The appendix adds practice-related case scenarios of cardiac problems.

College students can present unique challenges when possible cardiology issues exist, such as palpitations, activity-related orthopnea or dizziness, obesity, weight-related problems, and changing lifestyle modifications. Some student concerns originate from prior congenital and acquired cardiac problems. Physician guidance may be needed for short-term issues such as sports training or conditioning and obstetric cardiac complications. Long-term lifetime cardiac concerns exist in college students with hyperlipidemia, hypertension, and surgically corrected or palliated congenital or acquired heart lesions. Physicians caring for college students with valid cardiac issues must be aware of the latest interventional techniques such as stents, angioplasty, advancing pacemaker technology, electrophysiologic dysrhythmia detection, mapping, and improved ablation techniques.

More than one million young adult patients with congenital heart disease now lead normal or near normal lifestyles [2,3]. Most congenital cardiac patients as young adults are asymptomatic; fewer than 4% take cardiac medications

E-mail address: gene.luckstead@ttuhsc.edu

[4]. However, some students have significant residual congenital and acquired heart problems.

One also must appreciate the impact any cardiac problem has on social and psychologic aspects of patient care. Significant noncompliance cardiac care issues exist in the student population. A 30% to 40% noncompliance factor was noted by Gersony et al [5] in his large cardiac long-term follow-up study. Reminders on endocarditis precautions, safe activity-level guidance, and other restrictions are necessary when college students are in denial. Good communication among primary care physicians, cardiologists, and college physicians is critical for accurate information transfer and guidance [6,7]. When knowledge gaps include severity and classification of prior heart problems, reliable past medical information is mandatory [8,9].

College students with congenital heart anomalies can be classified into different groups. Doroshow [2] described three types of such cardiac patient care groups. Group one included mild congenital heart anomalies or well-tolerated defects like small ventricular septal defects (VSD), small patent ductus arteriosus (PDAs), mild aortic stenosis (AS), mild pulmonic stenosis (PS), and mitral valve prolapse. Group two had surgically or interventionally corrected VSDs, atrial septal defects (ASD), PDA, PS, or aortic coarctation patients. Patients with prior interventional, surgical palliation or correction for tetralogy of Fallot, transposition of great vessels (TGV), AS, or atrio-ventricular (A/V) canal defects made up group three. Additional reference information is also available from several other publications relevant for the college students with cardiac disease [1,3,10,11].

An increased risk for atrial dysrhythmias occurs after surgical ASD repair and possibly after interventional ASD closure [11]. Aortic valve stenosis patients often need further medical intervention later in life, such as angioplasty, surgical artificial valve replacement, or a Ross procedure [1]. College-aged students with an A/V canal defect (endocardial cushion defect) surgery need follow-up of their A/V valves (mitral or tricuspid) residual defects.

Although cardiac surgery for congenital heart anomalies is now successful in most instances, monitoring for persisting cardiac problems is needed. Such problems include abnormally high residual right or left ventricular pressures, significant residual ventricular septal defects, and pulmonary or aortic insufficiency. Also, ventricular arrhythmias, pacemaker implantation and follow-up after surgical complete heart block, and greater risk for sudden death warrant such monitoring in this college-aged group [1,10–13]. Closer scrutiny of older TGV patients with prior surgical atrial switch (Senning) or Mustard procedures is needed because of unpredictable long-term outcomes. By contrast, arterial switch (Jatene) corrective surgery for TGV has shown excellent outcomes [1,11]. Other forms of complex cyanotic lesions and single-ventricle spectrum anomalies have palliative operative procedures; most have either arterial shunts or Glenn or Fontan venocaval shunt operations and need individual or specialty physician monitoring.

Growth failure is uncommon in the young adult after correction or palliation of their cardiac anomalies and their pubertal growth. Obesity is a greater problem for these cardiac patients, similar to their noncardiac peer group [14]. Although other complaints such as chest pain and dyspnea occur more frequently, when compared with their noncardiac peers they usually are just as benign.

Bacterial endocarditis and exercise restriction is individualized depending on the congenital heart problem especially in the higher risk groups [1,11]. Most documented endocarditis cases occur in patients with cardiac abnormalities. Significant endocarditis in children with VSD, AS, or PS occurred in one large natural history study [5,11]. Bacterial endocarditis does not occur in ASD unless associated valve defects occur 6 months after complete repair for VSD and PDA and is uncommon with PS. However, be suspicious in the college-aged cardiac patient presenting with fever without a source, unexplained weight loss, malaise, chronic myalgia, and joint pain; obtain two to three blood cultures before starting antibiotics. Echocardiography can be especially helpful for right-sided heart lesions, VSD, and aortic valve lesions.

Psychosocial overlay occurring in college students with cardiac concerns mirrors emotional adjustments seen in others with chronic diseases. Anxiety, isolation, poor self-esteem, and depression occur in such cardiac patients. Sport participation is individualized; most can safely participate in various sport activities including elite-level athletics [1,11]. Intellectual function and levels of educational attainment are similar to their noncardiac peers. When they have mild or corrected heart disease, involvement in college activity is similar to that of peers without cardiac issues; some data suggest little difference occurs with the more severe forms of heart disease [15].

Chest pain in the college student

College students with chest pain complaints do fear an underlying cardiac cause for their chest pain [16,17]. Two types of chest pain are seen—one type is sharp and the other dull. The chest pain described as sharp and stabbing can be elicited by changing position, touching, or eating. [18] Other chest pain is more vague, nondescript, diffuse, and described as feeling pressure or dull. There are five major chest pain categories: musculoskeletal, pulmonary, gastrointestinal, psychologic, and cardiac. Noncardiac types of chest pain make up about 95%; only about 5% are actually cardiac in origin [11,19].

Most musculoskeletal chest pain is idiopathic; the pain is burning, pinprick, or stabbing. This pain is made worse with any increased intrathoracic pressure. Musculoskeletal pain can be chronic and recur over several weeks or months. The history should include questions on trauma, asthma, and allergies. Physical exam includes skin inspection for bruising, chest palpation for localized tenderness, and chest auscultation. One may need radiographs for possible rib fractures. EKGs and echocardiograms are indicated when cardiac problems are suspected. As musculoskeletal chest pain is self limited, only reassurance is needed. For some, a nonsteroidal anti-inflammatory or analgesic drug will relieve the pain. Heat application to the pain site alternating with moist and dry (heating pad) applications may also be helpful [11].

Chest pain from pulmonary causes such as asthma and infection is common [20]. This chest pain is secondary to inflammation of the pleura, pneumonia, or from a noninfectious cause. When pain complaints are severe, consider a pneumothorax. Spontaneous pneumothorax occurs more frequently in adolescents and young adults. When a tension pneumothorax results, severe chest pain and significant respiratory distress occur, requiring intubation or emergency insertion of a chest tube. Unless antecedent or other precipitating factors exist, acute dyspnea, fever, and severe chest pain from a pulmonary embolism are rare in college-aged students.

Upper gastrointestinal problems simulating chest pain occur in college students. Such pain results from esophagitis, gastritis from dietary or alcohol-related indiscretion, but occasionally peptic ulcers are present [21]. Typically those with peptic ulcers experience pain at night, which is exacerbated by eating, and will have mostly epigastric tenderness. Many students will have a family history of peptic ulcers.

Psychogenic chest pain origin accounts for approximately one fourth of college-aged students seen for chest pain complaints. Two thirds of these cases are associated with deaths in the family, separation anxiety, or some type of physical disability. About half of these patients have a family history of a similar condition. Often these students will have chest pain associated with hyperventilation syndrome or adolescent and young adult depression [11].

Cardiac chest pain

Although uncommon in the college student, several cardiac disease entities have chest pain as their clinical presentation. A history of exercise-related syncope or dizziness, recurrent syncope, severe chest pain, palpitations, and a family history of sudden death in young relatives should heighten cardiac concerns of hypertrophic cardiomyopathy. Arrhythmias can present as chest pain with most patients having some type of supraventricular or ventricular tachycardia. Additionally, cardiac-associated syndromes (eg, Marfan syndrome, Turner syndrome) present with a chief complaint of chest pain. Subtle congenital abnormalities of the coronary arteries can remain asymptomatic until chest pain or death occurs during exercise or sport activity. These anomalies include anomalous left coronary artery with the left coronary artery originating from the pulmonary artery, a single coronary artery, or other anomalies; most are recognized only after exercise and sudden death [22].

Acquired coronary artery abnormalities can occur in college-aged students and cause chest pain complaints. The potential for acquired coronary artery injury exists from Kawasaki disease. Twenty percent of untreated cases develop coronary aneurysms typically after the second or third week of the illness. Will many people with a Kawasaki history eventually develop a premature coronary artery problem? The answer is unknown. College students with homozygous type II hypercholesterolemia have an increased risk for developing coronary artery disease.

A source of chest pain can be pericardium involvement either primary or secondary from an infection (viral, bacterial, or fungal), autoimmune diseases, or inflammatory reaction. The myocardium is affected by many disease entities. Such myocardial involvement includes infectious agents (Cocsackie B virus, diphtheria, and other bacteria, fungal, or parasitic agents), drugs (cocaine), autoimmune reactions, or malignancies. These patients can present with congestive heart failure and chest pain or be surprisingly asymptomatic. Patients with anomalies of their cardiac valves clinically may have chest pain (ie, patients with severe aortic stenosis or mitral valve prolapse). About 10% to 15% of patients with mitral valve prolapse do complain of recurrent chest pain episodes; however, their pain cause appears to be idiopathic. Severe aortic valve stenosis-related chest pain is likely coronary artery ischemia related [11].

College-age atherosclerosis risk factors

Can risk factors for cardiovascular atherosclerosis in older adults be modified or changed during the adolescent and young adult years? The answer is largely unknown. Such risk factors in college students include obesity, smoking, sedentary lifestyle habits, and increased dietary fat intake. Essential hypertension may begin in adolescence or young adulthood and increases the risk of cardiovascular death in later adulthood. Physicians caring for youth can detect factors that cause considerable morbidity and even mortality later in life. Therefore, careful evaluation and effective education that promotes healthy adult life styles could pay big dividends in the adolescent and young adult.

The two basic lesions of atherosclerosis are the "reversible" fatty streak or spot present in all infants and children and the "nonreversible" atheromatous plaque usually present after puberty. Most fatty streaks remain unchanged or disappear during adolescence, but some may instead progress and become precursors of the atheromatous plaques. By contrast, most atheromatous plaques are extracellular, derived from plasma lipoproteins and are not reversible [23–27]. A multi-center cooperative study of Pathological Determinants of Atherosclerosis in Youth (PDAY) [28–30] performed autopsies on 2876 accident victims from 15 to 34 years of age; one half were black and one fourth were women. Boys aged 15 to19 years had about 20% fatty streaks in the aorta; plaques were only 0.35% in the aorta. The right coronary artery had fatty streaks in 1.8% of boys; plaques occurred in 0.2% of girls and 0.5% of boys. Atheromatous plaque development is similar for boys or girls until 15 years of age. No correlation was found between serum cholesterol level, aortic, or right coronary atheromatous plaques between the ages of 15 to 24 years; only largely reversible fatty streaks were seen until 15 years of age [23,28–32]. Significant numbers of atheromatous plaques do not occur in coronary arteries of boys until after 19 years of age. Although high blood cholesterol levels increase fatty streak formation, they don't enhance atheromatous plaque formation. [28–30,33] Actual progression in some instances does occur from arterial large vessel fatty streaks to nonreversible atheromatous plaques after puberty in males and after menopause in most females [28–31, 34,35].

Can cardiac risk factors such as high plasma lipids, hypertension, smoking, abdominal girth obesity, physical inactivity, and high dietary fat intake be changed in college youth? Regular exercise causes decreased LDL-C and increased HDL-C, reduces high blood pressure, and improves overall glucose metabolism. Some have postulated that regular exercise actually retards atherosclerosis progression or possibly causes a mild reversal. However, experimental evidence confirming that beneficial effects from exercise slowing the process of atherosclerosis is lacking. Physical activity or exercise has a positive effect on obesity factors and decreases mild or moderate systemic hypertension [36,37]. As obesity is partially responsible for the clustering of many cardiovascular risk factors, increased physical activity is a critical part of any youth obesity management program. Diet-induced weight loss alone without exercise or weight-training results in both fat and undesired "fat-free" muscle loss.

The apparent effect of diet, exercise, drugs, and genetics on all these parameters provides interesting results, which can be interpreted differently by physicians, cardiovascular experts, nutritionists, and other international groups [38–43]. The importance of long-term studies on such modifiable cardiovascular risk factors is being tracked by prospective cardiovascular long-term lipid study groups [44–47]. Although risk factors for atherosclerosis such as high cholesterol, hypertension, hypercystinemia, smoking, and obesity were low-risk factors in the past for children and young adults, now obesity, smoking, less physical activity, and type 2 diabetes mellitus are becoming more prevalent [48]. Pediatric obesity has increased about 30% in prevalence the last decade. Smoking also seems to be increasing in the adolescent and college ages [11]. If diet alone isn't the answer, what direction should physicians be providing for our youth? One obvious answer is the need for increased and sustained physical activity options for all college students. Students should opt for at least 40 to 60 minutes of moderate to vigorous physical activity per day. This need not be sport related. Increased physical activity levels when coupled with prudent dietary habits enhance all weight control issues, reduce marginal or high blood pressure, and promote long-term healthy lifestyle behaviors.

When should physicians screen for hyperlipidemia in young adults; especially LDL and HDL cholesterol? A multi-step process has been recommended by the Expert Panel on Blood Cholesterol Levels in Children and Adolescents [49]. Health assessment involves obtaining a family history for hyperlipidemia (one or both parents has a cholesterol level at or over 240 mg/dL) and premature cardiovascular events; if there is a positive family history, the youth is screened with a total cholesterol or fasting lipoprotein profile. The results of two fasting profiles can be averaged. A positive family history concerns a parent or grandparent with documented coronary artery disease before age 55 years. A positive history will document a myocardial infarction, sudden death, cardiac catheterization documenting coronary artery disease, angina pectoris, peripheral vascular disease, or cerebrovascular disease. Some clinicians do screen patients with an unknown family history but secondary hyperlipidemia exists and the cardiovascular risk factors of hypertension and obesity (Box 1).

Initial management for elevated lipids starts with dietary education. Mild elevations of LDL cholesterol and triglycerides usually are from secondary hyperlipidemia and one treats the underlying disorder along with dietary counseling. Primary hyperlipidemia is an uncommon genetic disorder affecting lipoprotein metabolism. Familial hypercholesterolemia, an autosomal dominant conditionm has very high LDL levels, decreased HDL levels, and normal triglyceride levels [11].

All youth should eat healthy diets, whether they have hyperlipidemia or not [50,51]. Their total cholesterol intake should be 300 mg a day, and total dietary fats about 30% of their caloric intake with saturated fats (including trans-unsaturated fats) less than 10%. This is the American Heart Association Step I diet. One should also stress youth promotion of proper exercise, avoidance of smoking, and decreasing exogenous obesity. If the total cholesterol is 170 to 199 mg/dL or LDL-C is 110 to 129 mg/dL, further dietary change is recom-

---

Box 1. Some examples of secondary hyperlipidemia

Alcohol
Anabolic steroids
Anorexia nervosa
Antihypertensive medication
Chronic renal disease
Diabetes mellitus
Glucocorticoids (hypercortisolism)
Hypothyroidism
Hypopituitarism
Isoretinoin
Nephrotic syndrome
Obesity (major factor)
Oral contraceptives
Obstructive liver disease
Pregnancy
Systemic lupus erythematosus

Adapted from Rowlett JD, Greydanus DE. The cardiovascular system in adolescent medicine. 3rd edition. Hoffmann AD, Greydanus DE, editors. Stamford, CT: Appleton and Lange; 1997. p. 147–73.

mended and advised to stay on the Step I diet. The lipoprtein panels are followed annually. When total cholesterol is 200 mg/dL or higher or the LDL-C is > 129 mg/dL, stricter dietary guidelines are needed. Total daily cholesterol intake is restricted < 200 mg and saturated fats less than 7%. This is the American Heart Association Step II diet.

Lipoprotein values normally change markedly from birth to early infancy; further changes continue into childhood, adolescence, and young adults until 32 years of age [23]. The average serum cholesterol from ages 1 year to 15 years is 150 mg/dL.; LDL-C level average is 100 mg/dL, and HDL-C average 50 mg/dL for both sexes.

Statin therapy is used when other measures fail, especially if the LDL is very high. These medications are now routinely used in adults, but side effects may limit their use during the adolescent and college-age years. Statin or HMG-CoA reductase inhibitors affect the hepatic LDL receptors while inhibiting the production of cholesterol; cholesterol (total and LDL) and triglycerides are lowered while HDL cholesterol increases. Side effects from statins include liver dysfunction-damage, myalgia, rash, and headaches.

Accurate hypertension diagnosis and proper management are important issues in adolescents and young adults. Apply the standard blood pressure reference values and guides published previously and cited in several recent texts [52–55]. These blood pressure guidelines are standardized from age 1 to 17 years and for female and male young adults. The blood pressure systolic, diastolic > 90 and > 95 percentiles are plotted against their referenced age and height standard percentiles during the pediatric, adolescent, and adult years. Blood pressure findings >140 systolic and > 90 diastolic usually are suspect for hypertension in the older ages, and > 120 systolic and > 80 diastolic suspect in younger ages, assuming proper blood pressure measurement techniques are used [52,55]. Management factors depend on the patient diagnosis of mild, moderate, or severe hypertension. Whether it is acute, subacute, or chronic systolic or diastolic, systemic hypertension also influences treatment measures. Anxiety, illness, drug side effects or abuse, obesity factors, renal, cardiac, and endocrine-related hypertension causes will need further study. Essential hypertension occurs in families in a high percentage where there is no known cause. Ambulatory blood monitoring or exercise stress testing can unmask labile or anxiety-related sources of hypertension. Severe hypertension requires close observation and treatment in a hospitalized setting; potent beta-blockers, vasodilators and other intravenous (IV) medications are used. An individualized approach to each case is preferred by most physicians instead of the previous use of a step-wise medication sequence with diuretics, beta-blockers, angiotensin-converting enzyme (ACE) inhibitors, calcium channel blockers, and other agents [52,53,55].

In summary, college students must understand the importance of increasing exercise and physical activity, improving weight control, decreasing smoking, and reducing hypertension to reduce cardiac risk factors. Safe and effective drug intervention for the high-risk atherosclerosis college students at this time appears possible but unproven for long-term use. College physicians can help address these short and long-term lifestyle challenges and cardiovascular and medical concerns for college students.

Heart murmurs and selected congenital heart anomalies in college students

One can detect a heart murmur in 50% of adolescents but such murmurs are much less frequent in young adults. Actual congenital or acquired heart disease is present in only 1% of those with murmurs. Of the large number of benign or "innocent" murmurs, two are most commonly noted. One is the pulmonary or high-pitched right ventricular origin outflow murmur and the second is the vibratory or musical quality early and midsystolic left ventricular murmur (Still's murmur). Usually the murmurs are grade 2 or 3, based on the 1–6 Levine murmur scale; thrills (with grade 4–6 murmurs) are uncommon (see additional murmur descriptions in the following sections) [52,56–58].

Advances in surgery over the past 30 years have significantly altered the natural history of many congenital cardiac disorders and most such children now are healthy and thriving in the adolescent and adult years [11,59–61]. However, some congenital cardiac disorders do escape childhood detection and are not be diagnosed until later; some of these are listed in Box 2 [52,61,62].

Aortic stenosis

AS clinically has a grade 2 or 3/6 systolic ejection murmur noted over the aortic area—second right and third left intercostal space. The murmur and associated systolic ejection click (valve only) is referred to the upper precordium, cardiac apex, and neck vessel areas. A thrill is palpable at the aortic valve and referral areas with grade four or greater murmurs (more common with subaortic

---

Box 2. Possible congenital heart anomalies in young adults

Anomalous coronary artery
Atrial septal defect
Aortic stenosis (bicuspid valve most common)
Coarctation of the aorta
Mitral valve prolapse
Pulmonary valve stenosis
Ventricular septal defects
Patent ductus arteriosus
Endocardial cushion defects (A/V canal types)

stenosis) [52,56,57,59] Isolated AS occurs in 3% to 5% of congenital heart anomalies, but AS is associated with 20% of other heart defects. Students have symptoms of chest pain, syncope, dyspnea, and fatigue if moderate or severe stenosis is present. Most students with mild or moderate AS are asymptomatic. EKG left ventricular hypertrophy is uncommon with AS; most have normal EKGs [11,56,63]. Blood pressure taken properly shows a narrow pulse pressure [64]. Progressive aortic valve stenosis often occurs; moderate or severe aortic stenosis may lead to exercise-related sudden death in ~1%. Youth with aortic stenosis can participate in specific sports with guidance and clearance provided by experts in cardiology and sports medicine by using national guidelines [65–67]. Surgical and medical issues include early diagnosis, subacute bacterial endocarditis (SBE) prophylaxis, interventional palliative measures, or surgery (eg, surgical valvotomy, balloon angioplasty, valve replacement) or the eventual use of the Ross surgical procedure [11].

Atrial septal defect

ASDs have no specific murmur; but their RV volume overload amplifies the functional pulmonary outflow murmur at the second left intercostal space. When pulmonary blood flow is greater than 2:1, experienced physicians hear a late (scratchy) diastolic tricuspid murmur or diastolic flow rumble (a functional tricuspid stenosis). A helpful clinical sign is a widely split and fixed second heart sound. Secundum ASDs are most common atrial defect in young adults; incomplete endocardial cushion (ostium primum ASD) defects are a distant second. A superior or left electrocardiographic QRS axis and mild RVH occurs more with ostium primum defects than secundum defects; echocardiograms usually delineate the ASD type. Occasionally sinus venosus type ASDs are encountered. Mild right ventricular enlargement on chest radiograph with mildly increased vascularity and an enlarged pulmonary artery segment are noted. Most ASD secundum types are closed interventionally today. There are recent reports of occasional dysrhythmias after interventional closure [68]. Except for bicuspid aortic valve defects, ASDs remain the most common defect seen in adolescent, young, and older adults [11,56,62,67].

Coarctation of the aorta

Mild or moderate aortic coarctation can go undiagnosed until adolescence or young adulthood. Coarctation of the aorta is often associated with a bicuspid aortic valve. Leg pain complaints, weakness, or cramps in the legs occur during or after exercise. A systolic ejection murmur can occur over the back, inter-scapular, and left chest supraclavicular regions. Coarctation causes arm hyper-tension with leg hypotension and delayed or absent femoral pulses. The phenotype of increased upper extremity musculature along with "stork-like" or thin legs occurs more frequently in older patients. Patients with coarctation of the aorta will have systolic bruits over the chest from collateral vessel circulation; chest radiographs show a dilated ascending aorta and posterior rib notching. If untreated or unrecognized, premature death in adults occurs from coarctation complications such as a dissecting aortic aneurysm rupture or cebrovascular accident (CVA) type complications from Circle of Willis aneurysm rupture. Management involves surgical or interventional palliation or correction of the aortic coarctation and associated defects. Excessive collateral vessel bleeding complications in older age coarctation of the aorta surgery occurs and spinal cord special perfusion is needed [11,56,59].

Mitral valve prolapse

Mitral valve prolapse (MVP) was initially diagnosed by echocardiographic studies in 5% to 10% of the general population; 20% were female adolescents and young women. When later revised MVP criteria were applied, mitral valve prolapse incidence was lowered to ~2% of the general population [69]. This anomaly usually is identified after ten years of age as an isolated finding; however, it can be seen earlier with certain cardiac-related syndromes like Marfan or Ehlers-Danlos syndrome (Box 3).

MVP typically has a mid-systolic click from prolapse of the posterior mitral valve leaflet into the left atrium. A late systolic murmur of mitral regurgitation

---

Box 3. Cardiac conditions/anomalies seen with mitral valve prolapse

Anorexia nervosa
Anxiety disorders
Atrial septal defects
Ehlers-Danlos syndrome
Marfan syndrome
Pectus carinatum or excavatum
Rheumatic fever
Rheumatoid arthritis
Scoliosis
Straight back syndrome
Systemic lupus erythematosus

Modified from Greyandus DE, Patel D, Pratt H, Bhave S, editors. India manual of adolescent medicine; review of adolescent medicine: cardiovascular disorders. Delhi, India: Cambridge Press; 2002.

follows the mid-systolic click. Examining the patient in an upright or standing position or performing a Valsalva maneuver decreases left ventricular volume and may enhance the MVP [11]. Some cardiologists advocate not diagnosing MVP unless actual evidence of myxomatous degeneration of the mitral valve exists [69]. A loud holosystolic murmur suggests the presence of moderate to severe mitral regurgitation with degeneration (similar to the Rheumatic Carey-Coombs murmur). A careful evaluation (including EKG, two- and three-dimensional echocardiography, three-dimensional MRI) is used to identify mitral valve dysfunction and clinically significant mitral regurgitation. There is a higher MVP incidence in females than males; frequently other family members have MVP [11].

MVP may be asymptomatic and noted on routine cardiac examination; one third have chest pain, tachycardia, palpitations, or fainting spells. Theories for chest pain origin include chordae tendinea stretching, myocardial ischemia, or arrhythmias. The pain can be a stabbing, precordial pain lasting hours to days; severe pain and cardiac arrhythmias can develop. Management depends on MVP severity. Youth without clinical findings of mitral insufficiency or symptoms have a benign course and need periodic evaluation for the development of mitral insufficiency. If chest pain develops, evaluate for other causes (see chest pain section). Beta-blockers may control chest pain in MVP especially when it is associated with arrhythmias. Patients with mitral valve insufficiency need SBE prophylaxis, whereas significant arrhythmias need cardiologic specialty evaluation and anticipatory management. Long-term studies have shown MVP to be a mild or benign condition unless serious arrhythmias occur or significant myxomatous valve degeneration occurs [70]. Sudden death rarely results from MVP and associated arrhythmias. Most students with MVP can participate safely in all sport and exercise activities with no or minimal restrictions. Females with MVP should not be on estrogen-containing contraceptives, due to the increased possibility of venous thromboembolism [56].

Patent ductus arteriosus

Patent ductus arteriosus (PDA) if small or moderate in size may go undiagnosed until later childhood and occasionally the adolescent or young adult years [62]. Clinically, patients have a continuous murmur, which peaks or "spills over" the second heart sound at the second left intercostal space or left upper chest area; occasionally it's heard over the back. PDAs are commonly associated with coarctation of the aorta, aortic valve stenosis, or both. When PDA is an isolated lesion, pulses are increased in both the arms and legs. When pulmonary blood flow is more than twice the systemic blood flow, one has an apical flow rumble or murmur (a resultant functional mitral stenosis from LV volume overload). EKG may be normal or show LVH; echocardiograms are usually diagnostic. Treatment is interventional or surgical, but risk of SBE or shortened life span or complications is increased without treatment [11,56].

Pulmonic stenosis

Pulmonic stenosis at the valve, infundibulum, and supravalvar levels can be undiagnosed until later childhood, adolescence, or adulthood. Pulmonic valve stenosis is the most common site; a systolic ejection click often precedes the systolic ejection murmur. A click is not heard in other types of pulmonic stenosis. The murmur refers to the upper chest from the valve level, is maximal at the valve site, and refers more to the left than right axilla. The amount of EKG right ventricular hypertrophy correlates with the degree of pulmonic stenosis in contrast to aortic stenosis where EKG correlation is poor. Echocardiography offers excellent diagnostic correlation for pulmonic stenosis severity. Increasing murmur intensity also correlates with increased pulmonic stenosis. Balloon angioplasty is an effective treatment for moderate or severe valve pulmonic stenosis. Some still require surgical relief, but most moderate or severe cases are recognized and treated in early childhood. Pulmonary stenosis is the principal heart anomaly in specific syndromes (Noonan, Leopard, and Rubella) and involves the valve and peripheral pulmonary artery or suprapulmonic levels [11,52, 56,60,71].

Tetralogy of Fallot

Children treated surgically for cyanotic congenital heart disorders now function well and survive well past young adulthood. Some have had Blalock-Taussig (subclavian artery to pulmonary artery) and other palliative shunts or total repair for their ventricular septal defect and infundibular pulmonic stenosis. A good predictive factor for long-term complications is their residual degree of right ventricular dysfunction. As college students, they will have a systolic ejection murmur at the right upper sternal border radiating to the back, chest, and axilla from pulmonary stenosis or residual right ventricular outflow dynamics. They often have pulmonary valve regurgitation, causing a protodiastolic murmur at the left upper sternal border. Both murmurs are common in youth after prior tetralogy of Fallot repair [11,56].

Major postoperative problems for such students include arrhythmias, sudden death, endocarditis, and myocardial failure. These youth are still encouraged to lead an active lifestyle but need SBE prophylaxis according to published standards [52,56,72,73]. Those with a history of cyanotic congenital heart disease and palliative cardiac surgery have greater risk for thromboembolism. Low-dose estrogen oral contraception is a safe option for sexually active youth who wish effective contraception [56]. The female adolescent with a good hemodynamic repair has the same risk of pregnancy complications as the general population. However, the risk of an infant with congenital heart disease is higher; genetic counseling is recommended and studies like a fluorescent in situ hybridization (FISH) for microdeletion on chromosome 22 (22 q11-) [74]. Fetal echocardiography is performed during the second trimester.

Ventricular septal defects

Murmurs from ventricular septal defects (VSDs) are usually holosystolic or pansystolic, medium to high in pitch, and grade 2 to 3 in murmur intensity. The smaller defects are actually louder than the bigger defects because of their restrictive nature (pressure differences between their left and right ventricles). When ventricular septal defects become smaller, they often have late attenuation of the murmur and attain higher pitch before spontaneous closure. Most VSDs are heard maximally at the left lower sternal border; some are heard best at the base of the heart. Larger defects have an associated diastolic flow rumble at the apex if the pulmonary blood flow is over twice the systemic blood flow ("functional" mitral stenosis from left atrial volume overload). Apical defects are least likely to close spontaneously, but 70% of small and medium sized ventricular septal defects do close by 5 to 6 years of age and another 10% by adolescence [1,11,56]. Thus, one expects to find about 10% to 20% of young adults and adolescents with persistent VSDs.

Other cyanotic cardiac anomalies

Surgically treated cyanotic lesions such as transposition of great vessels (TGV), total anomalous pulmonary return (TAPVR), tricuspid atresia, and single ventricle are seen in college students. Those with arterial switch correction for TGV are doing very well; similarly, TAPVR also do well. Other college students that have the cardiac anomalies of tricuspid atresia and single ventricle will be at various stages of palliation and need individual management guidelines and modification as they proceed through college life and into adulthood [11].

Syncope, dizziness, and possible cardiac problems

The evaluation of the college student with syncope must be thorough. An accurate description of the syncope event is very helpful. Prior cardiac problems, family history of syncope, associated illnesses, medication or drug use/abuse are obtained from the history [75–79]. There is a definite association with syncope during exercise and sudden death in both college-aged athletes and nonathletes. Syncope was associated with sudden death in nearly 25% of the cases [52,78]. However, most causes of syncope still are neurocardiac or vasovagal; physicians must search diligently for those that are more likely cardiac in origin.

EKG, Holter, and event monitors are helpful with dyrhythmia-related syncope, and echocardiographic studies or exams will help diagnose muscle function, valve and abnormal coronary, systemic, and pulmonary vessel abnormalities [52,80]. Exercise stress testing, electrophysiologic conduction mapping, and cardiac catheterization and angiography are needed in the higher risk syncope diagnostic dilemmas [52,78]. Students with exercise-related severe dizziness or syncope warrant further cardiovascular evaluation. This is especially true if planning to participate in sport or exercise-related activities [11].

Hypotension-associated dizziness episodes are relatively common in the adolescent and young adult, but most are orthostatic. Table 1 lists some of the underlying factors that may lead to such phenomena in youth. The most common factor is syncope or near-syncopal episodes. Neurocardiogenic syncope is diagnosed largely by history; some may need confirmation by a positive Tilt-Table Test. The evaluation includes a thorough history, including specifics such as amount of sleep, type of fluid intake, medication taken, and eating patterns. A careful physical examination and urine-specific gravity test also help to assess fluid volume status; other tests may be indicated by the findings. Management focuses on the perceived underlying cause [75–79].

Syncope during exercise is very different from syncope that occurs after extreme exercise or aerobic activities. One must diligently search for an underlying cardiac, CNS, or metabolic cause when syncope occurs during exercise as there is a higher risk of life-threatening events (see Table 1) [52]. Exercise-induced syncope without structural heart disease confirmed by Tilt-Table testing to be hypotension related is usually correctable by medical measures alone [52–76]. The recently described Brugada Syndrome has a high risk of

Table 1
Pathophysiology: syncope in college students

Vasomotor CV	Cardiac structural	Noncardiac causes
Neurocardiac system	Obstructive anomalies	Central nervous
-vaso-vagal	-Aortic stenosis	-Seizures
(most common)	-HCM (cardiomyopathy)	-Migraine
Increased vagal tone	-Coarctation of aorta	Metabolic-Endocrine
-fear, anxiety	Dysrhythmias	-Hypoglycemia
-adolescents	-Long or Short QT interval	-Hyperglycemia
-athletes	-SVT; VT; AF	-Toxins-poisoning
	-W-P-W; Heart block	
Psychiatric/psychological		
	-Pacemaker dysfunction	-
Hyperventilation/hysterical		
Reflex	Cardiac LV dysfunction	-Drug abuse
-Cough, hair grooming	-CHF	
-Positional, micturation	-Coronary artery anomalies	
Orthostatic		
-Dehydration		
-blood loss		

Abbreviations: AF, atrial fibrillation; CHF, congestive heart failure; HCM, hypertrophic cardiomyopathy; SVT, supraventricular tachycardia; VT, ventricular tachycardia; WPW, pre-excitation syndrome or Wolff-Parkinson-White syndrome.
Modified from Luckstead EF. Cardiovascular evaluation of the young athlete. Adolescent Med (STARS) 1998;9:441–55.

sudden death with exercise preceded by a syncopal event in ~80% of cases. Most reported cases were male adolescent and young adults [52,81].

Sudden death, dysrhythmias, palpitations and anxiety panic attacks

Hypertrophic cardiomyopathy, coronary artery anomalies, long QT syndromes, and Marfan syndrome remain the top four causes of exercise-associated sudden cardiac death in adolescents and young adults. All four can have syncope and chest pain as presenting symptoms or they can remain entirely asymptomatic until their sudden death episode [52,82]. Sport participation, training, and other exercise-related activities often precipitate symptoms of severe dizziness or syncope; unfortunately, some have sudden unexpected death. Exercise-related tachyarrhythmias occur with pre-excitation syndromes, long and short QT syndromes, Brugada syndrome, coronary artery anomalies, and other cardiac entities [52,81]. Diagnosis of only 20% of coronary artery anomalies occurs before sudden death. Exertional chest pain or syncope with exercise-related EKG changes was the only warning signs in these patients. Basilico's review of multiple sudden death studies in athletes demonstrated that between 42% and 57% of sudden deaths were cardiomyopathy related [67]. Patients with Long QT syndrome (QTc: > 460 msec; preferably > 500 msec) can achieve significant reduction in their sudden death risk by using beta-blocker medication. Several series have reported reductions from a 60% to 70% sudden death to 6% in Long QT patients [52]. Unfortunately, some undiagnosed youth with Long QT syndrome have sudden death as their first and only event. Routine EKGs only diagnose about 10% of Long QT individuals. Long QT syndrome patients will present with a history of syncope (30%), palpitations (15%), seizures (10%), and cardiac arrest (9%) [52,75,76]. There is a 30% positive family history for Long QT syndrome. Incidence in general population is one per 5000 population [83]. Recent genetic-phenotype correlations have been studied closely in Long QT syndromes trying to help predict those with a greater risk with swimming and increased exercise; other have sleep-related and auditory triggers for sudden death [84]. Intense aerobic activity and competitive sports can be lethal, but if a patient is on selected medication, recreational activities are usually permissible.

Acquired heart problems in the college student

Rheumatic fever and rheumatic heart disease

Rheumatic fever remains the leading cause of acquired heart disease in the world for children, adolescents, and young adults but is now second to Kawasaki syndrome in the pediatric ages (birth to 18 years) in America. The peak occurrence is late childhood age 7 to 10 years and late adolescence age 18 to 21 years. It is a collagen vascular disease affecting various systems in the body and involves an antigen-antibody immunologic hypersensitivity reaction that occurs within 2 to 3 weeks after either untreated or partially treated pharyngitis due to group A, beta-hemolytic streptococcus. Those with one episode are at greater risk for reccurence especially in the first year and the following five years. Rheumatic fever does not develop from streptococcal skin diseases, such as impetigo. Approximately 2% to 3% of untreated pharyngitis due to group A, beta-hemolytic streptococcus result in the sequelae of acute rheumatic fever.

Major clinical manifestations based on the revised Jones Criteria for acute rheumatic fever are carditis, polyarthritis, chorea, erythema marginatum, and subcutaneous nodules. Minor manifestations include arthralgia, fever, and positive laboratory tests (elevated erythrocyte sedimentation rate or elevated C-reactive protein). The presence of two major manifestations or one major (exceptions: Sub Q nodules or eythema marginatum alone) with two minor criteria strongly suggest rheumatic fever as the diagnosis [11,56,85–87]. Evidence of a preceding Group A beta-hemolytic streptococcal infection includes a positive throat culture, a positive rapid streptococcal antigen test and elevated streptococcal antibody titers of antistreptolysin O (ASO: above 250 to 300 Todd units), anti-streptokinase, anti-hyaluronidase, Anti-DNase B (antideoxyribonuclease B), or Anti-DPNase (antidiphosphopyridine nucleotidase) (Box 4 includes a differential diagnosis list for rheumatic fever) [11,56,88–90].

Carditis occurs in approximately 50% of rheumatic fever patients; children have this complication more than young adults do. The endocardium is more

---

Box 4. Differential diagnosis of rheumatic fever

Infective endocarditis
Infectious mononucleosis
Chorea
Henoch-Schonlein Purpura
Lyme disease
Myocarditis or pericarditis
Mixed collagen-vascular disease
Rheumatoid arthritis
Rubella arthritis
Septic arthritis
Serum sickness
Systemic lupus erythematosus
Uremia

Adapted from Greyandus DE, Patel D, Pratt H, Bhave S, editors. India manual of adolescent medicine; review of adolescent medicine: cardiovascular disorders. Delhi, India: Cambridge Press; 2002.

commonly involved, followed by myocardium and pericardium. Carditis develops within 3 weeks of the streptococccal infection and may follow the arthritis. If both major criteria occur, one is typically more severe than the other is. If chorea develops, carditis (usually mild) is present 30% of the time. Rheumatic fever patients with severe carditis have tachycardia and moderate to severe endocardial valve inflammation (usually with a so-called Carey-Coombs murmur suggestive of severe mitral regurgitation) and mild to moderate aortic regurgitation. When both aortic valve and mitral valve insufficiency occur together clinically or by echocardiographic studies, this strongly suggests acute rheumatic fever. Acute rheumatic fever is easier to diagnose when it is moderate to severe in degree; particularly in the 7- to 10-year-old or adolescent to young adult age ranges. Congestive heart failure can occur when the myocardium is primarily involved. Myocarditis can present with a broad range of clinical features, ranging from significant prolonged PR interval delay to clinical myocarditis with congestive heart failure. Sub Q nodules and erythema marginatum (or annulare) often accompany severe carditis in acute rheumatic fever patients [11,56].

Pericardial involvement with rapidly developing effusion with impending cardiac tamponade represents the greatest acute rheumatic fever lethal risk factor and must be aggressively treated. Pericarditis also can vary clinically, including distant heart sounds, friction rub, chest pain ,and specific EKG findings. Youth with pericardial effusion but no valvulitis may not have rheumatic fever but other disorders instead such as systemic lupus erythematosus, mixed collagen vascular disease, infectious pericarditis, or juvenile rheumatoid arthritis [87]. Usually nonrheumatic fever disorders with pericardial effusions are less severe and unlikely to have tamponade [11].

Arthritis is the most common major criteria of acute rheumatic fever and seen in 80% of adolescents and 95% of adults. Typically, one or more joints are swollen, tender, and warm; large joints are involved (knees, ankles, elbows, wrists) in a migratory fashion. Back pain and a preference to not move about in bed are common clinical acute rheumatic fever presentations. Abdominal pain sometimes accompanies the clinical symptoms of arthritis and other complaints. Any joint may be affected, but less than six are usually involved at any one time. Joint symptoms may last from several days to weeks if untreated; however, often salicylates or nonsteroidal medication dramatically improves the clinical symptoms and signs within 1 to 2 days. The arthritis of rheumatic fever is generally a benign acute condition and permanent joint sequelae not seen. When salicylates or nonsteroidal medication do not cause major and rapid joint symptom improvement, consider other possibilities such as collagen vascular diseases like SLE, rheumatoid arthritis, *Neisseria gonorrhea* arthritis, septic arthritis, and reactive arthritis. If septic joint is suspected, arthrocentesis is needed to obtain a joint cell count, Gram's stain, and bacterial culture [11,56,86].

Chorea (Sydenham's Chorea; St. Vitus Dance) may develop several months after the throat infection, during or without infection history and presents with choreiform movements of the extremities and trunk. There are involuntary, sudden, and purposeless motions that cease during sleep and may be unilateral (hemichorea). Muscle weakness and emotional lability are also common. Snapping or hyperreflexic deep tendon knee reflexes are typically noted. Chorea may be an isolated manifestation or occur in 25% to 30% with mild carditis; the latter is usually mild mitral valve regurgitation appearing with the chorea or as late as 2 to 3 months after the chorea develops. An echocardiogram provides confirmation of subtle aortic and mitral valve insufficiency evidence of rheumatic heart disease. College students with "isolated chorea" may not have serologic evidence of a recent streptococcal infection. A cross-reaction of antibodies has been postulated to develop, directed at both brain tissue and streptococci, causing the CNS changes. An MRI may reveal an increase in the patient's basal ganglia. Box 5 lists the differential diagnosis of chorea. Chorea can be a serious manifestation of rheumatic fever and last many weeks to months, ultimately resolving without complications [11,56].

One must simplify the sleeping and hospital environment by minimizing external stimuli and limiting visitors and TV, and so forth. Severe cases often need drugs such as Haloperidol to modify and shorten the chorea. Sedation and joint padding to prevent injury are helpful management principles. The family and particularly the school and teachers must have guidance as these patients go through recovery. Handwriting deterioration is often an early school sign with the emotional lablity; teachers often recognize symptoms before the parents. Recovery is monitored to some degree by the handwriting and emotional labilty improvement as ESR and other tests are not helpful [11].

Box 5. Differential diagnosis of chorea

    Ataxia/athetosis
    Benign familial chorea
    Chorea
    Conversion reactions
    Drug reactions
    Gilles de la Tourette syndrome
    Habit tics
    Huntington's chorea
    Hyperthyroid chorea
    Simple restlessness
    Systemic lupus erythematosus
    Wilson's disease

Adapted from Greyandus DE, Patel D, Pratt H, Bhave S, editors. India manual of adolescent medicine; review of adolescent medicine: cardiovascular disorders. Delhi, India: Cambridge Press; 2002.

Erythema marginatum occurs in less than 10% of those with rheumatic fever. This skin manifestation presents as an intermittent or transient pink, circular or macular rash with normal central skin involving the trunk and proximal extremities; the face is not involved. Erythema marginatum is a nonpruritic rash, not indurated, blanches with pressure, and increases with heat. This vasomotor phenomenon appears transiently for several weeks or months. When it is circular, it is called erythema annulare. One should never use this as the only major criterion for the diagnosis of acute rheumatic fever.

Subcutaneous nodules are firm, usually not tender (some are tender), and freely mobile in subcutaneous tissue; the skin is not involved. They range in size from 0.1 to 2.0 cm and may be single or multiple; they usually disappear in 1 to 2 weeks. The subcutaneous nodules of rheumatic fever are typically located over the extensor regions of the wrists, elbows, and knees; other locations include the back vertebral spinous processes (thoracic or lumbar), the occiput, buttocks, and Achilles tendons. Sub Q nodules are an uncommon feature of rheumatic fever, but when present are typically found only with acute carditis or subacute carditis (may not be seen until several weeks after the carditis appears). If these nodules are isolated without carditis and do not disappear in a few weeks, other disorders should be suspected, such as rheumatoid arthritis, sarcoidosis, collagen-vascular disorders, and neoplastic disease. One should never use this as the only major criterion for the diagnosis of acute rheumatic fever.

In summary, the major long-term sequelae from rheumatic fever is chronic rheumatic heart disease, especially from patients who had acute carditis or chorea. Prevention of rheumatic heart disease is most successful with the appropriate treatment of Group A beta-hemolytic streptococcal pharyngitis in all patients [95]. Recurrence rates of rheumatic heart disease are the greatest during the first year and the succeeding 5 years after the first episode. Highest risk periods are from ages 5 to15 years old with peaks at 7 to 10 years and 18 to 21. Children between the ages of 3 to 5 years will have severe carditis as their acute disease. Acute rheumatic fever does not occur below 3 years of age. There are known familial predilections for rheumatic fever. Anyone with rheumatic heart disease needs SBE and daily prophylactic antibiotics for life [11,56,88].

Systemic lupus erythematosus (SLE) is a multisystem disease that has widespread inflammation and immunologic abnormalities including autoantibodies. A set of revised criteria for diagnosis and classification is helpful for SLE. Four of more criteria should be present for a diagnosis of SLE. The criteria include malar or discoid rash, photosensitivity, oral or nasopharyngeal ulcerations, arthritis, serositis, renal-neurologic-hematologic, or immunologic disorder and antinuclear antibody [90]. The joint findings may precede the multisystem disease findings by years. Renal involvement occurs in 60% to 80%. Cardiac abnormalities are reported in 50% to 80% with pericarditis—up to 30% of children. Despite massive effusions, tamponade occurred less than 1% of one large series [91]. Tamponade is more likely with drug-induced lupus syndromes. NSAIDS and steroid therapy are used with larger effusions; mild effusions usually require no treatment. Myocarditis is less common and seen in about 8%; some may be a combination of myopericarditis. Endocardial involvement occurs at the aortic or mitral valve sites similar to acute rheumatic fever. Aortic valve insufficiency is the more serious problem with mitral insufficiency usually milder and less severe. Libman-Sacks verrucous vegetations occurred in about 50% of patients at autopsy in SLE patients. Heart block and arrhythmias can occur in young adults but are not common. Over 40 drugs have been linked to lupus-induced SLE with Procainamide, Hydralazine, and Isoniazid most prominently linked. Chorea although uncommon, may be a neurologic association of SLE.

Infective endocarditis

Infective endocarditis occurs when bacterial or fungal vegetations infect heart tissue, typically endothelial valves (damaged or prosthetic) or sites opposite a ventricular septal defect. Underlying factors are congenital or acquired heart disease, drug use, central venous catheters, mitral valve prolapse with MR. Acute endocarditis develops rapidly in heart tissue and presents as a toxic-looking patient with fever and evidence of embolic phenomena [92,93]. Subacute endocarditis may occur in youth with pre-existing heart disease and the subtle presentation may take weeks or months; minimal fever and occasional embolic events may be seen. However, the line between clinical presentations of acute versus subacute disease may be mixed. Infective endocarditis causes in youth often from Streptococcus viridans, Staphylococcus epidermidis, or Staphylococcus aureus. Staphylococcus aureus and Candida albicans occurs at the tricuspid valve disease from those using drugs intravenously [93]. Many other organisms are possible, including pneumococci, enterococci, Gram-negative bacilli, anaerobes, and fungi.

Box 6 lists some of the infective endocarditis signs or symptoms. The differential diagnosis includes rheumatic heart disease and systemic lupus erythematosis (SLE). Blood cultures taken during periods of elevated temperature increase the chances of identifying the causative organism; multiple (at least three) cultures are recommended. Echocardiography will help diagnose the valve or septal defect lesions of infective endocarditis. There can also be anemia, leukocytosis, elevated erythrocyte sedimentation rate, and microscopic hematuria. Aggressive bacterial-sensitive antibiotic treatment is important to sterilize the blood and reduce the vegetative lesion; occasionally surgical removal of the vegetations may be necessary. Complications such as embolization are frequent and the mortality rate can approach 20% [94,95].

Clinicians need to follow published SBE standards for endocarditis prophylaxis when patients at risk have various invasive-type procedures [72,73,94,95]. High-risk populations for endocarditis include those with previous endocarditis, prosthetic valves, complex forms of cyanotic congenital heart disease, high pressure left to right shunts like ventricular septal defects and A/V canal, aortic or pulmonic valve stenosis and surgical aortic-pulmonary shunts (like Blalock-Taussig shunts). Those at moderate risk include patients with acquired valvular

---

Box 6. Signs and symptoms: infective endocarditis

Arthritis
Fever
Fatigue and malaise
Nail bed splinter hemorrhages
Osler's nodes (tender subcutaneous embolic lesions in
   distal extremities)
Janeway and Roth nodes
Changing heart murmurs (mitral, aortic, and tricuspid valve sites)
Retinal hemorrhages
Splenomegaly
Clubbing
Abscesses or infarctions due to septic embolic to the brain,
   lungs or kidneys
Congestive heart failure
Cerebrovascular accident

Adapted from Greyandus DE, Patel D, Pratt H, Bhave S, editors. India manual of adolescent medicine; review of adolescent medicine: cardiovascular disorders. Delhi, India: Cambridge Press; 2002.

---

dysfunction (like chronic rheumatic heart disease), hypertrophic cardiomyopathy, mitral valve prolapse and other congenital heart disease.

Those with the same risk as the general population and not requiring SBE precautions include youth with repaired atrial septal defects, patent ductus arteriosus, or ventricular septal defect without residual after 6 months endothelization of the operative site. Others anomalies include isolated secundum atrial septal defect, mitral valve prolapse without mitral insufficiency, pacemakers, and those with Kawasaki disease or rheumatic fever without valvular heart disease. Not all procedures require SBE prophylaxis (eg, filling cavities, local dental anesthesia, incision, or biopsy of surgically scrubbed skin). However, many procedures causing bleeding do need SBE precautions, including body piercing [95].

Myocarditis in college youth

Myocarditis occurs mostly from viral infections; most are enteroviruses but also adenovirus, cytomegalovirus, and other viruses. Other causes include toxins, bacteria (Corynebacterium diphtheria in nonimmunized youth), syphilis (Treponema pallidum), rickettsial (Q fever; Rocky Mountain Spotted Fever), protozoal (Chagas'; malaria), collagen vascular disorders (SLE, juvenile rheumatoid arthritis [JRA]), sarcoidosis, rheumatic fever, dilated cardiomyopathy, mitochondrial disorders, storage disorders and others [56,96]. Myocarditis has a spectrum from asymptomatic to the more severe manifestations of congestive heart failure, arrhythmias, and sudden death. Any youth presenting with congestive heart failure or ventricular tachycardia of unknown origin is assumed to have myocardial involvement. The erythrocyte sedimentation rate (ESR), C-reactive protein (CRP), and cardiac enzymes are usually elevated; viral cultures, IgM, and IgG studies may isolate the specific virus. The chest radiograph and EKG may be normal or very abnormal in myocarditis; echocardiograms also may show mild to severe myocardial dysfunction. An endomyocardial biopsy increases the chances of identifying a specific causative agent. Management includes anti-arrhythmic drugs, pericardiocentesis, analgesics, and high-dose gamma-globulin. The prognosis is guarded, ranging from compete recovery to the need for heart transplantation [11,56].

Pericarditis

Infectious types of pericarditis include viral, tuberculosis, or other bacteria (*Staphylococcus aureus*, *Hemophilus influenza*, *Neisseria meningitidis*, *Neisseria gonorrhea*, *Salmonella*), and fungal (histoplasmosis and others in an immune-compromised host). Noninfectious pericarditis occurs with rheumatic fever, (during an acute attack), postpericardiotomy (postoperative in cardiac patients 5 to14 days after surgery), collagen vascular disorders (SLE, JRA), uremia and malignancies (lymphoma and metastatic) disease. Pericarditis may occur in collagen vascular disorders from the medication-induced or so-called idiopathic autoimmune pericarditis [11,56].

Symptoms from pericarditis include fever, chest pain (worse when supine), respiratory distress, abdominal pain, and, if tamponade is present, shock. On physical examination, cardiac auscultation reveals a friction rub (absent when there are moderate-large effusions), pulsus paradoxus (over 13 mm Hg BP changes), jugular venous distension, and diminished heart sounds. The chest radiograph shows a globular, "water bottle"-shaped heart, whereas the EKG reveals ST segment elevation and low voltages. Both EKG and chest radiograph may be normal in milder pericarditis cases.

The echocardiogram confirms that a pericardial effusion exists. Management depends on the underlying etiology and pericarditis severity. A pericardiocentesis is indicated for cardiac tamponade, as a diagnostic tool when an infectious or malignant origin is suspected and for treatment for bacterial or mycobacterial disease. Nonsteroidal anti-inflammatory drugs (NSAIDs), acetylsalicylic acid (ASA), Indomethacin or steroids are used for surgical postpericardiotomy syndrome or for rheumatic fever or collagen vascular disease. Intravenous immune globulin is used for sepsis-related pericarditis or idiopathic autoimmune pericarditis. Dialysis measures are used for pericarditis secondary to uremia. If an underlying malignancy causes the pericarditis, that also needs to be treated [11,56].

Sudden cardiac death

Box 7 lists sudden cardiac death causes in college youth; an occurrence rate of 1:100,000 to 1:300,000 exists. A complete family and personal history for cardiac disease is important in seeking to identify youth with a cardiac-induced sudden death potential; a careful medical examination is also important, especially if there is a history of dyspnea, syncope, angina, or in the family, sudden death [11,97,98].

The most common cause of sudden death in the adolescent or young adult athletes in the United States is hypertrophic cardiomyopathy (HCM) (36%) with or without obstruction; echocardiograms are necessary to make this diagnosis [61,98–101]. Coronary artery anomalies include coronary artery aneurysms and abnormal left coronary artery (absence or anomalous origin); they represent 24% of sudden death cases [102,103]. Increased left ventricular cardiac mass (not CHM) causes 10% of cases, whereas a ruptured aorta in Marfan syndrome

---

Box 7. Sudden cardiac death in youth

Aortic stenosis
Arrhythmia
Atrial septal defect (post-surgical or post-interventional closure)
Blunt trauma (Commotio Cordis)
Brugada syndrome
Coarctation of aorta
Congenital coronary artery anomalies
Congenital heart block (*Third Degree > Moebius Type 2*)
Drug-induced arrhythmias (cocaine with or without alcohol or heroin)
Ehlers-Danlos Syndrome
Hypertrophic cardiomyopathy (CHM)
Increased cardiac LV mass (not CHM)
Long Q-T syndrome (congenital; acquired)
Short QT syndrome
Marfan syndrome
Mitral valve prolapse
Myocarditis
RV arrhythmogenic cardiomyopathy
Tetralogy of Fallot (postoperative arrhythmias)
Transposition of great vessels (postoperative arrhythmias)
Wolff-Parkinson-White syndrome

Adapted from Luckstead EF. Cardiac risk factors and participation guidelines for youth sports. Pediatr Clin N Am 2002;49:681–707.

Box 8. Cardiac aspects of Marfan syndrome

Aortic root dissection, thoracic aortic aneurysm, and abdominal
  aortic aneurysm
Aortic insufficiency
Aortic root dilatation
Arrhythmias
Endocarditis
Mitral regurgitation
Mitral valve prolapse (often first sign in pediatric age)
Pulmonary artery dilation
Tricuspid valve prolapse

Data from [11,56,89,107]

(see next topic) represents about 5% of sudden death cases. Those with aortic stenosis (4%) usually have a classic loud systolic murmur at the right sternal border with radiation to the neck. Various lethal arrhythmias may occur, as noted with the Long Q-T syndrome Short QT syndrome [104] and the Wolff-Parkinson-White syndrome [55]. Cocaine can invoke lethal cardiac arrhythmias, especially when combined with alcohol or heroin to enhance the euphoria sought by the drug abuser (Box 8).

Syndromes with cardiac features

Marfan syndrome

This autosomal dominant connective tissue disorder has a wide phenotypic expression; prevalence is 4 to 10 per 100,000; a glycoprotein mutation of the fibrillin gene on chromosome 15 has been identified; spontaneous mutation occurs in 25% [105]. These are tall and slender youth with very long extremities; arm span is greater than the height. A common feature is arachnodactyly or "spider" fingers along with dolichostenomelia (long, narrow head) and a high arched palate. Major hand and feet joints are hyperextensible and joint dislocations are common even in the hip joint. About 75% have scoliosis with or without kyphosis. Other noncardiac defects include: eye defects (ectopia lentis, myopia with retinal detachment, strabismus, nystagmus, megalocornea, cataracts, coloboma, iris tremor), chest wall defects (pectus excavatum or carinatum), pulmonary defects (spontaneous pneumothorax, apical blebs), hernias (inguinal, diaphragmatic, umbilical, incision), striae cutis distensae, pes planus, renal ectopy, and others [11,56,105,106].

Marfan syndrome requires diagnosis by physical assessment and the family history. The cardiac features of Marfan syndrome will determine the sudden death risk and sport and activity safety restrictions (see Box 8). The diagnosis of Marfan syndrome requires one major criterion in one organ system and one minor criterion in a separate organ system with a positive family history. Without a positive family history, one major criterion in two different organ systems and another minor criterion if third organ system are required [104,107–110]. Box 9 lists these major Marfan diagnostic criteria. The differential diagnosis includes: Homocystinuria, Ehlers-Danlos syndrome, Marfanoid hypermobility syndrome, and familial MVP syndrome. An echocardiogram, chest radiograph, and slit lamp examination are important parts of the diagnostic assessment and are repeated as needed in patients with Marfan syndrome. The most recent mean survival age for males with Marfan syndrome in the United States was 43 years; it was 46 years of age for females. However, the positive effects now derived from earlier and increased use of higher dose beta-blockers in children and adolescents and earlier aggressive aortic vascular surgery decreases vascular catastrophic complications and should increase age survival ranges significantly [11,109,111].

Box 9. Diagnosis of Marfan syndrome

Cardiovascular system*
-Ascending aorta dilatation > dissection (involves sinuses
   of Valsalva)
Ophthalmologic system*
-Ectopia lentis
Central nervous system
-Dural ectasia
Musculoskeletal system*
-Pectus excavatum or carinatum
-Decreased upper to lower segment ratio or abnormal arm span
   to height ratio
-Pes planus
-Scoliosis (over 20 degrees) or spondylolisthesis
-Protusio acetabulae
Other (pulmonary-skeletal related)
-Increased superior-inferior lung parenchyma
-Spontaneus pneumothorax

* Major criteria.
Adapted from Greyandus DE, Patel D, Pratt H, Bhave S, editors. India manual of adolescent medicine; review of adolescent medicine: cardiovascular disorders. Delhi, India: Cambridge Press; 2002.

Comprehensive medical and surgical cardiology management for Marfan youth is required to attain maximal longevity. For example, surgical correction of aortic root dilation is performed when it reaches 6 cm on echocardiography and decreases premature death. Beta-blocker medications are recommended early before significant aortic dilation occurs and after prophylactic graft replacement for aortic dilation; many now use these medications when the aortic root is questionably enlarged [109,111]. Aortic rupture during sports-related or other exertion can occur, especially in sports or exercise activity with a high static (isometric) demand activities and those with possible acceleration-deceleration impact injury [66]. Marfan syndrome remains the fourth leading cause of sudden death in athletes [97,98]. Pregnant adolescents and young adults with Marfan syndrome who have aortic regurgitation or aortic root dilatation (over 4.0 cm) face increased risk for aortic dissection. College students with this syndrome who have chest pain need careful evaluation to rule out dissecting aortic aneurysms. Yearly ophthalmologic evaluation is mandatory to detect minor lens dislocation and other eye findings. Subacute bacterial endocarditis prophylaxis is important if structural aortic and mitral valve defects are present. Genetic counseling is important for all families because this is an autosomal dominant disorder.

Noonan syndrome

Noonan and Emke initially described Noonan syndrome in 1963. Many Noonan patients were included in Turner's original series as "male Turner syndrome" and have similar phenotypic appearances with short stature, webbed neck, and broad shield-shaped chests. The most common cardiac anomaly is pulmonic valve stenosis or pulmonic valve dysplasia. Additional anomalies include ASDs, and new reports over the past several years that 34% of Noonan cases have A/V canal defects and hypertrophic cardiomyopathy [55,76,85]. Identification recently of the chromosome abnormality from mutations of the 12q22-qter gene called PTPN11, the protein-tyrosine phosophatase 11 gene causes 50% of the Noonan cases particularly those with cardiac pulmonary stenosis [11,112].

Turner syndrome

Turner syndrome, an X-O chromosome anomaly occurs in one in 2000 female births and most commonly has the cardiac defects of coarctation of the Aorta in ~30%. Other frequently associated cardiac anomalies are patent ductus arteriosus and aortic stenosis [113]. This syndrome can also present with systemic hypertension and may have an increased risk for aortic dissection and rupture. All patients with documented Turner syndrome should have a baseline echocardiogram—even those without apparent heart disease.

Obstetric risk factors in the college student with heart disease

The pregnant college student with cardiac abnormalities can be at high risk for serious short- and long-term complications. Such complications may have a negative impact on their known cardiac problems as an adult. The success of the pregnancy and the potential threat to the expectant mother with a cardiac problem and fetus must be anticipated. Unfortunately, there is often a lack of insight by the adolescent cardiac who may become or is pregnant; at-risk behavior is often the norm rather than the exception. Patients with aortic stenosis, dilated cardiomyopathy, hypertrophic cardiomyopathy, Marfan syndrome, coronary artery disease, primary and secondary pulmonary hypertension, and uncorrected or poorly palliated congenital and acquired heart diseases are particularly at risk [114]. Cardiac problems such as arrhythmias, endocarditis, myopericarditis may occur during pregnancy in previously healthy adolescents. There also appears to be a risk for infection during pregnancy. Hypertension in the third trimester is a particular concern especially with pre-existing cardiac problems.

The risk to the fetus in maternal adolescent and young adult cardiac patients is higher with a reported 50% live birth rate, 35% abortion rate, and 14% miscarriage rate; prematurity rates are also higher [115,116]. Congenital heart lesions in pregnant adolescent patients include those with left to right shunts, obstructive lesions (many of which have been surgically or interventionally treated), and complex cyanotic defects with major correction or palliation. Patients with a history of rheumatic heart disease will usually have mitral or aortic valve insufficiency. Such patients usually tolerate pregnancy well unless there is severe valve insufficiency due to the afterload reduction from pregnancy vasodilatation [114]. It is important to prevent pregnancy effectively and safely in those adolescent patients with pulmonary hypertension and dilated cardiomyopathy. Arrhythmias such as supraventricular tachycardia and ventricular tachycardia may occur during pregnancy for the first time in both patients with or without heart problems. One should be particularly aware of secondary arrhythmias in college-aged students with prior congenital heart surgical or interventional repair (ASD, coarctation of aorta, or tetralogy of Fallot), congenital or acquired valve anomalies, and known cardiomyopathies. One should also remember that most cardiovascular medications given to pregnant adolescent mothers would also be present in breast milk or the fetus itself in lower concentrations. Some drugs such as ACE inhibitors are contraindicated during pregnancies; calcium channel blockers are also suspect and better not given [11,114].

Appendix A

Case #1

A 19-year-old male college student with moderate pectus excavatum complains of chest pain and dizziness with running. Paternal uncle is 6 feet

9 inches tall; several other family members are 6 feet 2 inches and 6 feet 5 inches tall. Father also has pectus; not operated. Sister also tall; mother and other brother are short like mother who is 5 feet 4 inches tall. All family members that are tall have hyper-flexible joints. No history of sudden death in family but a cousin had some type of emergency cardiac operation. Patient also has significant myopia in addition, wears glasses. He is tall measuring 6 feet 4 inches even with his mild thoracic scoliosis. Arm wingspan is two inches greater than body height. Cardiac exam reveals no murmur but a systolic ejection click is noted. Cardiac echocardiogram shows mild aortic root dilation above the 99% for age group peers. Diagnosis?

Case #2

Twenty-year-old college junior female has past history diagnosis of cyanotic heart disease associated with an ASD and VSD. She had two palliative operations as an infant and a Fontan veno-caval shunt at age 4 years. She takes Digoxin and Furosemide daily but is relatively asymptomatic. She is a good student and attains high grades. She is of normal height (5 feet 4 inches) and weighs 115 lbs. Her blood pressure and pulse are normal. She is minimally cyanotic with mild clubbing of her fingers and toes. EKG shows QRS Left Axis Deviation and mild LVH. She has no murmurs but has a single second heart sound. She has hepatomegaly of 1 to 2 cm but is not tender on palpation. She follows SBE precautions and is not short of breath for routine class attendance. What is the likely cardiac diagnosis?

Case #3

Eighteen-year-old college student presents to your clinic with severe chorea. She has had several days offever (102° to 103° Fahrenheit), a pruritic and transient recurrent rash, sore throat, and joint arthalgia for the past 2 to 3 weeks. Her arthralgia was migratory from her feet to her ankles, knees, and fingers, hands, and elbow areas. She had a syncopal event while talking on the phone to a friend before her clinic visit. There was a similar history of recurrent rash, fever, and arthalgia at age 10 years that resolved with analgesics over several days. She smoked marijuana to attempt to control her choreiform motions and to try to calm herself emotionally. (This only made her worse.) Her primary care doctor had prescribed her steroids over the phone, and this had improved her arthalgia and malaise somewhat. She had a grade two mitral insufficiency murmur clinically but no S-3 gallop. There was no pericardial friction rub or aortic valve insufficiency clinically. Her presenting lab studies: C reactive protein (CRP) = 6 and initial erythrocyte sedimentation rate (ESR) = 31; a subsequent ESR was 105 3 days later; ASO titer was 50 Todd units; rheumatoid antibody (RA) factor was strongly positive; antinuclear antibodies (ANA) was positive, as were the homozygous pattern anticardiolipin and Beta Z Glycoprotein studies. She had normal hemoglobin and hematocrit values but slight elevation of her white blood cell count; in addition, a shift to the left was increased neutrophils. An MRI and echocardiogram were obtained. Mild mitral valve insufficiency was confirmed by echocardiogram; Libmann-Sacks nodules were apparent on the ECHO. The MRI showed basal ganglia "brightening" but no other abnormalities. Diagnosis?

Case #4

Nineteen-year-old male college student comes to the clinic complaining of occasions of dizziness with exercise and some chest pain. He had complete repair of his cardiac problem at age 13 years but developed complete heart block during the surgery and had a permanent pacemaker placed at that time. He has had a recent pacemaker pack replacement due to pacemaker failure; now he has a demand pacemaker. He also had moderate thoracic scoliosis repaired with an orthopedic Herrington rod. Although he attains passing college grades, he has a diagnosis of attention deficit syndrome for which he takes medication. EKG shows a pacemaker rhythm; he has mild pulmonary insufficiency and mild residual pulmonic stenosis both clinically and by echocardiography studies. His general noncardiac examination was normal and he clinically appeared to be without any signs of distress but is anxious. Cardiac diagnosis?

Case #5

A twenty-year-old college junior on summer studies internationally has recently returned from a 3-week trip to Brazil. While in that country he had two separate episodes of illness with associated sore throat symptoms. The most recent also had associated generalized arthalgia and overall body stiffness. A college friend with him described his appearance as that of an "old man." The physician examining him said he had a virus causing his problems without any lab tests. The student complains of recurrent chest pain, generalized joint stiffness, problems walking and an unending backache. He has trouble sleeping comfortably. On physical examination, he elicited a circular nondistinct rash over chest and back areas but no other noncardiac abnormalities. Cardiac exam elicits a grade 2/6 high-pitched mitral insufficiency murmur at the apex and a grade 1-2/6 protodiastolic aortic valve insufficiency. No friction rub was noted or S-3 gallop, but sinus tachycardia was present. Lab studies had a ESR of 50; ANA was negative and CRP was less than one (negative). ASO titer was 2622 Todd units. Echocardiogram confirmed the clinical findings of aortic and mitral valve insufficiency; LV function was normal. Complete clinical resolution of the ar-thalgia and stiffness occurred 24 to 48 hours after starting aspirin. Diagnosis?

Case #6

A 21-year-old male college football player had a syncopal episode during conditioning drills and was brought to clinic for examination. This is the second time this has happened; a similar episode happened in high school during a football game scrimmage. His diagnosis at that time was "heat intolerance." A paternal uncle died suddenly in his early forties with some type of heart problem. General physical exam detects a 250-pound, 6-feet 4-inch, highly muscular physique. Blood pressure is elevated to 160 systolic; diastolic is 90. No murmurs are detected on three-position auscultation but the EKG does show LVH with T wave ischemia changes. An additional test confirms the suspected diagnosis in this patient and subsequently two of his four siblings. Diagnosis?

Select your likely diagnosis from the list below

1. Acute rheumatic fever
2. Hypertrophic cardiomyopathy
3. Systemic lupus erythematosus
4. Pacemaker for cmplete A/V block in tetralogy of Fallot patient
5. Long QT syndrome
6. Surgically pated Fontan for tricuspid atresia cyanotic heart disease
7. Marfan syndrome

References

[1] Luckstead EF. Cardiovascular evaluation of the young athlete. Adolesc Med 1998;9:441–55.
[2] Doroshow RW. The adolescent with simple or corrected congenital heart disease. Adol Med STARS 2001;12(1):1–22.
[3] Perloff JK. 22nd Bethesda Conference: Congenital heart disease after childhood: an expanding patient population. Circulation 1991;84:1881–90.
[4] Allen HD, Gersony WM, Tauert KA. Insurability of the adolescent and young adult with heart disease: fact or artifact? Circulation 1992;86:703–10.
[5] Gersony WM, Hayes CJ, Driscoll DJ, et al. Second natural history study of congenital heart defects. Circulation 1993;87:152–65.
[6] McInerny T. The role of the general pediatrician in coordinating the care of children with chronic illness. Pediatr Cl NA 1984;31:199–209.
[7] Somerville J. Management of adults with congenital heart disease; an increasing problem. Annu Rev Med 1997;48:283–93.
[8] Kaden GG, McCarter RJ, Johnson SF, et al. Physician-patient communication; understanding congenital heart disease. Am J Dis Child 1985;139:995–9.
[9] Cetta F, Podlecki DD, Bell TJ, et al. Adolescent knowledge of bacterial endocarditis prophylaxis. J Adolesc Health 1993;540:540–2.
[10] Moller JH, Anderson RC. 1000 consecutive children with a cardiac malformation with 26-to 37-year follow-up. Am J Cardiol 1992;70:661–7.
[11] Luckstead EF, Noubani H, In: Greydanus DE, Hoffman AD, editors. Chapter; Essentials of adolescent medicine. 4th edition. Cardiovascular disorders in the adolescent. Chapter 11. New York: Medicine McGraw-Hill Publishers, in press.
[12] Walsh CA. Syncope and sudden death in the adolescent. Adol Med STARS 2001;12(1): 105–32.
[13] Cullen S, Celermajer DS, Franklin RC, et al. Prognostic significance of ventricular arrhythmia after repair of tetralogy of Fallot. J Am Coll Cardiol 1994;23:1151–5.
[14] Shuurmans FM, Pulles-Heintzberger CFM, Gerver WJM, et al. Long-term growth of children with congenital heart disease. Acta Pediatr 1998;87(12):1250–5.

[15] Manning JA. Congenital heart disease and the quality of life. In: Engle ME, Perloff JK, editors. Congenital heart disease after surgery: benefits, residua, sequelae. York Medical Books; 1983. p. 347–61.

[16] Brenner JI, Ringel RE, Berman MA, et al. Cardiologic perspectives of chest pain in childhood: a referral problem? to whom? Pediatric Clin North Am 1984;31:1241–58.

[17] Lam JC, Tobias JD. Follow-up survey of children and adolescents with chest pain. South Med J 2001;94:921–4.

[18] Selbst SM, Ruddy RM, Clark BJ, et al. Pediatric chest pain: a prospective study. Pediatrics 1988;82:319.

[19] Magarian GI, Hickham DH. Non-cardiac causes of angina-like chest pain. Prog Cardiovasc Dis 1986;29:65–80.

[20] Wiens L, Sabath R, Ewing L, et al. Chest pain in otherwise healthy children and adolescents is frequently caused by exercise- induced asthma. Pediatrics 1992;90:350–3.

[21] Sabri MR, Ghavanini AA, Haghighat M, et al. Chest pain in children and adolescents: epigastric tenderness as a guide to reduce unnecessary workup. Pediatr Cardiol 2003;24:3–5.

[22] Luckstead EF, Greydanus DE. In cardiac evaluation: medical care of the adolescent athlete. Los Angeles, CA: Practice Management Information Corporation; 1993.

[23] Olson RE. Atherosclerosis in children: implications for the prevention of atherosclerosis. Adv Pediatr 2000;47:55–78.

[24] Haust MD. The genesis of atherosclerosis in the pediatric age group. Pediatr Pathol 1990; 10:253–71.

[25] Stary HC. Regression of atherosclerosis in primates. Virchows Arch A Pathol Anat 1979; 383:11–6.

[26] Stary HS. The sequence of cell and matrix changes in atheroscleric lesions of coronary arteries in the first forty years of life. Eur Heart J 1990;11:3E–19E.

[27] Bouziota C, Koutedakis V. A three year study of coronary heart disease risk factors in Greek adolescents. Ped Exerc Sci 2003;15:9–18.

[28] The Pathological Determinants of Atherosclerosis in Youth (PDAY) Research Group. A preliminary report on the relationship of atherosclerosis in young men to serum lipoprotein cholesterol concentrations and smoking. JAMA 1990;264:3018–24.

[29] McGill HC, for the PDAY Research Group. Effect of serum lipoproteins and smoking on atherosclerosis in young men and women. Arterioscler Thromb Vasc Biol 1997;17:95–106.

[30] Holman RL, McGill HC, Strong JP, et al. The natural history of atherosclerosis: the early aortic lesions seen in New Orleans in the middle of the 20th century. Am J Pathol 1958;34: 209–29.

[31] Strong JP. The PDAY Research Group: prevalence and extent of atherosclerosis in adolescents and young adults: implications for prevention from the pathobiological determinants of atherosclerosis in youth studies. JAMA 1999;281:727–35.

[32] Berenson GS, Wattigney WA, Tracy RE, et al. Atherosclerosis of the aorta and coronary arteries and cardiovascular risk factors in persons aged 6 to 30 years and studied at necropsy (The Bogalusa Heart Study). Am J Cardiol 1992;70:851–8.

[33] Strobl WA, Widhalm K. The natural history of serum lipids and lipoproteins during childhood. In: Widhalm K, Naito HK, editors. Detection and treatment of lipid and lipoprotein disorders of childhood. Alan Liss Publishers; 1985. p. 101–21.

[34] Robbins SL, Cotran RS, editors. Arteriosclerosis: pathological basis of disease. 2nd edition. WB Saunders; 1979. p. 598–611.

[35] Ginsburg BE, Zetterstrom R. Serum cholesterol concentrations in early infancy. Acta Pediatr Scand 1980;69:581–5.

[36] Morrison JA, Barton BA, Biro FM, et al. Overweight, fat patterning and cardiovascular disease risk factors in black and white boys. J Pediatr 1999;135:451–7.

[37] Morrison JA, Sprecher DL, Barton BA, et al. Overweight, fat patterning and cardiovascular disease risk factors in black and white girls. J Pediatr 1999;135:458–64.

[38] National Cholesterol Education Program. (NCEP). Report of the expert panel on blood cholesterol levels in children and adolescents. Pediatrics 1992;89:525S–84S.

[39] Kwiterovich PO, Barton BA, McMahon RP, et al. Effects of diet and sexual maturation on low-density lipoprotein cholesterol during puberty: The Dietary Intervention Study of Children (DISC). Circulation 1997;96:2526–33.

[40] American Heart Association. Committee on Nutrition, Central Committee for Medical and Community Program. Diet and heart disease. New York: American Heart Association; 1968.

[41] NIH Consensus Development Conference Statement. Lowering blood cholesterol. JAMA 1985;253:2080–6.

[42] Olsen RE. Mass screening vrersus screening and selective intervention for the prevention of coronary artery disease. JAMA 1986;255:2204–7.

[43] Newman TB, Garber AM, Holtzman NA, et al. Problems with the report of the expert panel on blood cholesterol levels in children and adolescents. Arch Pediatr Adolesc Med 1995;49: 241–7.

[44] Berenson GS, Srinivason SR, Cresanta JL, et al. Dynamic changes in serum lipoproteins in children during adolescence and sexual maturation. Am J Epidemiol 1981;113:157–70.

[45] Lauer RM, Lee J, Clarke WR. Factors affecting the relationship between childhood and adult cholesterol levels: the Muscatine study. Pediatrics 1988;82:309–18.

[46] Widhalm K, Strobl W, Westphal G. Age dependency and tracking of serum lipids and lipoproteins in healthy children 11–14 years. Atherosclerosis 1981;38:189–96.

[47] Anonymous. Lipid Research Clinic Data Book. Bethesda, MD: National Institutes of Health; 1980 [NIH Publication No 80–1527].

[48] Berenson GS. for The Bogalusa Heart Study. Association between multiple cardiovascular risk factors and athersclerosis in children and young adults. N Engl J Med 1998;338:1650–66.

[49] Osganian SK, Stampfer MJ, Speigelman D, et al. Distribution of and factors associated with serum homocysteine levels in children; child and adolescent trial for cardiovascular health. JAMA 1999;281:1189–96.

[50] Krauss RM, Eckel RH, Howard B, et al. AHA dietary guidelines. Revision 2000: a statement for healthcare professionals from the Nutrition Committee of the American Heart Association. Circulation 2000;102:2284–99.

[51] American Academy of Pediatrics National Cholesterol Education Program. Report of the expert panel on blood cholesterol levels in children and adolescents. Pediatrics 1999;89: 525–84.

[52] Luckstead EF. Cardiac risk factors and participation guidelines for youth sports. Pediatr Clin N Am 2002;49:681–707.

[53] Wells T, Stowe C. Approach to use of antihypertensive drugs in children and adolescents. Curr Ther Res Clin Exp 2001;62:329–50.

[54] National High Blood Pressure Education Program Working Group on Hypertension Control in Children and Adolescents. Update on the 1987 task force report on high blood pressure in children and adolescents: a working group report from the national high blood pressure education program. Pediatrics 1996;98:649–58.

[55] National High Blood Pressure Education Program Working Group on High blood Pressure in Children and Adolescents. The fourth report on the diagnosis, evaluation and treatment of high blood pressure in children and adolescents. Pediatrics 2004;114(2):555–76.

[56] Rowlett JD, Greydanus DE. In: Hoffmann AD, Greydanus DE, editors. The cardiovascular system in adolescent medicine. 3rd edition. Stamford, CT: Appleton and Lange; 1997. p. 147–73.

[57] Etchells E, Bell C, Robb K. Does this patient have an abnormal systolic murmur? JAMA 1997;277:564.

[58] Sapin SO. Recognizing normal heart murmurs: a logic-based mnemonic. Pediatrics 1997; 99:616–9.

[59] Brickner ME, Hillis LD, Lange RA. Congenital heart disease in adults. N Engl J Med 2000; 342:256–63.

[60] Allen HD, Franklin WH, Fontana MC. The adolescent and young adult: cardiac problems in the adolescent and young adult. In: Emmanouilides GC, Riemenschneider TA, Allen HD,

Gutgesell HP, editors. Moss and Adams' heart disease in infants, children and adolescents, including the fetus and young adults. 5th edition. Baltimore, MD: Williams & Wilkins; 1994. p. 657–64.

[61] Hagler DJ. Palliated congenital heart disease. In: Walsh CA, Doroshow RW, editors. Adolescent cardiology; adolescent medicine (STARS). Philadelphia: Hanley & Belfus, Inc. Med Publishers; 2001. p. 23–34.

[62] Hannoush H, Younes H, Arnaout S, et al. Patterns of congenital heart disease in unoperated adults: a 20-year experience in a developing country. Clin Cardiol 2004;27:236–40.

[63] Swenson JM, Fischer DR, Miller SA, et al. Are chest radiographs and electrocardiograms still valuable in evaluating new pediatric patients with heart murmurs or chest pain? Pediatrics 1997;99:1–3.

[64] Park MK, Menard SW, Yuan C. Comparison of auscultatory and oscillometric blood pressures. Arch Pediatr Adol Med 2001;155:50–3.

[65] Luckstead EF, Greydanus DE. The sport-specific physical examination and cardiovascular examination; in medical care of the adolescent athlete. Los Angeles, CA: Practice Management Information Corporation; 1993.

[66] The 26th Bethesda Conference. Recommendations for determining eligibility for competition in athletes with cardiovascular abnormalities. J Am Coll Cardiol 1994;24:845–99.

[67] Basilico FC. Cardiovascular disease in athletes. Am J Sports Med 1999;27(1):108–20.

[68] Suda K, Raboisson MJ, Piette E, et al. Reversible atrioventricular block associated with closure of atrial septal defects using the amplatzer device. J Am Coll Cardiol 2004;43(9): 1677–82.

[69] Perloff JK, Child JS, Edwards JE. New guidelines for the clinical diagnosis for mitral valve prolapse. Am J Cardiol 1986;57:1124–9.

[70] Nisimura RA, McGoon MD, Shub C, et al. Echocardiographic documented MVP: long term follow-up of 237 patients. N Engl J Med 1985;313:305–9.

[71] Danford DA, Salaymeh KJ, Martin AB, et al. Pulmonary stenosis: defect-specific diagnostic accuracy of heart mumurs in children. J Pediatr 1999;134:76–81.

[72] Dajani AS, Taubert KA, Wilson W, et al. Prevention of bacterial endocarditis: recommendations by the American Heart Association. JAMA 1997;277:1794–801.

[73] Anonymous. Prevention of bacterial endocarditis. Med Lett 2001;43:1116–7, 1998.

[74] Feit LR. Genetics of congenital heart disease: strategies. Adv Pediatr 1998;45(10):267–92.

[75] Narchi H. The child who passes out? Pediatr Rev 2000;21:384–9.

[76] Grubb BP, Olshansky B. Syncope: mechanisms and management. Armonk, NY: Futura Publishers; 2001.

[77] Moak JP, Bailey JJ, Makhlouf FT. Simultaneous heart rate and blood pressure variability analysis: mechanisms underlying neurally mediated cardiac syncope in children. J Am Coll Cardiol 2002;40:1466–72.

[78] Kosinski DJ. Syncope in the athlete. In: Grubb BP, Olshansky B, editors. Syncope: mechanisms and management. Armonk, NY: Futura Publishers; 2001. p. 317–36.

[79] Ross R, Grubb BP. Syncope in the child and adolescent. In: Grubb BP, Olshansky B, editors. Syncope: mechanisms and management. Armonk, NY: Futura Publishers; 2001. p. 305–16.

[80] Pellica A, Maron BJ, Culasso F, et al. Clinical significance of abnormal echocardiographic patterns in trained athletes. Circulation 2000;102:278–84.

[81] Priori SG, Aliot E, Blomstrom-Lundquist C, et al. Task force on sudden death of the European Society of Cardiology. Eur Heart J 2001;22:1418.

[82] Wever EFD, Robles de Medina EO. Sudden death in patients without structural heart disease. J Am Coll Cardiol 2004;43(7):1137–44.

[83] Keating MT, Sanuinetti MC. Molecular and cellular mechanisms of cardiac arrhythmias. Cell 2001;104:569–80.

[84] Zaeba W, Moss AJ, Schwartz PJ, et al. Influence of the genotype on the clinical course of the Long QT syndrome. N Engl J Med 1998;339:960–5.

[85] Jones TD. Diagnosis of rheumatic fever. JAMA 1944;126:481.

[86] Sondheimer HM, Lorts A. Cardiac involvement in inflammatory disease: systemic lupus erythematosus, rheumatic fever and Kawasaki disease. Adolesc Med 2001;12:69–78.

[87] Special Writing Group of the Committee on Rheumatic Fever, Endocarditis, and Kawasaki Disease of the Council on Cardiovascular Disease in the Young of the American Heart Association. Guidelines for the diagnosis of rheumatic fever; Jones criteria, 1992 update. JAMA 1992;268:2069.

[88] Berrios X, del Camp E, Guzman B, et al. Discontinuing rheumatic fever prophylaxis in selected adolescents and young adults. Ann Intern Med 1993;118:401.

[89] Greydanus DE, Patel D, Pratt H, Bhave S, editors. India manual of adolescent medicine; review of adolescent medicine: cardiovascular disorders. Delhi, India: Cambridge Press; 2002.

[90] Danjani A, Taubert K, Ferrieri P, et al. Treatment of acute streptococcal pharyngitis and prevention of rheumatic fever: a statement for health professionals. Pediatrics 1995;96:758.

[91] Doherty N, Siegel R. Cardiovascular manifestations of SLE. Am Heart J 1985;110:1257–65.

[92] Bayer AS, Bolger AF, Taubert KA, et al. Diagnosis and management of infective endocarditis and its complications. Circulation 1998;98:2936–48.

[93] DeWitt DE, Paauw DS. Endocarditis in injection drug users. Am Fam Phys 1996;53:2045–52.

[94] Wilson WR, Karchmer AW, Dajani AS, et al. Antibiotic treatment of adults with infective endocarditis due to Streptococci, Enterococci, Staphylococci, and HACEK microorganisms. JAMA 1995;274:1706–13.

[95] Cetta F, Podlecki CD, Bell TJ. Adolescent knowledge of bacterial endocarditis prophylaxis. J Adolesc Health 1994;14:540.

[96] Towbin JA. Myocarditis and pericarditis in adolescents. Adolesc Med 2001;12:47–68.

[97] Maron BJ, Shirani J, Poliac LC, et al. Sudden death in young competitive athletes. JAMA 1996;1276:199.

[98] Maron BJ, Thompson PD, Puffer JC, et al. Cardiovascular preparticipation screening of competitive athletes. A statement for health professionals from the Sudden Death Committee (Clinical Cardiology) and Congenital Cardiac Defects Committee (Cardiovascular Disease in the Young), American Heart Association. Circulation 1996;94:850–6.

[99] Shaddy RE. Cardiomyopathies in adolescents: dilated, hypertrophic, and restrictive. Adolesc Med 2001;12:35–45.

[100] Spirito P, Seidman CE, McKenna WJ, et al. The management of hypertrophic cardiomyopathy. N Engl J Med 1997;366:775.

[101] Liberthson RR. Sudden death from cardiac causes in children and young adults. N Engl J Med 1996;334:1039.

[102] Basso C, Maron BJ, Corrado D, Thiene G. Clinical profile of congenital coronary artery anomalies with origin from the wrong aortic sinus leading to sudden death in young competitive athletes. J Am Coll Cardiol 2000;35(6):1493–501.

[103] Rowland TW. Screening for risk of cardiac death in young athletes. Sports Science Exchange 1999;12(3):1–5.

[104] Gaita F, Giustetto C, Bianchi F, et al. Short QT Syndrome: pharmacological treatment. J Am Coll Cardiol 2004;43(8):1494–9.

[105] Dietz HC, Cutting GR, Pyertiz RE, et al. Marfan syndrome caused by a recurrent de novo missense mutation in the fibrillin gene. Nature 1991;352:337.

[106] Marfan M. Un cas de deformation congenitale des quatre membres plus prononcee aux extremites characterisee par l'allongement des os avec un certain degre d'amincissement. Bull Mem Soc Med Hop Paris 1896;13:220.

[107] De Paepe A, Devereux RB, Dietz HC, et al. Revised diagnostic criteria for the Marfan syndrome. Am J Med Genet 1996;62:417.

[108] Pyeritz RE. Disorders of vascular fragility: implications for active patients. PSM 2001; 29(6):53–60.

[109] Salim MA, Alpert BA. Spors and Marfan syndrome: awareness and early diagnosis can prevent sudden death. PSM 2001;29(5):80–93.

[110] Kainulainen K, Pulkkinen L, Savolainen A, et al. Location on chromosome 15 of the gene defect causing Marfan syndrome. N Engl J Med 1990;323:935.

[111] Shores J, Berger KR, Murphy EA, et al. Progression of aortic dilatation and the benefit of long term beta-adrenergic blockade in Marfan's syndrome. N Engl J Med 1994;330:1335.

[112] Cunniff C. Turner syndrome. Adolesc Med 2002;13:359–66.

[113] Taraglia M, Mehler EL, Goldberg R, et al. Mutations in PTPN11, encoding the protein tyrosine phosphatase SHP-2, cause Noonan syndrome. J Med Genet 2001;29:465–8.

[114] Mendelson MA. Gynecologic and obstetric issues in the adolescent with heart disease. Adolesc Med 2001;12:164–74.

[115] Simon-Stevens C. Providing effective reproductive health care and prescribing contraceptives for adolescents. Pediatr Rev 1996;19:124–31.

[116] Whitemore R, Hobbins JC, Engle MA. Pregnancy and its outcome in women with and without surgical treatment for congenital heart disease. Am J Cardiol 1982;50:641–51.

ELSEVIER
SAUNDERS

PEDIATRIC CLINICS
OF NORTH AMERICA

Pediatr Clin N Am 52 (2005) 279–305

Diabetes on the College Campus

Manmohan K. Kamboj, MD

Pediatrics Program, Division of Pediatric Endocrinology, College of Human Medicine,
Michigan State University–Kalamazoo Center for Medical Studies, 1000 Oakland Drive,
Kalamazoo, MI 49008-1284, USA

Diabetes mellitus (DM) is a metabolic syndrome characterized by hyperglycemia caused by defects in insulin secretion, insulin action, or both. Because insulin is needed by the body to convert glucose into energy, these defects result in abnormally high levels of glucose accumulating in the blood. The lack of effective insulin action leads to alterations in carbohydrate, fat, and protein metabolism. The chronic hyperglycemia of diabetes is associated with long-term damage, dysfunction, and failure of various organs, especially the eyes, kidneys, nerves, heart, and blood vessels. The main types of diabetes to be aware of in this context are type 1 DM (T1DM), type 2 DM (T2DM), maturity onset of diabetes of the youth (MODY), and diabetes secondary to other conditions (Table 1). Students on the college campus may have pre-existing diabetes or may develop it after their arrival. College life is a period of great adjustment for this group of older adolescents and young adults in many areas, and management of diabetes is no exception.

Incidence and prevalence

The incidence and prevalence of various kinds of diabetes are highly variable in different ethnic populations. T1DM is one of the most common chronic illnesses of adolescence, with a frequency in the United States of 1 in 360 at the

E-mail address: kamboj@kcms.msu.edu

Table 1
Common names for different types of diabetes

Type	Common names
T1DM:	Insulin-dependent diabetes mellitus, or IDDM; juvenile diabetes, or JD; diabetes mellitus 1, or DM1; type 1 diabetes, or T1D; ketosis prone
T2DM	Non–insulin-dependent diabetes mellitus, or NIDDM; maturity onset diabetes; adult onset diabetes; ketosis resistant
MODY	Formerly MODY 1, 2, and 3 with mutations on chromosome 20, chromosome 7, and chromosome 12, respectively

age of 16 years. The annual incidence decreases after the age of 20 years. Although T1DM accounts for only 5% to 10% of patients with this form of diabetes, there are approximately 150,000 people younger than 20 years and 400,000 people older than 20 years with this condition in the United States [1]. The first incidence peak occurs at the age of approximately 5 to 7 years, with a second peak noted at puberty. The incidence is much lower in African Americans, American Indians, Asian Americans, and Hispanics as compared with the white population; in addition, gender distribution is similar for men and women. T1DM is associated with a higher risk in a genetically or HLA similar family member. The incidence of T2DM is increasing at an epidemic proportion in adolescents and young adults, with African Americans constituting approximately 70% of the patients with T2DM. A tenfold increase in incidence of T2DM has been observed in 10- through 18-year-olds in the past decade [1]. A high incidence has been reported in Native American youth, Hispanics, and white adolescents as well. The T2DM epidemic curve seems to closely parallel the obesity epidemic curve. A large proportion of T2DM in adolescents remains undiagnosed during the prolonged preclinical phase of the disease [2].

Classification of diabetes mellitus

Based on different pathogenetic mechanisms, DM may be classified into T1DM, T2DM, MODY, or DM from secondary causes [3,4]. T1DM is an autoimmune disease characterized by destruction of the pancreatic β cells and consequent insulin deficiency. Environmental factors superimposed on a genetic predisposition seem to initiate the autoimmune process. Some patients, however, have no evidence of autoimmunity or any other known causal factor and are labeled idiopathic. These patients are mostly from an African or Asian background, exhibit a strong inheritance pattern, and have no HLA association. T1DM is otherwise HLA linked and has evidence of autoimmunity in the form of islet cell antibodies, anti-insulin antibodies, and antibodies against other islet cell antigens (eg, glutamic acid decarboxylase, islet tyrosine phosphates IA2 and IA2β). The presence of antibodies seems to be predictive of T1DM, and impairment of the first phase of insulin secretion is the first detectable abnormality [3].

T2DM is the most prevalent form of diabetes in adults. It is a result of the inability of the body to properly use insulin, a condition which subsequently may develop into insulin deficiency. The presentation of T2DM is more insidious than T1DM; T2DM may be incidentally picked up on routine physical examination, or found on investigations for obesity or acanthosis nigricans. There is usually a relative hyperinsulinemia at the time of diagnosis [5,6].

MODY encompasses several forms of diabetes caused by defects in the β-cell function, and is characterized by impaired insulin secretion, but normal insulin action, and a strong family history of diabetes, implying an autosomal-dominant inheritance. Defects in six chromosomes involving more than 200 mutations have been identified thus far [1]. Diabetes can also occur secondary to exocrine pancreatic conditions, such as cystic fibrosis, and other endocrine disorders

---

Box 1. Etiologic classification of diabetes

Type I diabetes
  Immune-mediated
  Idiopathic
Type 2 diabetes
MODY
  Genetic defects of β-cell function
Secondary type of diabetes
  Genetic defects in insulin action (e.g., lipoatrophic diabetes)
  Diseases of the exocrine pancreas (e.g., cystic fibrosis)
  Endocrinopathies (e.g., Cushing's syndrome, acromegaly,
    glucagonoma, pheochromocytoma)
  Drug- or chemical-induced (e.g., glucocorticoids, N-3
    pyridylmethyl-N'4 nitrophenyl urea [Vacor] rodenticide)
  Infections (e.g., congenital rubella, CoxSackievirus B, Cyto-
    megalovirus, adenovirus and mumps)
  Uncommon forms of immune-mediated diabetes (Stiffman
    syndrome, anti-insulin receptor antibodies)
  Other genetic syndromes sometimes associated with
    diabetes (e.g., Prader-Willi syndrome, Down's syndrome,
    Klinefelters syndrome, Turner's syndrome,
    Wolfram's syndrome)
Gestational diabetes mellitus (GDM)

Adapted from: American Diabetes Association: Type 2 diabetes in children and adolescents (Consensus Statement). Diabetes Care 2000;23:381–9.

(eg, Cushing's syndrome) or on exposure to certain exogenous toxins, drugs, or poisons (Box 1) [7].

Impaired glucose tolerance (IGT) is the intermediate stage between normal glucose homeostasis and DM. Patients with IGT exhibit hyperglycemia on oral glucose tolerance test, but not at levels diagnostic of diabetes; they usually have a normal or near normal hemoglobin A1c (HbA1c), and the hyperglycemia may be precipitated under stress conditions in some individuals. IGT is a risk factor for future diabetes and cardiovascular disease; in addition, it is associated with the insulin resistance syndrome (syndrome X or the metabolic syndrome).

Diagnosis

The initial presentation may be acute, classic, or subtle. About one third of the patients with T1DM present in an acute emergency in the state of severe decompensation, which is referred to as diabetic ketoacidosis (DKA) and requires emergency resuscitative measures. The remaining patients may present almost equally with either the classic presentation, including polyuria, polydipsia, polyphagia, and weight loss, or they may be asymptomatic and their condition may be detected on a routine urinalysis. There may be a variable preclinical period, and the condition tends to be precipitated by an intercurrent illness. There may be history of abdominal pain, nausea, or vomiting, with a differential diagnosis of acute abdomen or gastroenteritis. Evidence of candidal vaginitis or persistent dermatologic infections because of the presence of chronic hyperglycemia may be seen. Patients in severe or late stages of DKA may even present with Kussmaul's breathing or frank coma, which may steer the initial workup toward pulmonary or neurologic issues.

T2DM, however, may have a prolonged preclinical phase and should be looked for in adolescents and young adults with obesity, pseudoacanthosis

Table 2
Diagnostic criteria for diabetes mellitus

Criterion	Fasting plasma glucose (mg/dL)	2-h postprandial glucose (mg/dL)
Normoglycemia	< 100	< 140
Impaired fasting glucose	≥ 100 but < 126	—
Impaired glucose tolerance	—	≥ 140 but < 200
Diabetes	≥ 126	≥ 200
	Symptoms of diabetes and random blood glucose ≥ 200 (repeated on two separate occasions)	

Adapted from American Diabetes Association. Screening for diabetes (position statement). Diabetes Care 2004;27(Suppl 1):S11–4.

Box 2. Testing for type 2 DM in children and adolescents

WEIGHT–BMI $>85^{th}$ percentile for reference standards
RISK FACTORS–Presence of two risk factors:
- Presence of signs of insulin resistance – acanthosis nigricans, PCOS, hypertension, dyslipidemias
- Race and ethnicity : with high incidence of type 2 DM – African-American, Latin American, Hispanic, Pacific Islander, Asian American
- Family history of type 2 DM in first or second degree relative

TESTING RECOMMENDATIONS
- should be started at 10 years or at pubertal onset
- repeated every 2 years
- testing with fasting plasma glucose should be done

Adapted from: American Diabetes Association: Standards of medical care in diabetes (Position Statement). Diabetes Care 2004; 26(Suppl 1):S15–35.

---

nigricans, hypertension, hyperlipidemia, hyperandrogenism, and polycystic ovary syndrome (PCOS). The classic triad of polyuria, polydipsia, and polyphagia may be present. Alternatively, the patients may present in DKA or in nonketotic hyperosmolar coma because of "glucose toxicity," in which there may be a state of functional insulin deficiency caused by prolonged hyperglycemia [3]. The diagnostic criteria are summarized in Table 2 [2,3]. The findings must be confirmed on two separate occasions in case of absence of unequivocal hyperglycemia. The use of HbA1c as a diagnostic criterion is still not recommended. Box 2 outlines the testing recommended for individuals with T2DM [3].

Management of diabetes

The management of DM requires a comprehensive, multidisciplinary approach involving the diabetes care team, which is composed of the primary care physician, endocrinologist, clinic nurse, diabetes nurse educator, nutritionist, psychologist, and social worker [8]. Regular and close monitoring of glycemic control, along with management of multiple other issues involved on an ongoing basis, is essential for optimization of intensive diabetes management [9]. Initial therapy is tailored toward management of the individual presentation.

Patients with T1DM and T2DM in DKA exhibit multiple metabolic derangements because of hypoinsulinemia and resultant hyperglycemia, dehydration, lipolysis, proteolysis, metabolic acidosis, fluid, and electrolyte derangements; these patients are managed in a similar manner [10,11]. The degree of decompensation is assessed by obtaining baseline levels of electrolytes, blood urea nitrogen, creatinine, venous blood gas, plasma glucose, urine dip (for specific gravity, pH, sugar, ketones), and urine microscopy. An assessment is made of the severity of dehydration, mental status, Kussmaul's breathing, and ketosis. Most patients in DKA exhibit moderate to severe dehydration requiring appropriate fluid correction over 36 to 48 hours, whereas a resuscitative fluid bolus of normal saline of 10 to 20 mL/kg should be reserved for patients with circulatory compromise. Judicious fluid replacement is essential to avoid cerebral edema, which is associated with a high mortality rate. Appropriate electrolyte monitoring and replacement of sodium, potassium, phosphate, and magnesium should be undertaken as indicated by laboratory results. Insulin drip is initiated at 0.1 units/kg per hour, and dextrose is added to the intravenous (IV) fluids once serum glucose falls to approximately 250 mg/dL. The insulin and glucose infusion rates are closely titrated to maintain blood glucose levels between 100 and 200 mg/dL, normalize electrolytes, correct acidosis, and clear ketonuria [12]. Each institution should have a standardized protocol in place to minimize errors and to facilitate management; close monitoring is the key for success. The protocol at the current author's institute includes hourly vital signs and neurologic assessment, hourly capillary blood glucose monitoring, and two hourly electrolytes; there is also strict intake–output recording and assessment of all urine specimens for glucose and ketones. IV insulin therapy is continued until the patient is able to tolerate oral intake and the urine is ketone-negative.

Transition to subcutaneous insulin

If the patient is not in ketoacidosis or once ketonuria clears, transition to subcutaneous insulin is initiated. A customized insulin regimen is initiated after consultation with the patient and family. Diabetes education is initiated as soon as the patient is able to participate along with the parents and close friends and roommates likely to be involved in diabetes care [8]. These older adolescents and young adult patients are educated in "basic survival skills," including capillary blood glucose and urine ketone testing and insulin injections. Dose adjustments in the insulin regimen are made taking into account the relative inactivity during hospitalization. Nutrition education is introduced, and patients are given food lists to facilitate carbohydrate and calorie counting. Patients start carbohydrate counting and learn to calculate the dose of the rapid-acting insulin according to the insulin–carbohydrate ratio, if using the intensive, flexible insulin regimen. They are discharged when clinically stable and proficient in basic survival skills, with adequate diabetes supplies and insulin; an appointment for a follow-up office visit is given along with contact information for the patients to call the follow-up primary care physician or endocrinologist. Daily phone contact by the patient is encouraged to monitor glycemic control, alter insulin-dosing/regimen if required, and answer questions. This process is continued until appropriate control is obtained; then, patients can be followed up on as required or on an emergency contact basis. The patient and parents are encouraged to call earlier on in case of a question or illness to avoid undue progression of complications.

Patients with T2DM who present with an acute condition are managed similarly; however, because of insulin resistance, they should additionally be started on metformin. This medication is started at 500 mg/day with dinner and then gradually increased to a maximum of 2 to 2.5 g/day in two or three divided doses with meals (or the long-acting form may be used once daily) along with the insulin regimen. Patients should be informed about the gastrointestinal side effects of metformin to avoid discontinuation of this medication for that reason. Over time, the insulin dose may be weaned if indicated according to the glycemic control.

Types of insulin and insulin regimens for type 1 diabetes mellitus

Patients who have T1DM depend on insulin for survival. Many insulin preparations are available today, allowing individualized management for each patient depending on specific needs. Based on duration of action, the various types of insulins may be divided into four main groups: rapid-acting, short-acting, intermediate-acting, and long-acting insulins [13]. Nevertheless, there is great variability in insulin action between individual patients and even within the same patient because of varied rates of absorption. Further adjustments in the insulin regimen are based on blood glucose values obtained from patients' self-monitoring of blood glucose (SMBG). Rapid- and short-acting insulin can be adjusted on a 2- to 3-day SMBG observation period; however, the intermediate- and long-acting insulin should be adjusted only after a 2- to 5-day observation period.

Extensive blood glucose monitoring needs be done before and after meals and during the night; this is recommended initially (at the start of therapy), when intensifying the insulin regimen, or when investigating the cause of hypoglycemia or hyperglycemia. The insulin dose usually begins with about 0.6 to 0.75 units/kg per day and may go up to an average of 1 unit/kg per day in older adolescents and young adults in college, based on SMBG. The two most commonly used insulin regimens are the three-injections-a-day regimen and the flexible-intensive insulin regimen (Box 3) [14]. Once- or twice-daily insulin regimens usually offer inadequate control. Achievement and maintenance of tight control is emphasized from the beginning, and the patient is preferably started directly on an intensive management regimen that has been discussed

Box 3. Two commonly used insulin regimens

Three-injections-a-day regimen

Intermediate-acting insulin (neutral protamine Hagedorn [NPH] or Lente), prebreakfast and before bedtime, plus rapid/short-acting insulin (Lispro, Aspart), prebreakfast and predinner

- Calculate total daily insulin dose (based on body weight)
- Two thirds of the dose prebreakfast (2 parts intermediate- + 1 part rapid-acting)
- One third of the dose in the evening (1 part rapid-acting predinner and 2 parts NPH at bedtime)
- Usually no lunchtime insulin required
- Consistency in meal timings required
- Consistency in carbohydrate content of meals required
- Meal content needs to be more or less similar from day to day

Flexible-dose regimen

Long-acting insulin (eg, Glargine/Lantus) once-a-day subcutaneous (usually at bedtime) for basal insulin coverage plus rapid-/short-acting insulin as bolus for meal coverage

- Calculate total daily insulin dose (based on body weight)
- 50% of dose as Lantus
- Insulin-to-carbohydrate ratio calculated initially using 1800 rule (1800 ÷ total daily insulin = correction factor)
- Correction factor ÷ 3 = insulin-to-carbohydrate ratio
- Correction factor is used to correct for hyperglycemia
- Insulin required with any carbohydrate ingestion (meal/snack)
- More flexible with regard to meal timings and content

with the family, whereas further fine-tuning and dose adjustments are made based on SMBG.

Insulin delivery devices

The basic insulin delivery devices are insulin preparations in vials, syringes, and needles. Syringes and needles are disposable and should not be reused. They are relatively inexpensive, but they require technical expertise and are cumbersome, with multiple items to carry. Insulin pen devices and pen needles

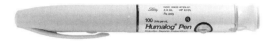

Fig. 1. Humalog Insulin pen. (Courtesy of Eli Lilly and Company, Indianapolis, Indiana.)

offer convenience, are capable of more precise dosing, do away with the need for carrying vials of insulin or drawing up doses, and are much quicker for adolescents to be able to use discretely in social situations. Patients should be advised about proper needle disposal (Figs. 1 and 2).

Continuous subcutaneous insulin infusion (CSII) by means of the insulin pump mimics normal insulin secretion by providing rapid-acting insulin over the 24-hour period at varying rates to mimic basal secretion [15–17]. The basal rates can be programmed appropriately to prevent nocturnal hypoglycemia or the dawn phenomenon (Fig. 3). Variable bolus options, depending on the meal content, are available in the form of immediate, square-wave, or dual-wave delivery. Therefore, patients with CSII have the potential and advantage of easily varying meal size, meal content, meal timing, and even skipping meals without compromising glycemic control. Pumps also have the option of being suspended during prolonged physical activity to avoid hypoglycemia. Despite these advantages in improving glycemic control when properly used, patients need to be extremely motivated and committed to achieve glycemic control and be willing to do frequent SMBG. They also have to develop technical expertise to deal with the pump and equipment, catheter insertion, and care of insertion site. In addition, they must be able to troubleshoot problems involving mechanical failures. Patients need adequate knowledge about carbohydrate counting to be able to make calculations for the amount of insulin for meals and snacks and correction for hyperglycemia.

Treatment of type 2 diabetes mellitus

For patients with T2DM, the treatment plan may vary depending on clinical circumstances at the time of diagnosis. If DKA is the presenting diagnosis, management is similar to that in patients with T1DM. These patients usually require a much higher dose of insulin and the addition of an insulin sensitizer, most commonly metformin, to improve insulin sensitivity. Gradually, the dose

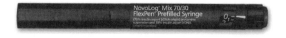

Fig. 2. Novo FlexPen. (Courtesy of Novo Nordisk, Bagsværd, Denmark.)

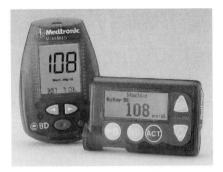

Fig. 3. Insulin pump. (Courtesy of Medtronic, Northridge, California.)

of metformin can be increased and insulin doses decreased. If the diagnosis is made either on routine physical examination or on investigations for obesity, PCOS, or hyperandrogenism, however, treatment may be initiated with metformin at 500 mg once a day and slowly built up to approximately 2 to 2.5 g/day; either long-acting preparations once a day or dividing the dose to twice a day with meals can be used [18]. Patients with T2DM associated with PCOS/metabolic X syndrome will additionally need assessment of and treatment for hyperlipidemia, hypertension, and hyperandrogenism. Medications available for use in T2DM act by means of different mechanisms. Different agents may be used alone or in combinations, and insulin may have to be added if there

Table 3
Oral medications for the treatment of type 2 diabetes mellitus

Medications	Usual daily dose (mg)
Sulfonylureas (act at the β cell, increase insulin secretion)	
Glimepiride (Amaryl)	1–4
Glipizide (Glucotrol)	10–20
Glyburide (Glynase)	5–20
Micronised glyburide (Micronase)	3–12
Glipizide extended release (Glucotrol XL)	5
α-Glucosidase inhibitors (act at the small intestine, increase insulin sensitivity)	
Acarbose (Precose)	50–100
Miglitol	50–100
Theazolidinediones (act at the muscle and fat, increase insulin sensitivity*)	
Rosiglitazone	4–8
Pioglitazone	15–45
Biguaides (act at the liver and muscle, increase insulin sensitivity)	
Metformin (Glucophage)	1000–2500
Others (act at the β cell; augment supply of insulin)	
Repaglinide (Prandin)	1–4

  * Probably by means of PPAR α.

is inadequate glycemic control with the oral agents alone [19]. Metformin is currently the most commonly used insulin sensitizer recommended for adolescents and adults with T2DM. Sibutramine has been approved for use in adolescents older than 16 years for weight control in obesity. The α-glucosidase inhibitors (acarbose and miglitol) are still not approved for use in younger adolescents; however, these agents may be used alone or in combination in older adolescents and young adults with T2DM. Oral agents commonly used are summarized in Table 3 [20].

Obese patients should be encouraged to lose weight and hence lower their BMI. Weight control and not gaining any additional weight may be initial steps in the right direction for these students, and deserve positive re-enforcement. Studies have shown the role of dietary interventions and modifications, and physical activity and exercise, to be of equivalent efficacy to that of metformin alone [21]. Lifestyle changes should be encouraged not only for the patient but for the whole family to be effective [22,23]. Dieticians should be involved from the onset to educate patients about different constituents of food, carbohydrate counting, making intelligent decisions about food choices, and making food exchanges. Varied levels of exercise activity have been recommended. Exercise improves insulin resistance in addition to its role in weight control.

Role of nutrition in diabetes

Individualized medical nutrition therapy (MNT) should be an integral part of diabetes education of each patient with diabetes on an ongoing basis, preferably by a dietician trained in diabetes. The aim of MNT is to improve health through healthy nutrition, achieve adequate metabolic control, and make appropriate dietary adjustments to deal with complicating factors; this therapy should be done in a framework to suit individual needs [24–26]. Healthy lifestyles are promoted in all patients, especially in individuals at high risk of developing T2DM, in the form of a healthy diet and adequate exercise to encourage weight loss or at least maintain stable weight [22,23]. In older adolescents and young adults with T1DM, insulin regimens should be adjusted for patients' normal dietary intake and physical activity to promote normal growth and development; for those with T2DM, nutrition should be modified along with increased physical activity to improve hyperinsulinemia and decrease insulin resistance [23]. Patients who have T1DM and who are on intensive insulin regimens (CSII or multiple daily injections [MDI]) adjust premeal short-acting insulin dose based on the carbohydrate content of their meal, hence the importance of carbohydrate counting. Patients on fixed-dose regimens need to be more consistent in the carbohydrate content of their meals and the timing of meals. Basic knowledge about the food pyramid, carbohydrate counting, and relative food content with regard to carbohydrates, protein, and fats is essential for achieving good glycemic control.

Role of exercise

Obesity and a sedentary lifestyle are predisposing factors for development of IGT and T2DM. Exercise has universal benefits for everyone, but it can be an important preventive and therapeutic tool in T2DM; the onset of T2DM can be delayed with regular exercise. Exercise programs need to be individualized. Potential benefits include weight reduction, improved insulin sensitivity, and lowering of hyperlipidemia and cardiovascular risk; in addition, there is a reduction in the dose of insulin and oral medications. Lifestyle changes consisting of dietary modifications as per the MNT and regular exercise program have been caused improvement in all of the previously described parameters [21–23].

Means of blood glucose monitoring

SMBG is done by measuring capillary blood glucose with blood glucose meters [27]. Many blood glucose testing meters present helpful features, including the ability to test alternative sites (besides fingertips), larger memory capacity for data storage (for many months), and the capability of being downloaded on computer programs. In one new system, the blood glucose meter and pump interact with each other, whereas other meters allow the patient to record data on carbohydrate ingestion and insulin dosing. Despite the capability of these meters to store, download, and offer data for evaluation, patients should still be encouraged to record SMBG data in logbooks, to detect patterns early.

Glucose sensors

Continuous and intermittent glucose sensing may be used as an adjunct to, not a replacement for, SMBG, and provides a method to optimize glycemic

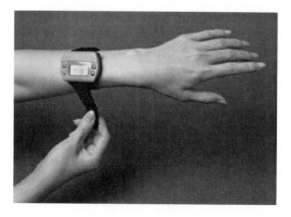

Fig. 4. GlucoWatch Biographer. (Courtesy of Cygnus, Inc., Redwood City, California.)

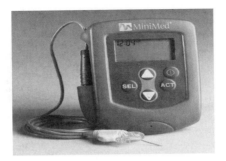

Fig. 5. The Continuous Glucose Monitoring System, or CGMS. (Courtesy of Medtronic, North-ridge, California.)

control. Two different devices are presently available: the Continuous Glucose Monitoring System, or CGMS (Medtronic MiniMed), and GlucoWatch Biographer (Cygnus; Figs. 4 and 5) [28–30]. Both devices are calibrated by finger-stick SMBG and then sense glucose in the subcutaneous interstitial fluid. Indications for monitoring by any of these systems include patients with elevated HbA1c, unexplained variability in glucose readings, and unexplained hypogly-cemia or hypoglycemia unawareness [31]. Other devices are under investigation.

Glycated hemoglobin (A1c)

HbA1c testing measures the chronic, nonenzymatic concentration-dependent binding of glucose to hemoglobin. This analysis has facilitated the follow-up of glycemic control of patients with diabetes [27,32,33]. It is the strongest statistically associated variable to predict risk of complications. Recent advances have made convenient finger-stick testing of HbA1c possible at the time of office visits. This development has greatly improved the ability to assess long-term glycemic control, authenticate SMBG data, discuss the results with the patient at the time of the visit, and make changes in the insulin/diet regimen to improve glycemia. Some hemoglobinopathies, anemias, and polycythemia may affect the results. The HbA1c test is done every 3 months at the time of office visits.

Ketone testing

Ketone testing offers a great tool for monitoring the progress during DKA management, to detect onset of ketosis during hyperglycemia or periods of illness at home; hence, it is incorporated into sick-day management [27]. Urine strips are commonly used to test for acetoacetate, and readings are reported as trace, small, medium, or large. Some newer blood glucose testing meters are capable of testing for beta hydroxy butyric acid in the blood, at home or in the office setting.

Diabetes management—the team approach

The intensive management of diabetes requires multidisciplinary care and support. This team comprises the primary care physician, endocrinologist, diabetes nurse, diabetes nurse educator, nutritionist, psychologist, and social worker. The team members need to focus on a common goal and expectations, with each member imparting the same message. Problems of each patient are identified, and individualized treatment plans are formulated and incorporated by all of the team members.

Adjustments to independence

Older adolescents and young adults have been used to having the family involved in their diabetes management, supervision, and care for years, as is highly recommended; however, when at college, they are on their own. Like multiple other issues of gradual independence at this age, they should gradually be given responsibility for self-care of diabetes with regard to performance skills and decision making about adjustments in insulin dose for different situations. These students will experience a change of health care providers on relocation, and they may take time getting comfortable with their new set-up and diabetes caregivers. Until this relocation successfully occurs, it is helpful for these patients to remain in contact with their previous health team. Earlier home experience in ability to deal with, and troubleshoot, minor and major problems in daily diabetes management and care builds the confidence of these young adults over time and helps them to become comfortable when faced with independent living, while successfully caring for their diabetes.

Sports and diabetes

Many management strategies have been developed to facilitate sports participation in patients with DM. Besides the usual benefits of regular exercise and physical activity, there are additional benefits for patients with diabetes, such as decreasing insulin resistance, improving insulin sensitivity, and improving glycemic control, which result in lowering of insulin requirements and weight reduction or weight control. The details of the activity are planned, and the necessary modifications in the insulin regimen are worked out by the diabetes caregivers and applied; necessary alterations are made to achieve the desired results. It is important to avoid hypoglycemia because it may prove to be life-threatening during active sports activity. Recommendations may include taking a lower-than-usual calculated dose of insulin at the meal before the scheduled activity or ingesting extra carbohydrate choices before or during the activity, depending on the blood sugars obtained pre-, mid-, and post activity. The dedication, meticulousness, and commitment required to succeed in sports also result in achieving successful intensive diabetes control management. Patient who have T1DM usually require closer observation and are more difficult to control in these scenarios than patients with T2DM. It is important to individualize each student's regimen and adjust it by trial and error until the desired control is obtained. Those with some diabetes complications, such as retinopathy, should not engage in heavy weight lifting and contact sports to avoid ocular consequences of high blood pressure. The presence of peripheral and autonomic neuropathy may also place the patient at risk to get injured. Therefore, taking up any high-risk sports activity in which the student with diabetes may be at risk or may be a risk to others around him or her needs careful assessment and evaluation [34].

Driving, drinking, drugs, and diabetes

As is commonly stated, "Driving is a privilege and not a right." Therefore, along with other responsibilities involved in being a responsible driver, it is mandatory for a person with diabetes to maintain euglycemia to be safe and alert, not only for him- or herself but for all others on the road. The driver with diabetes should know his or her blood sugar level before getting behind the wheel, have a rapidly acting source of carbohydrates on hand, and should carry medic alert information. Ideally, the driver's license should state that the driver is diabetic. The issue of responsible driving should be a component of the intensive diabetes education. In addition to diabetes care for the young driver, the concern with alcohol and driving is the same as that for any other driver. Drinking and driving or driving under the effect of alcohol is dangerous and illegal, and should be discouraged. These patients have the added risk of hypoglycemia because of interference with hepatic gluconeogenesis and glycogenolysis. At college parties, there should always be a designated driver to ensure a safe drive back.

Although alcohol is illegal for use in adolescents and young college students, street drugs are illegal for use at any age. Aside from the long-term devastating consequences of drug abuse and drug dependence, patients with diabetes may experience masking of symptoms of hypoglycemia or severe hyperglycemia when under the influence of these drugs. These drugs also affect judgment and decision making and compromise the ability to take optimal care of diabetes; therefore, use of all these agents should be discouraged.

Smoking and diabetes

Cigarette smoking has been recognized as one of the most important avoidable causes of premature death; it accounts for one in every five deaths in the United States. The high risk of morbidity and mortality caused by macrovascular complications associated with combined smoking and diabetes is now well recognized. Smoking under peer pressure in the college environment is a real danger, leading to an addictive behavior. Each health care provider in the college health service and other offices who sees the student with DM (and all students) should repeatedly emphasize the importance of not initiating smoking in nonsmokers. Smokers should be firmly urged to quit and should be provided with cessation counseling, referral to cessation programs, and assistance with cessation aids. The use of pharmacologic agents, such as nicotine replacement, bupropion, or nortriptyline, in addition to behavioral modifications, may enhance cessation rates. Motivated patients should be encouraged and fully supported through the process of quitting tobacco use [35].

Influenza and pneumococcal immunizations in diabetes

Influenza and pneumococcal disease have been noted to cause high risk of complications, hospitalizations, and mortality in patients with DM. Therefore, recommendations regarding immunizations with these vaccines include yearly influenza vaccination and at least a one-time pneumococcal vaccination in these patients [36]. Special considerations may be necessary for patients with a history of egg allergy.

Acute complications of diabetes

Acute complications may arise from hyperglycemia or hypoglycemia. Acute problems with glycemic control may be less severe in patients with T2DM versus in patients with T1DM. Careful monitoring of glycemic control needs to be maintained at all times to avoid hypoglycemia and hyperglycemia.

Hyperglycemia

Hyperglycemia may trigger the onset of DKA, with components of hyperglycemia, ketosis, and acidosis [9–12]. Although more commonly seen in T1DM, it has been well recognized in T2DM as well. The entity labeled nonketotic hyperosmolar coma (NKHC) also has been described in patients with T2DM. Cerebral edema is a life-threatening complication that may be seen during treatment of DKA, although it is more common in younger individuals than in adults [37]. The incidence of cerebral edema has been further lowered by careful fluid replacement protocols. Vigilant testing, adequate hydration, and intensification of insulin regimen according to the sick-day protocol need to be repeatedly emphasized to these students to minimize short-term side effects and hospital admissions.

Sick-day management

Intensive diabetes management protocols with rapid and accurate assessment of blood glucose and urine ketones have greatly lowered the rate of recurrent hospital admissions for patients with DKA. Diabetes programs usually have their own written protocols for sick-day management for use at home. Patients and their families are provided with these at the onset of diabetes, so that early recognition and timely intervention with the help of a health care provider (by means of telephone) can usually eliminate the progression of DKA and obviate the need for hospitalization. Patients are told to check for ketones if their blood glucose level is more than 250 mg/dL or if they feel ill. Emphasis is placed on maintaining adequate hydration, frequent monitoring of blood glucose (every 1–2 h) to check hyperglycemia, and avoiding hypoglycemia; in addition, the urine should be checked for urine ketones in each void. Noncaloric fluids are advised when blood sugars are more than 250 mg/dL, and caloric fluids are recommended when blood sugars are 200 mg/dL or show a downward trend. The basal insulin (NPH, Lantus, or basal rate on the pump) is continued at the same dose, whereas boluses of short-acting insulin are given at 2- to 4-hour intervals based on blood glucose, urine ketones, and oral intake. Insulin should never be withheld because this may lead to precipitation of DKA [37]. These basic principles of sick-day management are reinforced repeatedly at office visits and also at the time of phone contact, so that by the time these older adolescents are ready for college, they are prepared for managing a sick-day scenario on their own. It is critical to emphasize the importance of early physician phone contact and the need to recognize the failure of home/dormitory management early and seek timely emergency room care.

Hypoglycemia

Multiple abnormalities in the glucose, insulin, and counter-regulatory hormone (namely, glucagon, epinephrine, cortisol, and growth hormone) feedback system in DM lead to abnormalities in glucose homeostasis, causing hypoglycemia. Signs and symptoms depend on the severity of hypoglycemia and are usually obvious with blood glucose levels falling below 50 to 60 mg/dL. Symptoms include the following: tremors, palpitations, severe hunger, sweating, headaches, irritability, mood changes, drowsiness, unresponsiveness, unconsciousness, and even seizures [12]. The aim of intensive management is to achieve adequate glycemic control with minimal episodes of such hypoglycemia. Acute episodes of hypoglycemia may lead to accidents and injuries at work, on the street, while driving or swimming, or during sporting events. Repeated episodes of seizures are also associated with poor school performance and memory deficits, and may lead to permanent central nervous system compromise. Common causes of hypoglycemia are listed in Box 4.

Mild to moderate hypoglycemia is treated by ingesting 10 to 15 g of carbohydrate, preferably a simple sugar in the premeasured form or as in juice

---

Box 4. Common causes of hypoglycemia

Insulin errors (inadvertent or deliberate)

- Reversal of morning and evening dosage
- Reversal of short- or rapid-acting and intermediate- or long-acting insulin
- Improper timing of insulin in relation to food
- Excessive insulin dosage

Intensive insulin therapy

- Erratic or altered absorption of insulin
- More rapid absorption from exercising limbs
- Unpredictable absorption from lipohypertrophied injection sites
- Changing insulin preparations or regimens

Nutrition

- Omitted or inadequate amounts of food
- Timing errors: late snacks or meals

Exercise

- Unplanned activity
- Prolonged duration or increased intensity of activity

Alcohol and drugs

- Impaired hepatic gluconeogenesis associated with alcohol intake
- Impaired mentation associated with alcohol, marijuana, or other illicit drugs

Adapted from American Diabetes Association. Special situations. In: Bode WB, editor. Medical management of type 1 diabetes. 4th edition. Alexandria, VA: American Diabetes Association; 2004. p. 121–60.

---

or regular soda. If hypoglycemia occurs and it is not a mealtime, blood glucose should be rechecked in 15 to 20 minutes and, if normal, followed by a 15-g longer-acting mixture of complex carbohydrate and protein. For severe hypoglycemia or altered mental status, the student should be given IV glucose (10–25 g of 50% dextrose, diluted) or intramuscular or subcutaneous glucagon.

If these are unavailable, glucose gels applied between the gum and cheek may help, but this method is not a preferred method of treatment. It is recommended that the patient keep some source of carbohydrate and a glucagon kit with them at all times [38]. Roommates, friends, and family members should be educated about treatment of hypoglycemia and glucagon administration. It is also recommended that all patients with DM always wear a medic alert.

Chronic complications of diabetes

Chronic complications of DM appear after varying durations of the disease process. The timing of the onset of chronic complications is directly related to the level of hyperglycemia and the cumulative amount of time the tissues are exposed to the high levels of glucose. The prevalence of chronic complications, therefore, in younger patients is lower, and the incidence increases with an increase in duration of the disease. The main complications are as follows: retinopathy, nephropathy, neuropathy, macrovascular disease, and limited joint mobility. Patients with T2DM and T2DM may exhibit all kinds of complications depending on the duration of the disease. College students therefore may experience varied levels of chronic complications, depending on the age at diagnosis and the level of long-term glycemic control.

Retinopathy

In patients who have T1DM, significant retinopathy is usually not seen before 5 years' duration of DM. Twenty years after diagnosis, nearly all patients with T1DM have background retinopathy, whereas approximately 60% of patients with T2DM have the disease. The retinopathy may comprise macular edema, nonproliferative retinopathy, or proliferative retinopathy; it may not cause any visual symptoms until an advanced stage, therefore necessitating regular (yearly or more frequent, if required) expert ophthalmologic examinations. Prompt photocoagulation of proliferative retinopathy should be undertaken, even before visual symptoms develop, to preserve or restore vision [39]. In T1DM and probably T2DM, intensive insulin treatment to attain normoglycemia will prevent or ameliorate retinopathy [41]. Any visual symptoms, vitreal hemorrhages, macular edema, or neovascularization need to be referred immediately and photocoagulation undertaken at the earliest, if and when required; otherwise, there may be a 25% to 50% risk of severe visual loss within 2 years [42].

Nephropathy

Approximately 20% to 30% of patients with T1DM eventually develop end-stage renal failure requiring dialysis, whereas 5% to 10% of patients with T2DM develop this condition after having had the disease for 20 years [43–45]. Diabetic nephropathy therefore needs careful monitoring of urine by dipstick, blood pressure screening at every visit, and annual urine microalbuminuria measurements [46,47]. A microalbuminuria (urinary albumin excretion rate) of 30 to 300 mg every 24 hours may sometimes either spontaneously resolve or herald early nephropathy often associated with hypertension; this condition can gradually evolve to overt stages and subsequently to advanced nephropathy associated with compromised renal function, end-stage renal disease, hypertension, and uremia requiring dialysis and renal transplantation. All patients with T2DM and patients with pubertal T1DM with disease duration of 5 years or more are recommended to undergo yearly screening in any of the following three methods: (1) spot urine for albumin–creatinine ratio; (2) timed samples, overnight or 24-hour urine collection samples for the same are acceptable means of measuring albumin excretion rate [1]. Because of great variability in testing, repeat testing should be performed before labeling the level of nephropathy. Hypertension, which is usually secondary to renal disease, needs to be regularly screened for, diagnosed early, and treated aggressively. Multiple blood pressure measurements should be done before starting treatment. Many groups of drugs may be used, including angiotensin converting enzyme inhibitors, angiotensin II receptor blockers, diuretics, β-adrenergic blocking agents, or even calcium antagonists [48]. The treatment of diabetic nephropathy is generally supportive and preventive; therefore, it is essential to maintain adequate glycemic control and take care of factors that may predispose to or aggravate nephropathy, such as hyperlipidemia, protein restriction, urinary tract infection, neurogenic bladder, and use of radio contrast dyes. Once end-stage renal disease ensues, the only two options available are dialysis and renal transplantation.

Neuropathy

The prevalence of diabetic neuropathy again depends on the duration and severity of hyperglycemia in T1DM and T2DM. Neuropathy may involve peripheral, autonomic, or focal nerves and becomes one of the most troublesome complications of diabetes [40,49]. It is rarely seen within 5 years of the disease. In addition, it has been shown in the Diabetes Control and Complications Trial that intensive treatment may significantly delay the onset and progression of diabetic neuropathy [50]. Late complications of polyneuropathy include foot ulcerations and unrecognized trauma to the hands and feet because of loss of sensory perception, necessitating aggressive and early treatment of any infections. Autonomic neuropathy usually affects one or two organ systems (eg, cardiovascular, gastrointestinal, or genitourinary systems producing diffuse subclinical dysfunction). Neuroarthropathies or Charcot's joints are also seen [44].

Macrovascular complications

DM is a risk factor for cardiovascular and cerebrovascular diseases. These diseases occur earlier, are more severe, and have a worse prognosis in patients with DM. They are considered high risk and therefore any dyslipidemia and hypertension need to be aggressively treated [51]. Cigarette smoking should be highly discouraged.

Special situations in female college students with diabetes

Two clinical scenarios specific for older adolescent and young adult females on the college campus are pregnancy and PCOS.

Pregnancy with diabetes

All female adolescents, including college students, with diabetes need to practice effective methods of contraception consistently to avoid unplanned pregnancy because of the high risk for the mother. There is also a high risk of miscarriages, fetal anomalies, major malformations, and metabolic abnormalities caused by maternal hyperglycemia. No method of contraception method is contraindicated in diabetes and therefore the methods with higher rates of protection should be offered to these patients. In addition, precautions for protection from sexually transmitted diseases and HIV infections should always be practiced. All female college students should be routinely counseled about the previously mentioned risks and advised to use effective contraception at all times unless abstaining from sex or in good metabolic control and trying to conceive. In recognition of the importance of appropriate diabetes management in pregnancy, the American Diabetes Association recommends the "preconception care program once pregnancy is desired and planned." This program basically includes education about interactions of diabetes, pregnancy, and family planning; it also involves diabetes self-management skills, diabetes care by a physician, laboratory testing, with specialized psychologic counseling and support for stress reduction and improved compliance [52].

Polycystic ovarian syndrome

PCOS is being increasingly recognized in the adolescent female population. Older adolescents and young adult females with PCOS are hyperandrogenic and have approximately a 40% reduction in insulin-stimulated glucose disposal as compared with controls [53]. Improvement in hyperandrogenemia is also associated with improved insulin sensitivity. A history of intrauterine growth retardation and premature adrenarche are now being recognized as predisposing factors for insulin resistance and PCOS.

Psychosocial effects

Many aspects of intensive diabetes care are in direct conflict with the need for independence and peer acceptance in older adolescents and college students.

This situation may result in noncompliance with blood glucose testing, insulin administration, dietary indiscretions, seeking help with medical care, and keeping clinic appointments. Multiple issues therefore emerge leading to poor glycemic control, and depression may also result. Depression is an important comorbidity for patients with diabetes and requires careful management because of its severe impact on the quality of life [54–56]. If anticipated early, these issues can be addressed in advance by the diabetes caregivers and psychologist. Many of the newer treatment strategies and modalities are helpful in offering a more flexible lifestyle, although increased monitoring is still necessary.

Career selection

Today, most professions are open to persons with diabetes. Jobs involving situations where the safety of many others depends on this one individual may not be the best career choices for patients with diabetes; therefore, professions such as the military and commercial aviation are not career options. Generally speaking, with intensive management, students with DM should be able to enjoy most professions and be able to participate in most leisure activities and hobbies.

Emerging therapies

There are many new treatment options being developed in DM, which are presently in different phases of clinical trials and may soon be approved by the FDA for clinical use.

Newer insulins

Insulin Detemir is a new long-acting insulin analog for basal insulin coverage, which is obtained by altering the structure of the insulin molecule by omitting the amino acid at B30 and attaching a 14-carbon fatty acid side chain at B29. This change causes enhanced binding to albumin in subcutaneous tissue to delay absorption, and in plasma, it limits the amount of free insulin available for action, hence increasing its duration of action. Its pharmacokinetic profile seems to be superior to NPH and may have the option of use once or twice daily [57]. Insulin Glulisine (3^BLys – 29^B – GLU – human insulin) is a new rapid-acting insulin being developed and seems to have a profile similar to other rapidly acting insulins.

Alternative insulin delivery systems

Efforts have been made, and are ongoing, to find alternative insulin delivery systems besides the subcutaneous route. Pulmonary insulin delivery by means of inhalation, peritoneal insulin delivery by means of implantable pumps, transdermal insulin delivery, buccal insulin delivery, and oral insulin preparations are being developed and are in various stages of clinical trials. These newer forms promise more convenience for insulin administration. Closed-loop insulin delivery systems (eg, Medtronic MiniMed 2007 Pump, Medtronic, Northridge, California) involve continuous peritoneal insulin infusions by means of programmable implantable pumps, with specially formulated U-400 insulin allowing for refills every 2 to 3 months [58]. The intraperitoneal insulin is absorbed into the portal circulation, closely simulating physiologic insulin delivery and absorption. This insulin delivery may be programmed with accurate blood glucose measurements obtained from a long-term glucose sensor inserted in the superior vena cava and connected to the implantable pump [57]. Research in this area is being actively pursued and may soon revolutionize the management of diabetes, especially T1DM.

Other islet cell hormones

Amylin (analog Pramlintide) is a hormone cosecreted with insulin; it has effects complementary to insulin and is also deficient in patients with T1DM. Amylin regulates the inflow of glucose into circulation after meals, whereas insulin is involved in the regulation of glucose out of the circulation. It may be potentially helpful in patients with T1DM who have suboptimal control, when incorporated into the insulin regimen. Trials are ongoing, and it is not yet been approved for clinical use [59]. Islet neogenesis-associated protein, or INGAP, peptide has been shown to have the ability to stimulate islet cell neogenesis and hence improve glycemic control and even reverse diabetes (in the animal model). If there is evidence of a similar response in humans, it may have dramatic implications for patients with DM in the future [60].

Islet cell transplantation

Using modifications of the Edmonton protocol, hundreds of islet allotransplantations have been done worldwide [61]. The procedure still has difficulties with regard to sufficient islet cell yield and issues with immunomodulation and immune suppression. To expand the potential benefits of islet transplantation, there is intensive ongoing research on xenogenic islets, the use of stem cells, interventions to achieve islet regeneration and proliferation, and bioengineering techniques for insulin-producing cells; it is hoped that further research will allow the full benefit of this mode of intervention for a larger number of patients with diabetes [61,62].

Summary

Diabetes is a common chronic disease of the older adolescent and young adult age groups. T1DM and T2DM are most prevalent, with a much lower incidence of MODY and some types of diabetes secondary to other causes. The incidence of T2DM is much higher in certain ethnic groups and is presently increasing at an epidemic proportion, paralleling the obesity curve. Testing guidelines have been recommended for patients at high risk for early detection of T2DM. The initial presentation of diabetes may vary from asymptomatic to presentation with serious metabolic decompensation in DKA or NKHC. Multiple options are available for treatment of both T1DM and T2DM. Patients with T1DM may be treated with various insulin regimens and CSII. SMBG, glycated hemoglobin, and ketone testing offer excellent means of monitoring glycemic control. The risk of microvascular and macrovascular complications is directly proportional to level and duration of hyperglycemia. Comprehensive intensive management can normalize daily life and significantly decrease and delay the incidence of chronic complications. College students are exposed to many interfering/modifying factors, including increasing independence and exposure to high-risk behavior, such as drinking, driving, taking drugs, and having unprotected sex, predisposing to unplanned pregnancies; these factors contribute to inadequately controlled/monitored diabetes status. Intensive therapeutic regimens with ongoing comprehensive diabetes education can greatly improve these individuals' diabetes control. Newer and emerging treatment options continue to be developed to facilitate treatment modalities for diabetes and possibly to find a cure.

The information in this article is largely based on recommendations of the American Diabetes Association, which is not only a strong advocate for patients with diabetes but also is a comprehensive resource for information on all aspects of diabetes, both for patients and medical staff. Further information may be obtained at the organization's Web site: www.diabetes.org.

Acknowledgments

The author thanks Drs. Martin Draznin, Dilip Patel, and Donald Hare for their critical review of the manuscript and Ms. Amy Esman and Ms. Cori Edgecomb for their expert administrative assistance.

References

[1] American Diabetes Association. Medical management of type 1 diabetes. In: Bode BW, editor. Diagnosis and classification/pathogenesis. 4th edition. Alexandria, VA: American Diabetes Association; 2004. p. 5–18.

[2] American Diabetes Association. Epidemiology of type 2 diabetes and obesity in children. In: Rosenblum AL, Silverstein JH, editors. Type 2 diabetes in children and adolescents. Alexandria, VA: American Diabetes Association. p. 17–24.

[3] American Diabetes Association. Diagnosis and classification of diabetes mellitus (position statement). Diabetes Care 2004;27(Suppl 1):S5–10.

[4] Expert Committee on the Diagnosis and Classification of Diabetes Mellitus. Follow-up report on the diagnosis of diabetes mellitus. Diabetes Care 2003;26:3160–7.

[5] American Diabetes Association. Type 2 diabetes in children and adolescents (consensus statement). Diabetes Care 2000;23:381–9.

[6] American Diabetes Association. Type 2 diabetes in children and adolescents. Pediatrics 2000;105:671–80.

[7] American Diabetes Association. Screening for diabetes (position statement). Diabetes Care 2004;27(Suppl 1):S11–4.

[8] American Diabetes Association. Standards of medical care in diabetes (position statement). Diabetes Care 2004;26(Suppl 1):S15–35.

[9] Kaufman FR, Halvorson M. The treatment and prevention of diabetic ketoacidosis in children and adolescents with type 1 diabetes. Pediatr Ann 1999;28:576–82.

[10] American Diabetes Association. Hyperglycemic crisis in diabetes (position statement). Diabetes Care 2004;26(Suppl 1):S94–102.

[11] Kitabchi AE, Umpierrez GE, Murphy MB, et al. Management of hyperglycemic crises in patients with diabetes mellitus [technical review]. Diabetes Care 2001;24:131–53.

[12] American Diabetes Association. Special situations. In: Bode BW, editor. Medical management of type 1 diabetes. 4th edition. Alexandria, VA: American Diabetes Association; 2004. p. 121–60.

[13] American Diabetes Association. Insulin administration (position statement). Diabetes Care 2004;26(Suppl 1):S111–3.

[14] American Diabetes Association. Multiple component insulin regimens in therapy in intensive diabetes management. In: Klingensmith GJ, editor. Intensive diabetes management. 3rd edition. Alexandria, VA: American Diabetes Association; 2003.

[15] American Diabetes Association. Insulin infusion pump therapy in intensive diabetes management. In: Klingensmith GJ, editor. Intensive diabetes management. 3rd edition. Alexandria, VA: American Diabetes Association; 2003.

[16] Lenhard MJ, Reeves GD. Continuous subcutaneous insulin infusion: a comprehensive review of insulin pump therapy. Arch Intern Med 2001;161:2293–300.

[17] Pickup J, Keen H. Continuous subcutaneous insulin infusion at 25 years: evidence base for the expanding use of insulin pump therapy in type 1 diabetes. Diabetes Care 2002;25:593–8.

[18] Bristol-Meyers Squibb. Glucophage (metformin) [package insert]. New York: Bristol-Meyers Squibb; 1999.

[19] White JR. The pharmacological reduction of blood glucose in patients with type 2 diabetes mellitus. Clin Diabetes 1998;16:58–67.

[20] American Diabetes Association. Overview of medications used to treat type 2 diabetes. In: Campbell RK, White JR, editors. Medications for the treatment of diabetes. 3rd edition. Alexandria, VA: American Diabetes Association; 2000. p. 23–43.

[21] Diabetes Prevention Program Research Group. Reduction in the incidence of type 2 diabetes with lifestyle intervention or metformin. N Engl J Med 2003;346:393–403.

[22] Tuomilehto J, Lindstrom J, Eriksson JG, et al. Prevention of type 2 diabetes mellitus by changes in life-style among subjects with impaired glucose tolerance. N Engl J Med 2001; 244:1343–50.

[23] Stone NJ. Focus on lifestyle change and the metabolic syndrome. Endocrinol Metab Clin N Am 2004;33:493–508.

[24] American Diabetes Association. Nutrition principles and recommendations in diabetes (position statement). Diabetes Care 2004;27(Suppl):S36–46.

[25] Franz MJ, Bantle JP, Beebe CA, et al. Evidence-based nutrition principles and recommendations for the treatment and prevention of diabetes and related complications [technical review]. Diabetes Care 2002;25:148–98.

[26] American Diabetes Association. Management. In: Kelley DB, editor. Medical management of type 2 diabetes. Alexandria, VA: American Diabetes Association; 1998. p. 27–85.

[27] American Diabetic Association. Tests of glycemia in diabetes (position statement). Diabetes Care 2004;26(Suppl. 1):S91–3.

[28] Schiaffini R, Ciampalini P, Fierabracci A, et al. The continuous glucose monitoring system (CGMS) in type I diabetic children is the way to reduce hypoglycemic risk. Diabetes Metab Res Rev 2002;18:324–9.

[29] Eastman RC, Chase HP, Buckingham B, et al. Use of the GlucoWatch Biographer in children and adolescents with diabetes. Pediatr Diabetes 2002;3:127–34.

[30] Sachedina N, Pickup JC. Performance assessment of the Medtronic-MiniMed Continuous Glucose Monitoring System and its use for measurement of glycaemic control in Type I diabetic subjects. Diabet Med 2003;20(12):1012–5.

[31] Speiser PW. Continuous glucose monitoring in managing diabetes in children. Diabetes Metab Res Rev 2002;18:330–1.

[32] Goldstein DE, Little RR, Lorenz RA, Malone JL, Nathan D, Peterson CM. Tests of glycemia in diabetes [technical review]. Diabetes Care 1995;18:896–909.

[33] Sacks DS, Bruns DE, Goldstein DE, Maclaren NK, McDonald JM, Parrott M. Guidelines and recommendations for laboratory analyses in the diagnosis and management of diabetes mellitus. Diabetes Care 2002;25:750–86.

[34] Draznin MB. Type I diabetes and sports participation—strategies for training and competing safely. Phys Sports Med 2000;28(12):49–56.

[35] American Diabetes Association. Smoking and diabetes (position statement). Diabetes Care 2004;27(Suppl 1):S74–5.

[36] American Diabetes Association. Influenza and pneumococcal immunizations in diabetes (position statement). Diabetes Care 2004;26(Suppl 1):S111–3.

[37] American Diabetes Association. Tools of therapy in medical management of type 1 diabetes. In: Bode WB, editor. Medical management of type 1 diabetes. 4th edition. Alexandria, VA: American Diabetes Association; 2004.

[38] Cryer PE, Davis SN, Shamoon H. Hypoglycemia in diabetes. Diabetes Care 2003;26:1902–12.

[39] Aiello LM. Perspectives on diabetic retinopathy. Am J Ophthalmol 2003;136:122–35.

[40] Diabetes Control and Complications Trial Research Group. The effect of intensive treatment of diabetes on the development and progression of long-term complications in insulin-dependent diabetes mellitus. N Engl J Med 1993;329:977–86.

[41] Diabetes Control and Complications Trial Research Group. The relationship of glycemic exposure (HbA1c) to the risk of development and progression of retinopathy. The Diabetes Control and Complications Trial. Diabetes 1995;44:968–83.

[42] American Diabetes Association. Diabetic retinopathy (position statement). Diabetes Care 2004;27(Suppl 1):S84–7.

[43] American Diabetes Association. Diabetic nephropathy (position statement). Diabetes Care 2004;27(Suppl 1):S79–83.

[44] American Diabetes Association. Complications. In: Bode BW, editor. Medical management of type 1 diabetes. 4th edition. Alexandria, VA: American Diabetes Association; 2004. p. 183–233.

[45] Jacobson HR, Striker GE. Report on a workshop to develop management recommendations for the prevention of progression in chronic renal disease. Am J Kidney Dis 1995;25:103–6.

[46] Mogensen CE, Keane WF, Bennett PH, et al. Prevention of diabetic renal disease with special reference to microalbuminuria. Lancet 1995;346:1080–4.

[47] Bennett PH, Haffner S, Kasiske BL, et al. Screening and management of microalbuminuria in patients with diabetes mellitus. Am J Kidney Dis 1995;25:107–12.

[48] Remuzzi G, Ruggenenti P, Perico N. Chronic renal diseases: renoprotective benefits of renin-angiotensin system inhibition. Ann Intern Med 2002;136:604–15.

[49] Vinik AI, Park TS, Stansberry KB, Pittenger GL. Diabetic neuropathies. Diabetologia 2000;43:957–73.

[50] Diabetes Control and Complications Trial Research Group. The effect of intensive treatment of diabetes on the development and progression of long-term complications in insulin-dependent diabetes mellitus. N Engl J Med 1993;329:977–86.

[51] American Diabetic Association. Treatment of hypertension (position statement). Diabetes Care 2004;27(Suppl 1):S65–7.

[52] American Diabetes Association. Preconception care of women with diabetes (position statement). Diabetes Care 2004;27(Suppl 1):S76–83.

[53] American Diabetes Association. Epidemiology of type 2 diabetes and obesity in children. In: Rosenbloom AL, Silverstein JH, editors. Type 2 diabetes in children and adolescents. Alexandria, VA: American Diabetes Association; 2003. p. 25–45.

[54] Goldney RD, Phillips PJ, Fisher LJ, Wilson DH. Diabetes, depression, and quality of life. Diabetes Care 2004;27:1066–70.

[55] Lin EHB, Katon W, Von Korff M, et al. Relationship of depression and diabetes self-care, medication adherence, and preventive care. Diabetes Care 2004;27:2154–60.

[56] Lustman PJ, Anderson RJ, Freedland KE, de Groot M, Carney RM, Clouse RE. Depression and poor glycemic control: a meta-analytic review of the literature. Diabetes Care 2000; 23(7):934–42.

[57] American Diabetes Association. Emerging therapies. In: Bode BW, editor. Medical management of type I diabetes. 4th edition. Alexandria, VA: American Diabetes Association; 2004. p. 233–48.

[58] Steil GM, Blumauer N, Leech J, Long K, Panteleon AE, Rebrin K. Closed loop insulin delivery using subcutaneous (SC) glucose sensing and SC insulin delivery [abstract]. Diabetes 2001;50(Suppl 2):A132.

[59] Buse JB, Weyer C, Maggs DG. Amylin replacement with pramlintide in type 1 and type 2 diabetes: a physiological approach to overcome barriers with insulin therapy. Clin Diabetes 2002;20:137–44.

[60] Gagliardino JJ, Del Zotto H, Massa L, Flores LE, Borelli MI. Pancreatic duodenal homeobox-1 and islet neogenesis-associated protein: a possible combined marker of activateable pancreatic cell precursors. J Endocrinol 2003;177(2):249–59.

[61] Shapiro AMJ, Lakey JRT, Ryan EA, et al. Islet transplantation in seven patients with type 1 diabetes using a glucocorticoid-free immunosuppressive regimen. N Engl J Med 2000;343:230–8.

[62] Ryan EA, Lakey JR, Rajotte RV, et al. Clinical outcomes and insulin secretion after islet transplantation with the Edmonton protocol. Diabetes 2001;50(4):710–9.

ELSEVIER
SAUNDERS

Pediatr Clin N Am 52 (2005) 307–319

PEDIATRIC CLINICS
OF NORTH AMERICA

Substance Abuse on the College Campus

Mary Ellen Rimsza, MD, FAAP[a,b,*],
Karen S. Moses, MS, RD, CHES[a]

[a]School of Health Services Administration and Policy, W.P. Carey School of Business,
Student Health and Wellness Center, Arizona State University, PO Box 872104, Tempe,
AZ 85287-210, USA
[b]Mayo Clinic College of Medicine, Scottsdale, AZ, USA

Substance abuse is a major health and behavioral concern in college students. Alcohol and marijuana are the most commonly abused drugs on college campuses. Others include tobacco, 3,4-methylenedioxymethamphetamine, gamma-hydroxybutyrate, flunitrazepam (Rohypnol), lysergic acid, ketamine, methamphetamine, phencyclidine, cocaine, and psilocybin mushrooms. This article reviews the use of these drugs by college students. Substance use is a major contributing factor in poor academic performance and failure to successfully complete a college education.

Alcohol

Approximately 80% of college students drink alcohol and over 40% of college students are heavy episodic (binge) drinkers; binge drinking is usually defined as having 5 or more drinks in a row for men and 4 or more drinks for women. Although their noncollegiate peers drink more often, college students tend to drink more heavily when they do drink [1,2]. Indeed, college students binge drink more often than age-matched peers and focus on "drinking to get drunk" more than other 18- to 22-year olds [3].

Drinking rates vary by living arrangement. Rates are highest in fraternities and sororities, followed by on-campus housing (eg, dormitories, residence halls)

---

* Corresponding author. School of Health Management and Policy, W.P. Carey School of Business, Arizona State University, PO Box 874506, Tempe, AZ 85287-4506.

E-mail address: mrimsza@asu.edu (M.E. Rimsza).

0031-3955/05/$ – see front matter © 2005 Elsevier Inc. All rights reserved.
doi:10.1016/j.pcl.2004.10.008

pediatric.theclinics.com

[4]. The percentage of sorority and fraternity students who report binge drinking is approximately 80%, whereas the percentage of students who live in residence halls who report binge drinking is approximately 45%. Students who live independently off-site (eg, in apartments) drink less, while commuting students who live with their families drink the least [5].

Binge drinking is more common at the beginning of the school year, but also peaks during examination periods, spring break, and home football week-ends. Because many students initiate heavy drinking during their first days of college, excessive alcohol consumption can interfere with a successful transition to the college setting. Some experts feel that binge drinking is a product of the college environment where campus, community, peers, and individual devel-opmental factors lead to episodic heavy drinking. Excessive drinking is more likely to occur at schools located in the Northeastern United States and where fraternities and sororities are prominent [5].

The tradition of drinking is entrenched on college campuses. Environmental factors, such as low alcohol prices and easy accessibility to alcohol on or near college campuses, also encourage heavy drinking. Almost 50% of underage college students report that it is easy for them to obtain alcohol, and in 2001, approximately 43% of underage students reported binge drinking, a rate similar to that of all college students. Although some have suggested that the underage student's easy access to alcohol may be due to lax enforcement, over 70% of underage drinkers report that they obtain alcohol from another student who is of legal age rather than by direct purchase [6].

Approximately 1400 college students between the ages of 18 and 24 die every year as a result of hazardous drinking, and 500,000 more suffer alcohol-related unintentional injuries. Alcohol-related automobile injuries are one of the most common causes of death in this age group. Approximately 29% of college students who drink report driving after drinking and 21% report unplanned sexual activity associated with drinking. Thus, excessive drinking and risky behavior following the drinking of alcohol are significant health problems on the college campus.

Alcohol is absorbed quickly from the gastrointestinal tract and effects are noted within 10 minutes of ingestion, peaking at 40 to 60 minutes. Diluted alcoholic drinks are absorbed more slowly than highly concentrated alcohol. Alcohol that is mixed with carbonated liquids is absorbed more rapidly than noncarbonated alcohol-containing drinks. Consuming foods high in fat or protein delays the absorption of alcohol [7].

The most common serious adverse health effect of alcohol consumption for college students is injuries that occur when intoxicated. Injuries associated with alcohol use include motor vehicle crash injuries, drowning, and falls. In-deed, alcohol-related motor vehicle crashes are the most common cause of death for 15- to 24-year olds in the United States. Medical complications of acute intoxication include gastrointestinal irritation, aspiration pneumonia, pancreatitis, gastrointestinal bleeding, and coma. When large amounts of alcohol are ingested over a short period, respiratory arrest may occur. Alcohol is a central nervous system depressant that at low doses impairs judgment, short-term memory, and thought processing. Motor coordination, attention, and reaction time are also impaired.

The behavioral and physical consequences of alcohol use correlate well with the blood alcohol level, which is expressed as gram of alcohol per 100 mL of blood. A blood alcohol level of 0.05% is associated with a pleasant euphoric feeling, while a level of 0.20% indicates marked intoxication and 0.30% is associated with stupor. Death can occur when blood alcohol levels reach 0.35%. Blood alcohol levels correlate well with concentration of alcohol in the breath.

Heavy alcohol use also affects students who do not drink. These secondhand effects of drinking include serious offenses such as verbal, physical, and sexual assault, as well as more minor effects such as disturbed sleep, interrupted studying, and having to take care of a drunken student. Students who have been drinking physically assault approximately 600,000 students per year, and more than 70,000 students are sexually assaulted [8]. Almost 50% of residence hall students who do not drink report that they have had to take care of a drunken student, 10% have been assaulted by someone who has been drinking, and 19% have experienced unwanted sexual advances from someone who has been drinking. These secondhand effects are more common among students living in sorority and fraternity housing.

Although high school students who go on to college tend to drink less than their non–college-bound classmates, college drinking patterns are often a continuation of alcohol use that began during high school. Four out of five students have consumed alcohol by the end of high school, and 51% have done so by the eighth grade. Nearly two thirds (64%) of twelfth-graders report having been drunk at least once. Approximately 30% of twelfth-graders report binge drinking [9].

Many strategies to decrease alcohol consumption and associated risk-taking behaviors among college students have been proposed. Successful programs are associated with synergistic use of a variety of strategies, including student participation and involvement, educational and informational process, and changes in campus regulatory and physical environment [10]. Successful programs often combine cognitive–behavioral skills with motivational enhancement interventions as well as norms or values clarification. Social norms campaigns seek to alter students' perceptions about the number of students who drink excessively and the amounts of alcohol they consume.

Environmental strategies that have been used to decrease drinking among college students include increased enforcement of minimum legal drinking age law. Increasing the legal drinking age for purchase and consumption of alcohol has been the most successful effort to date in reducing underage drinking and alcohol-related problems [11]. Most studies have shown that raising the minimum legal drinking age decreases alcohol consumption and alcohol-related motor vehicle crashes. Even with minimal enforcement minimum legal drinking age laws have been shown to reduce alcohol consumption; increased enforcement can result in increased reduction of alcohol use by underage students [12].

Increased enforcement such as compliance checks on retail alcohol outlets are highly effective in reducing alcohol sales to minors [13,14]. Lowering legal blood alcohol content for drivers over 21 years of age as well as for younger drivers also has been shown to reduce alcohol-related injuries and deaths [15]. Another community approach that may be helpful is restricting alcohol retail outlet density near college campuses. Studies of the number of alcohol licenses or outlets per population size have found a relationship between the density of alcohol outlets, consumption, and related problems such as violence, other crime, and health problems [16]. Chaloupka and Wechsler [17] have reported that there are higher levels of drinking and binge drinking among college students when a larger number of businesses sold alcohol within 1 mile of campus.

Higher prices and increased taxes on alcohol also can help reduce alcohol consumption and alcohol-related problems. Responsible alcohol beverage service policies including checking identification, serving alcohol in standard sizes, limiting sales of pitchers, refusing to sell alcohol to intoxicated patrons, promoting alcohol-free drinks and food, and eliminating last-call announcements also may be helpful. To prevent sales to underage patrons, it is important to back identification policies with penalties for noncompliance. These approaches recognize that the excessive drinking by college students is a community problem, not just a college problem, and that it requires community support and collaboration to be successful.

Although the consequences of alcohol abuse during the college years may not end with graduation and some college students will continue to be problem drinkers, most college students do not continue their binge drinking after their college years. This suggests that prevalence of binge drinking is strongly influenced by living in the college environment and the developmental stage of most college students [3]. Although binge drinking decreases with increasing age, adolescents who binge drink are more likely than those who do not binge drink to still be binge drinkers in adulthood. A recent study showed that 50% of men and 33% of women who were binge drinkers at 17 to 20 years of age continued to be binge drinkers at 30 to 31 years of age. In contrast, among 30- to 31-year-olds who did not binge drink when they were 17 to 20 years of age, only 20% of men and 8% of women were binge drinkers. Thus problem drinking in adolescence predicts problem drinking in adulthood [18].

Tobacco

Each year, more than 1 million children and adolescents become regular smokers. Indeed, children and adolescents are the primary source of new smokers for the tobacco industry, because few people initiate tobacco smoking after reaching adulthood [19]. Half of smokers die prematurely of tobacco-related disease, and tobacco use is the leading preventable cause of death in the United States [20,21].

According to the Centers for Disease Control and Prevention (CDC), smoking prevalence among young adults 18 to 24 years of age increased between 1991 and 2002 [22]. The CDC defines current smokers as those who reported both having smoked 100 or more cigarettes during their lifetimes and who currently smoke every day or some days. From 1991 to 2002, the prevalence of current smoking among young adults increased, whereas the prevalence decreased among other age groups studied. Young adults identified as current smokers increased from 22.9% in 1991 to 28.5% in 2002 in the United States [23]. In contrast, adults identified as current smokers decreased from 25.7% in 1991 to 22.5% in 2002. Young adults ages 18 to 24 years started this period in 1991 with lower smoking prevalence (22.9%) than those who were 25 to 44 years of age (30.4%) and those who were 45 to 64 years of age (26.9%). Young adults ended this period in 2002 with higher smoking prevalence than these age groups, with 18- to 24-year-olds at 28.5%, 25- to 44-year-olds at 25.7%, and 45- to 64-year-olds at 22.7% [23]. These increases have occurred despite the known risks related to tobacco use, the many programs to reduce tobacco use rates, the increase in laws and policies prohibiting smoking in public places, and the growing stigma against smoking among adults.

Since 1983, CDC reports consistently indicate that educational attainment is inversely related to adult smoking prevalence. For example, smoking prevalence is lowest among those with undergraduate (12.1%) and graduate degrees (7.2%), and highest among adults who had earned a General Educational Development diploma (42.3%) and those with a grade 9 to 11 education (34.1%). From 1983 through 2002, the largest decreases in smoking prevalence occurred among adults with a college degree (10.0% decrease) and those with some college education (9.3% decrease) [23]. This might lead one to believe that smoking rates among current college students are lower than in the rest of the young adult population. However, smoking rates among college students ages 18 to 24 years are similar to their noncollege peers, and the rates appear to be increasing.

Current cigarette smoking prevalence among college students was reported at 29% in the 1995 National College Health Risk Behavior Survey [24], 28.5% in the 1999 College Alcohol Study [25], and 28.2% in the 2000 Monitoring the Future Study [26]. Thus, it appears that the prevalence of current smoking among college students is similar to that of young adults in general.

Although the percentage of college students who had smoked in the last 30 days remained unchanged between 1997 and 1999 at 28.5%, the number of cigarettes smoked by current smokers increased. In 1997, 24.2% of current student smokers had between 1 and 9 cigarettes a day; in 1999 this proportion rose to 43.6% [27].

Smoking rates among white college students were higher than among African American, Hispanic, and Asian–Pacific Islander students, although African American student smoking rates are increasing faster than the other groups [23]. In 1999, 36.1% of white students, 25.6% of Hispanic students, 23.0% of Asian college students, and 15.9% of African American students were identified as current smokers [27]. These data reflect an increase in current smoking rates between 1993 and 1999 of 42.7% among African American students, 31.2% among white students, 22.5% among Asian–Pacific Islander students, and 12.0% among Hispanic students.

The College Alcohol Study identified other factors that appeared to influence current smoking rates among college students. The proportion of current smokers was greater among students living in housing where smoking was permitted (30.6%), compared with students living in housing where smoking was not permitted (21.0%) [27]. Membership in a fraternity or sorority increased the likelihood of smoking, with men 30% more likely to smoke and women 50% more likely to smoke if they were members in a fraternity or sorority [28]. This study also demonstrated that current college student smokers were more likely to use alcohol and other drugs. Smokers were nearly 5 times more likely to report heavy episodic drinking behavior and over 6.5 times more likely to be current marijuana users [28].

A study by DeBarnardo and colleagues [29] examines college students' motivation for smoking. In this study, 49.3% of the subjects smoked as a result of stress, and 31.9% smoked as a result of depression. The National College Health Assessment provides evidence that depression and stress are increasing among college students. Results of this assessment in spring 2000 indicate that 10% had been diagnosed with depression, compared with 14.9% in spring 2004 [30]. The proportion of students who report that their level of stress has affected their academic performance increased from 29.0% in spring 2000 to 32.4% in spring 2004 [30]. This may partailly explain the increase in smoking among college students.

Although college student smokers are motivated to quit smoking because of their concerns about their current and future health, they have difficulty in doing so. Indeed, the College Alcohol Study indicates that 20% of smokers made 5 or more quit attempts in the past year [31]. Lack of knowledge about the adverse effects of smoking is not a factor, because 98.4% of both smokers and non-smokers considered themselves knowledgeable about the adverse health effects of smoking; also, 89.9% did not want to receive more information about the health consequences of smoking [29].

The active ingredient in cigarettes is nicotine, which is well absorbed in the lungs through inhalation. Tolerance develops with continued use. Tobacco use fits all the criteria for drug dependence or addiction, thus treatment strategies need to address the complicated pharmacologic and behavioral factors. Smoking cessation programs have variable effectiveness, and adolescents who are oc-casional smokers are more likely to successfully quit than daily smokers. Con-sequently, physicians need to focus on preventing occasional smokers from progressing to daily smokers.

Colleges and universities can play an important role in identifying current smokers, providing cessation education and encouragement, and creating environments that discourage smoking behavior. Two approaches have strong evidence of effectiveness in smoking cessation: counseling and pharmacotherapy.

The highest rates of smoking cessation occur when these two approaches are combined. Adolescents who are trying to quit can benefit from nicotine replacement therapy. The US Food and Drug Administration has approved four types of nicotine replacement products (gum, nasal spray, transdermal patch, and inhaler). Nicotine replacement helps relieve withdrawal symptoms in the smoker who is abstaining from cigarettes and reduces cravings. Using nicotine replacement therapy in addition to counseling doubles the smoking cessation rates compared with placebo treatment. The efficacy of each of these forms of nicotine replacement is similar at 12 weeks of follow-up, but the transdermal patch has the highest rate of compliance [32]. The nicotine patch should be used for 8 weeks; there is little difference among the various brands [19].

Bupropion is an antidepressant that has also been shown to be effective in tobacco cessation when combined with counseling [33]. In one study that compared bupropion and the nicotine patch, bupropion was associated with higher rates of abstinence from tobacco use at 1-year follow-up. Cessation rates were not significantly improved by using both bupropion and nicotine patch [33].

Club drugs

"Club drugs" are a group of illicit drugs that are most commonly used at nightclubs and rave parties. These drugs include stimulants, depressants, and hallucinogens. Commonly used club drugs are 3,4-methylenedioxymethamphetamine, gamma-hydroxybutyrate, flunitrazepam (Rohypnol), lysergic acid, ketamine, methamphetamine, phencyclidine, and, occasionally, cocaine and psilocybin mushrooms. Rave parties began in England in the 1980s and spread to the United States in the early 1990s. These parties are marathon dances held in large makeshift dance halls. Party themes emphasize harmony, empathy, and a sense of belonging. Partygoers believe that the rave drugs enhance feelings of closeness with others and enjoy the sensory enhancement, visual distortions, and illusions created by the drugs.

3,4-Methylenedioxyethamphetamine

3,4-Methylenedioxymethamphetamine (MDMA) is a selective serotonergic neurotoxin and one of the most popular club drugs; it is a stimulant and a hallucinogen. Other street names for MDMA include ecstasy, XTC, E, X, and Adam. In the 1980s, it became a popular drug on college campuses. Because it reduces inhibitions and produces a feeling of empathy for others, it is sometimes called the "hug drug" or the "feel good drug." The drug is taken orally in tablet form; initial effects occur within 30 minutes to 1 hour after ingestion and its peak effect occurs in 90 minutes, with effects that last 4 to 8 hours. Signs of toxicity include sympathetic overactivity, disturbed behavior, and fever. MDMA suppresses the need to eat, drink or sleep, which enables partygoers to remain awake for prolonged periods, sometimes 2 to 3 days. Many of the serious side effects are related to hyperthermia and include delirium, rhabdomyolysis, acute renal failure, seizures, and coma. MDMA can also have hepatotoxic effects. Serotonin depletion may lead to depression and tolerance occurs with continued use [34]. MDMA can be detected by urine toxicology screening if very large quantities are ingested. In these cases, MDMA can result in a positive urine toxicology screen for amphetamines. The diagnosis can be confirmed by gas chromatography or mass spectrometry.

Gamma-hydroxybutyrate

Gamma-hydroxybutyrate is a central nervous system depressant with such street names as liquid X, liquid ecstasy, soap, easy lay, Georgia home boy, grievous bodily harm, G, and goop. It is easily manufactured at home using instructions available on the Internet. Gamma-hydroxybutyrate is available in liquid, powder, tablet, and capsule formulations; however, it is primarily taken in its liquid form, often added to bottles of water. It causes a sense of euphoria and intoxication. Low-dose side effects include drowsiness, dizziness, nausea, and visual disturbances; high doses can result in respiratory depression, coma, and seizures.

Flunitrazepam

Flunitrazepam (Rohypnol) is a benzodiazepine that has been legally used as a preanesthetic medication. It is now illegal in the United States, but is legally available in Latin America and Europe. Some of the street names for rohypnol are: roofies, rophies, roche, Mexican valium, and the forget-me-pill. It is available in both tablet and liquid form. Similar to other benzodiazepines, flunitrazepam has anxiolytic, sedative, and anticonvulsant properties. Side effects include hypotension, drowsiness, visual disturbances, dizziness, confusion, and gastrointestinal upset. Because it causes anterograde amnesia and decreases inhibitions, it is commonly used as a "date rape" drug. The drug is colorless, tasteless, and easily dissolved in liquid; the tablet form dissolves easily in water.

Ketamine

Ketamine, a veterinary anesthetic, is also used as a date rape drug. It induces a dissociative, dream-like state. Street names for ketamine include special K, vitamin K, and cat valium. At low doses, attention span, memory, and learning ability are impaired; at high doses, depression, delirium, hypertension, and respiratory depression can occur. The powder form can be placed in marijuana or tobacco cigarettes.

Methamphetamine

Methamphetamine is a central nervous system (CNS) stimulant that also may be taken at rave parties; street names include speed, ice, chalk, crystal, glass, crank, and fire. It is the *N*-methyl homolog of amphetamine and this *N*-methyl group increases penetration of the blood–brain barrier. Thus, methamphetamine has higher CNS stimulant activity along with less peripheral nervous system and less cardiovascular stimulation compared with amphetamine. In general, amphetamine drugs stimulate the CNS indirectly by increasing the release and inhibiting the breakdown and storage of catecholamines. Thus, the drug's effects depend on catecholamine stores so that continued use leads to depletion of catecholamine stores and the rapid development of tachyphylaxis.

Methamphetamine is available as a white, soluble, crystalline powder that can be smoked, snorted, injected, or ingested orally. Most adolescents snort or smoke the drug. If taken intravenously or smoked, methamphetamine quickly causes an intense euphoria that lasts only a few minutes. The rapid onset of action can result in an acute psychotic episode characterized by violent behavior, severe paranoia, and hallucinations. This "hyperviolence syndrome" may result in severe injury or death of family or friends of users [35]. In contrast, snorting the powder or taking the drug orally results in a pleasant high of longer duration.

Undesirable side effects result from methamphetamine's stimulation of peripheral alpha- and beta-receptors; these adverse effects include tachycardia, tachypnea, fever, hypertension, irritability, tremors, insomnia, and loss of appetite. Chronic use is associated with visual and tactile hallucinations, psychosis, paranoia, memory loss, and paranoid behavior. Aggression and agitation resulting in bizarre violent behavior may occur, especially after a heavy binge cycle [35].

Hallucinogens that may be ingested at raves include d-lysergic acid (LSD), phencyclidine (PCP), and psilocybin mushrooms. MDMA also has mild hallucinogenic properties. LSD is a potent hallucinogen that is derived from morning glory seeds. Street names include acid, blotter, cubes, dots, L, and sugar. It is available as a clear or white water soluble material and usually is distributed on a blotter paper, sugar cube, or stamp. LSD causes euphoria and hallucinations.

PCP is a white crystalline powder that is dissolved in water, pressed into tablets, or dipped into cigarettes. Street names for PCP include angel dust, crystal, hog, supergrass, and wack. PCP inhibits catecholamine reuptake, which leads to increased adrenergic symptoms. Psilocybin mushrooms, also known as shrooms and mushies, may be cooked and added to other foods or boiled in water to make a tea. Its hallucinogenic effect begins within 20 minutes of ingestion and last about 6 hours. Side effects include muscle weakness, drowsiness, and nausea.

Students who attend raves may ingest a variety of drugs, often with alcohol. Although urine toxicology tests can be used to detect cannabis, PCP, and amphetamines, other rave drugs are more difficult to detect. Rohypnol is quickly metabolized and can only be detected by specialized toxicologic testing using gas chromatography or mass spectrometry on urine specimens that are collected soon after ingestion. This makes it difficult to identify its use in sexual assaults. The usual urine toxicology screens also will fail to identify MDMA unless large doses are ingested.

Marijuana

Marijuana is an illicit drug that has been used by more than 50% of 17- to 18-year-olds in the United States [9]. However, in the 2002 National College Health Assessment, 59.7% of college students reported that they had never used marijuana and only 2.6% reporting daily use in the past 30 days; this suggests that college students are less likely to use marijuana that their peers who do not attend college. Among college students, men were more likely to be daily users than women (4.3% versus 1.5%) [36]. In a 1999 survey of college students, approximately 91% of students who used marijuana in the past 30 days also used other illicit drugs or smoked cigarettes or engaged in binge drinking [37].

The active ingredient in marijuana is delta-9-tetra-hydrocannabinol. Marijuana is usually smoked as a "joint" or using a water pipe (bong), but it can be taken orally. Within minutes of smoking marijuana users experience an intense relaxed feeling and euphoria that can last for several hours. Chronic users develop a tolerance for the drug and psychologic dependence. Frequent use interferes with cognitive function, shortens memory span, and alters time perception. Thus, chronic users have academic difficulties and lack interest in day-to-day activities. Adverse physical effects are chronic cough, bronchitis, and bronchospasm [38].

Cocaine

Cocaine is a central nervous system stimulant extracted from coca leaves. It can be taken orally, intravenously, intranasally, or by inhalation. Approximately 9% of American high school students have used some form of cocaine. It causes a profound but short-lived euphoria that lasts about 5 minutes if smoked and 10 to 30 minutes if snorted. Tolerance and addiction develop quickly. Because the drug causes arterial constriction, adverse effects include angina, myocardial infarction, and cerebral vascular events; sudden death may also occur. Other side effects include seizures, hypertension, abdominal pain, fever, irritability, and hypertension. Cocaine use may result in an extremely aggressive paranoia.

Anabolic steroids

Anabolic steroids are synthetic derivatives of testosterone. They are taken for nonmedical purposes to increase muscle mass and improve athletic performance.

Because they do increase muscle mass, strength, and training capacity, there is a powerful motivation for their use. It also is widely thought that when combined with proper training and diet, they improve athletic performance. Thus, coaches and trainers may encourage their use. Anabolic steroids can be administered orally or through intramuscular injection. The doses used to enhance athletic performance are 10 or more times the recommended therapeutic dose. Although there are no immediate behavioral effects of taking anabolic steroids, there is evidence of dependence among long-term users. [19]

There are many serious adverse effects of anabolic steroid use. These drugs impair hepatic function and are associated with cholestatic jaundice, hepatoma, and liver carcinoma. They also are associated with decreased high-density lipoprotein to cholesterol levels, which may increase the risk of coronary heart disease. Prolonged use can result in testicular atrophy, decreased sperm counts, and gynecomastia in men and menstrual irregularities, hirsutism, and clitoral hypertrophy in women. For both men and women, anabolic steroids also are associated with the development of acne, hypertension, and male-pattern baldness.

Studies on the behavioral effects of anabolic steroids have had conflicting results. While some studies have reported increased moodiness, aggression and mania, other placebo-controlled double-blind studies of men who were not athletes and had no underlying psychiatric disorder showed no increase in angry behavior [39,40].

Summary

Although substance abuse is less common among college students than their peers, it is still a major health and behavioral concern in this age group. Alcohol and marijuana are the most commonly abused drugs on college campuses. Drug use is a major contributing factor in poor academic performance and failure to successfully complete a college education.

References

[1] O'Malley PM, Johnston LD. Epidemiology of alcohol and other drug use among American college students. J Stud Alcohol Suppl 2002;14:23–39.

[2] Schulenberg J, O'Malley PM, Bachman JG, et al. The problem of college drinking: insights from a developmental perspective. Alcohol Clin Exp Res 2001;25:473–7.

[3] Bower AM. Are college students alcoholics? J Am Coll Health 2002;50:253–5.

[4] Wechsler H, et al. College binge drinking in the 1990s: a continuing problem. Results of the Harvard School of Public Health 1999 College Alcohol Survey. J Am Coll Health 2000;48:199–210.

[5] Wechsler H, et al. Trends in college binge drinking during a period of increased prevention efforts. J Am Coll Health 2002;50:203–17.

[6] Wechsler H, et al. Underage college students' drinking behavior, access to alcohol, and the influence of deterrence policies. J Am Coll Health 2002;50:223–36.

[7] American Academy of Pediatrics Committee on Substance Abuse. A guide for health professionals. 2nd edition. Elk Grove Village (IL): American Academy of Pediatrics; 2002.

[8] Task force of the National Advisory Council on Alcohol Abuse and Alcoholism. A call to action: changing the culture of drinking at US colleges. Bethesda (MD): National Institutes of Health. US Department of Health and Human Services. NIH Publication No. 02-5010, April, 2002.

[9] Johnston LD, O'Malley PM, Bachman JG, editors. Monitoring the future. In: National results on adolescent drug use: overview of key findings, 2001. Bethesda (MD): National Institute on Drug Abuse; 2002. p. 1–61.

[10] Ziemelia A, Bucknam RB, Elfessi AM. Prevention efforts underlying decreases in binge drinking at institutions of higher education. J Am Coll Health 2002;50:238–49.

[11] Task Force of the National Advisory Council on Alcohol Abuse and Alcoholism. A call to action: changing the culture of drinking at US Colleges. Bethesda (MD): National Institutes of Health; 2002.

[12] Wagenaar A, Toomey TL. Effects of minimum drinking age laws: review and analyses of the literature from 1960 to 2000. J Stud Alcohol Suppl 2002;14:206–25.

[13] Barry R, et al. Enhanced enforcement of laws to prevent alcohol sales to underage persons—New Hampshire, 1999–2004. MMWR Morb Mortal Wkly Rep 2004;53:452–4.

[14] Wagenaar A, O'Malley P, LaFond L. Communities mobilizing for change on alcohol: outcomes from a randomized community trial. J Stud Alcohol 2000;61:85–94.

[15] Shults R, et al. Review of the evidence regarding interventions to reduce alcohol impaired driving. Am J Prev Med 2001;48:66–88.

[16] Toomey TL, Wagenaar AC. Environmental policies to reduce college drinking: options and research findings. J Stud Alcohol Suppl 2002;14:193–205.

[17] Chaloupka FJ, Wechsler H. Binge drinking in college: the impact of price, availability, and alcohol control policies. Contemp Econ Policy 1996;14:112–24.

[18] McCarty CA, et al. Continuity of binge and harmful drinking from late adolescence to early adulthood. Pediatrics 2004;114:714–9.

[19] Coupey SM. Substance abuse: a guide for health professionals. Elk Grove Village (IL): American Academy of Pediatrics Committee on Substance Abuse; 2002. p. 191–8.

[20] Centers for Disease Control and Prevention. Tobacco use—United States, 1900–1999. MMWR Morb Mortal Wkly Rep 1999;48:986–93.

[21] Klein JD, Camenga DR. Tobacco prevention and cessation in pediatric patients. Pediatr Rev 2004;25:16–24.

[22] Center for Disease Control. Surveillance for selected tobacco-use behaviors—United States, 1900–1994. MMWR Morb Mortal Wkly Rep 1994;43:1–10.

[23] Center for Disease Control. Cigarette smoking among adults—United States, 2002. MMWR Morb Mortal Wkly Rep 2004;53:427–31.

[24] Center for Disease Control. Youth risk behavior surveillance. National College Health Risk Behavior Surve—United States, 1995. MMWR Morb Mortal Wkly Rep 1997;46:1–54.

[25] Rigotti N, Lee JE, Wechsler H. US college students' use of tobacco products: results of a national survey. JAMA 2000;284:699–705.

[26] Johnston LD, O'Malley PM, Bachman JG. Monitoring the future: national survey results on drug use, 1975–2000. Volume 2: college students and adults ages 19–40. Bethesda (MD): National Institute on Drug Abuse; 2001.

[27] Wechsler H, Lee JE, Rigotti NA. Cigarette use by college students in smoke-free housing: results of a national study. Am J Prev Med 2001;20:202–7.

[28] Emmons KM, et al. Predictors of smoking among US college students. Am J Public Health 1998;88:104–7.

[29] DeBernardo RL, et al. An email assessment of undergraduates' attitudes toward smoking. J Am Coll Health 1999;48:61–6.

[30] Baltimore American College Health Association Survey. National College Health Assessment: reference group executive summary. Baltimore (MD): American College Health Association; 2004.

[31] Wechsler H, et al. Increased levels of cigarette use among college students, a cause for national concern. JAMA 1998;280:1673–8.

[32] Rigotti NA. Treatment of tobacco use and dependence. N Engl J Med 2002;346:506–12.

[33] Jorenby DE, et al. A controlled trial of sustained-release bupropion, a nicotene patch, or both or smoking cessation. N Engl J Med 1999;340:685–91.

[34] Schwartz RH, Miller NS. MDMA (ecstasy) and the rave: a review. Pediatrics 1997;100:705–8.

[35] MacKenzie RG, Heischober B. Methamphetamine. Pediatr Rev 1997;18:305–9.

[36] American College Health Association. National College Health Assessment: reference group executive summary spring 2002. Baltimore (MD): American College Health Association; 2002.

[37] Gledhill-Hoyt J, et al. Increased use of marijuana and other illicit drugs at US colleges in the 1990s: results of three national surveys. Addiction 2000;95:1655–67.

[38] Greydanus DE, Patel DR. Substance abuse in adolescence: a complex conundrum for the clinician. Pediatr Clin North Am 2003;50:1179–223.

[39] Pope HG, Katz DL. Psychiatric and medical effects of anabolic-androgenic steroid use: a controlled study of 160 athletes. Arch Gen Psychiatry 1994;51:375–82.

[40] Tricker R, et al. The effects of supraphysiological doses of testosterone on angry behavior in healthy eugonadal men: a clinical research center study. J Clin Endocrinol Metab 1996; 81:3754–8.

ELSEVIER
SAUNDERS

PEDIATRIC CLINICS
OF NORTH AMERICA

Pediatr Clin N Am 52 (2005) 321–334

Index

Note: Page numbers of article titles are in **boldface** type.

A

Acyclovir, for herpes simplex virus infections, 223–224

Adam (3,4-methylenedioxyethamphetamine), in college environment, 313–314

Adequacy, promotion of, in depression, 113

ADHD. *See* Attention-deficit/ hyperactivity disorder.

Adjustment Disorder with depressed mood, in college students, 111

Airway
obstruction of, in infectious mononucleosis, 12
responsiveness of, in asthma, 14

Alcohol abuse, in college students, 37–38, 293, 307–310

Allergy
asthma in, 13–16
to tricyclic antidepressants, 121

Almotriptan, for migraine, 19

Alprazolam
for anxiety disorders, 102, 104
for panic disorder, 106–107
for social phobia, 107

Amenorrhea, in college students, 188–192
drug-induced, 191–192
in eating disorders, 189–190
in hypergonadotropic hypogonadism, 190–191
in polycystic ovary syndrome, 185–186
in pregnancy, 188–189

American Academy of Neurology, concussion grading system of, 33

Amitriptyline, for depression, 119–120

Amnesia, from benzodiazepines, 104

Amoxapine, for depression, 119–121

Amoxicillin, for prostatitis, 209

Amphetamines
abuse of, 38, 315
for attention-deficit/hyperactivity disorder, 74–75

Ampicillin, for prostatitis, 209

Amylin, for diabetes mellitus, 300

Anabolic steroid use, in college students, 37–39, 316–317

Androstenedione use, in college athletes, 40

Anemia, in infectious mononucleosis, 13

Anger, in depression, 111–112

Ankle sprains, in college athletes, 39, 41–44

Anogenital warts, human papillomavirus, 199–202

Anorexia nervosa. *See* Eating disorders (anorexia nervosa and bulimia nervosa).

Anovulation
bleeding in, 182
in polycystic ovary syndrome, 184–186

Anterior cruciate ligament, injury of, in college athletes, 45–46

Anterior drawer test, for ankle injury, 42

Anticholinergic effects, of tricyclic antidepressants, 120

Antidepressants
for attention-deficit/hyperactivity disorder, 75–77
for depression
discontinuation of, 127–128
indications for, 115–117
monoamine oxidase inhibitors, 116, 118, 121, 125–127
selection of, 117
selective serotonin reuptake inhibitors, 116–118, 121–124
tricyclic, 115, 118–121
types of, 115–117

Encephalitis, Japanese, immunization for,
in college students, 237

Endocarditis, infective, in college students,
263–264

Endometritis, menstrual disorders in, 186–187

Ephedrine and ephedra, college athletes
using, 40

Epididymitis, in *Chlamydia trachomatis*
infections, 219

Epilepsy, oral contraceptive use in, 145

Epstein-Barr virus infections, infectious
mononucleosis in, 9–13

Erectile dysfunction, 209–212

Erythema marginatum, in rheumatic fever, 262

Erythromycin
for *Chlamydia trachomatis*
infections, 220
for *Trichomonas vaginalis*
infections, 208

Erythropoietin, abuse of, in college athletes, 38

Escherichia coli, in urinary tract infections, 21

Ethinyl estradiol, in oral contraceptives, 139

Etonogestrel, in vaginal contraceptive ring,
148–149

Exercise. *See also* Athletes.
atherosclerosis and, 248
in diabetes mellitus, 290

Eye, disorders of, in diabetes mellitus, 297

F

FABER test, in back pain, 50

Famciclovir, for herpes simplex virus
infections, 223–224

Family
depression in, 112
eating disorders and, 88

Family therapy, for eating disorders, 91–92

Fatigue
from psychostimulants, 81
in infectious mononucleosis, 13

Fatty streaks, in arteries, of college students,
247–248

Feelings
expression of, in depression, 112–113
guilty, in depression, 111

Female Athlete Triad, 190

Flexibility, promotion of, in depression, 113

Fluid therapy, for diabetic ketoacidosis, 284

Flunitrazepam, abuse of, 314

Fluoxetine
for depression, 121
for eating disorders, 93

Flurazepam, for anxiety disorders, 103

Fluvoxamine, for obsessive-compulsive
disorder, 108

Fowler's sign, in shoulder impingement
syndrome, 54

G

Gaenslin test, in back pain, 50

Gamma-hydroxybutyrate, abuse of, 314

Garcinia camboga, college athletes using, 41

Gastrointestinal disorders, chest pain in, 246

Generalized anxiety disorder,
in college students, 106

Genetic factors
in depression, 111
in dyslipidemia, 249
in eating disorders, 87
in Marfan syndrome, 268
in panic disorder, 98

Genital herpes, 222–223

Genitourinary disorders, in male college
students, **199–216**
human papillomavirus infections,
199–202
prostatitis, 208–209
sexual dysfunction, 209–212
testicular cancer, 202–204
urethritis, 20–22, 206–208, 219–222
varicocele, 204–206

Glucose monitoring, in diabetes mellitus, 285,
290–291

Glucose tolerance, impaired, in college
students, 282

GlucoWatch Biographer, for glucose
monitoring, 291

Glutamine supplements, college athletes
using, 41

Glycated hemoglobin, testing for, 291

Glycoprotein G test, in herpes simplex virus
infections, 223

tobacco, 37, 293–294, 310–313
toxicology tests for, 315–316
with diabetes mellitus, 293

Sudden cardiac death, in college students, 29–32, 258, 266–267

Sumatriptan, for migraine, 19

Support groups, for eating disorders, 92

Supraspinatus test, in shoulder impingement syndrome, 53

Sydenham's chorea, in rheumatic fever, 260–261

Syncope, in college students, 256–258

Syphilis, in college students, 225–226

Systemic lupus erythematosus, in college students, 262–263

T

Talofibular ligaments, injury of, in college athletes, 42

Tension, reactions to, in depression, 112

Testicular cancer, in college students, 202–204

Testosterone
abuse of, in college athletes, 38
deficiency of, sexual dysfunction in, 210

Tetanus, immunization for, in college students, 238

Tetralogy of Fallot, in college students, 255

Thrombosis, from oral contraceptives, 144

Thyroid disease, menstrual disorders in, 187

Tobacco use, in college students, 37, 293–294, 310–313

Today contraceptive sponge, 151

Transdermal hormonal contraception, 145–146

Transition programs, for college-bound students with learning disabilities, 62–64, 66

Transplantation, islet cell, for diabetes mellitus, 300

Transposition of great vessels, in college students, 256

Tranylcypromine, for depression, 125, 127

Travelers, to foreign colleges, immunizations for, 236–237

Trazodone, for depression, 118

Tribulus terrestris, college athletes using, 41

Trichloroacetic acid, for anogenital warts, 201

Trichomonas vaginalis infections, in college students, 226–227
female, 186
male, 208

Tricyclic antidepressants, for depression, 115, 118–121

Trimethoprim-sulfamethoxazole
for prostatitis, 209
for urinary tract infections, 21–22

Trimipramine, for depression, 119–120

Tuberculosis, in international college students, 239

Turner syndrome, cardiovascular disorders in, 269

Typhoid fever, immunization for, in college students, 237

U

Ulcers
in herpes simplex virus infections, 222–223
in syphilis, 225–226

Urethritis, in college students, 20–22
in *Chlamydia trachomatis* infections, 219–220
in gonorrhea, 221–222
male, 206–208

Urinary tract infections, in college students, 20–22

Urine culture, in prostatitis, 209

Urine dipstick test, for infections, 21

V

Vaccinations. *See* Immunizations.

Vaginal bleeding, in college students
breakthrough, from oral contraceptives, 145
in pregnancy, 188–189
menstrual, excessive, 181–183

Vaginal ring, for contraception, 148–149

Valacyclovir, for herpes simplex virus infections, 223–224

Valgus stress test, for medial collateral ligament sprain, 47

Valproate, for migraine, 20

Receive your CME certificate immediately...

log on to www.pediatric.theclinics.com to take and score your test on-line.

THE PEDIATRIC CLINICS OF NORTH AMERICA

Sponsored by
The University of Virginia School of Medicine
Charlottesville, Virginia

Karen S. Rheuban, MD

ASSOCIATE DEAN FOR CONTINUING MEDICAL EDUCATION
MEDICAL DIRECTOR, OFFICE OF TELEMEDICINE
PROFESSOR OF PEDIATRICS
UNIVERSITY OF VIRGINIA HEALTH SYSTEM
CHARLOTTESVILLE, VIRGINIA

Based on the issue
College Health (Vol 52:1)

This activity has been planned and implemented in accordance with the Essential Areas and Policies of the Accreditation Council for Continuing Medical Education (ACCME) through the joint sponsorship of the University of Virginia School of Medicine and Elsevier. The University of Virginia School of Medicine is accredited by the ACCME to provide continuing medical education for physicians.

The University of Virginia School of Medicine designates this continuing medical education activity for a maximum of 90 category 1 credits per year, 15 credits per issue toward the AMA Physician's Recognition Award. Each physician should claim only those credits that he/she actually spent in the activity.

The American Medical Association has determined that physicians not licensed in the US who participate in this CME activity are eligible for AMA PRA category 1 credit.

Test expires 12 months following publication date.

Publication Date: February 2005   Test expires: March 31, 2006

TEST NO. PD0502 • FEBRUARY 2005

W. B. SAUNDERS COMPANY
An imprint of Elsevier, Inc.

The Curtis Center
Independence Square West
Philadelphia, PA 19106–3399

http://www.us.elsevierhealth.com

CONTINUING MEDICAL EDUCATION
SUPPLEMENT TO THE PEDIATRIC CLINICS OF NORTH AMERICA
ISSN 0031–3955   FEBRUARY 2005

CHANGE OF ADDRESS
We cannot score tests submitted after the 12-month deadline has expired. Please notify us immediately of any change in address to ensure that your test booklet reaches you in a timely manner. Send address changes, along with a copy of the mailing label from your test booklet, to:

W. B. Saunders Company
Periodicals Fulfillment
6277 Sea Harbor Drive
Orlando, FL 32887–4800

Customer Service: 1-800-654-2452 (US). From outside of the US, call 1-407-345-1000.
E-mail: elspcs@elsevier.com

TEST NO. PD0502 • FEBRUARY 2005

GOAL

The goal of *The Pediatric Clinics of North America* is to keep practicing pediatricians and pediatric residents up to date with current clinical practice in pediatrics by providing timely articles reviewing the state of the art in patient care.

OBJECTIVES

- describe the common sexually transmitted diseases in college students
- identify the incidence and risks of human papilloma virus infection in young women
- recognize common menstrual disorders in young women
- define the appropriate limitations to be placed on activities related to acute and chronic injuries and medical conditions

ACCREDITATION

The Pediatric Clinics of North America is planned and implemented in accordance with the Essential Areas and Policies of the Accreditation Council for Continuing Medical Education (ACCME) through the joint sponsorship of the University of Virginia School of Medicine and W. B. Saunders Company. The University of Virginia School of Medicine is accredited by the ACCME to provide continuing medical education for physicians.

The University of Virginia School of Medicine designates this continuing medical education activity for a maximum of 90 category I credits per year, 15 credits per issue toward the AMA Physician's Recognition Award. Each physician should claim only those credits that he/she actually spent in the activity.

The American Medical Association has determined that physicians not licensed in the US who participate in this CME activity are eligible for AMA PRA category I credit.

Category I credit can be earned by reading the text material, taking the CME examination online at http://www.theclinics.com/home/cme, and completing the evaluation. After taking the test, you will be required to review any and all incorrect answers. Following completion of the test and evaluation, your credit will be awarded and you may print your certificate.

DISCLOSURES

As a provider accredited by the Accreditation Council for Continuing Medical Education (ACCME), the Office of Continuing Medical Education of the University of Virginia School of Medicine must ensure balance, independence, objectivity, and scientific rigor in all its individually sponsored or jointly sponsored educational activities. All authors/editors participating in a sponsored activity are expected to disclose to the readers any significant financial interest or other relationship (1) with the manufacturer(s) of any commercial product(s) and/or provider(s) of commercial services discussed in an educational presentation and (2) with any commercial supporters of the activity (significant financial interest or other relationship can include such things as grants or research support, employee, consultant, stock holder, member of speakers bureau, etc.) The intent of this disclosure is not to prevent authors/editors with a significant financial or other relationship from writing an article, but rather to provide readers with information on which they can make their own judgments. It remains for the readers to determine whether the author's/editor's interest or relationships may influence the article with regard to exposition or conclusion.

Disclosure of discussion of non-FDA approved uses for pharmaceutical products and/or medical devices: The University of Virginia School of Medicine, as an ACCME provider, requires that all authors/editors identify and disclose any "off label" uses for pharmaceutical products and/or for medical devices. The University of Virginia School of Medicine recommends that each reader fully review all the available data on new products or procedures prior to instituting them with patients.

Please note the disclosure information in the front of the *Clinics* issue.

TEST NO. PD0502 • FEBRUARY 2005

INSTRUCTIONS FOR COMPLETING THE EXAMINATION FOR CREDIT

The test booklet has been mailed to you for your convenience; however, all examinations must be taken online in order to receive credit.

Please register online at www.theclinics.com/home/cme using the account number provided on the mailing label of this test booklet. Instructions for completing the test are provided on the website. With the online service, readers will benefit from the convenience of instant scoring and credit.

Test questions will be available online for 12 months.

Technical support is available Monday through Friday during the hours of 7:30 am to 6:00 pm EST:

Customer Service Department
6277 Sea Harbor Drive
Orlando, FL 32887 USA
(800) 654-2452 (Toll Free US & Canada)
(407) 345-4299 (Outside US & Canada)

FAX: (407) 363-9661
E-mail: elspcs@elsevier.com

If you do not have access to a computer, please call Customer Service to obtain an answer sheet and envelope. Please return your answer sheet via mail in the envelope provided; *faxed answer sheets will not be accepted*. Remember to complete both the test and the subsequent program evaluation. Please allow 4 to 6 weeks for processing and scoring answer sheets submitted in this manner.

1. States that do not authorize prescribing by physician assistants include:

   A. Louisiana
   B. Indiana
   C. Ohio
   D. all of the above

2. Issues related to ongoing care for college students with heart disease include which of the following?

   A. prophylaxis against bacterial endocarditis
   B. exercise limitations in high-risk patients
   C. concerns regarding self-image
   D. all of the above

3. Common causes of chest pain in college-aged students include all of the following EXCEPT:

   A. reactive airways disease
   B. gastroesophageal reflux disease
   C. rheumatic fever
   D. costochrondritis

4. Cardiac causes of chest pain include:

   A. myocarditis-pericarditis
   B. marfan syndrome/aortic dissection
   C. Kawasaki disease/coronary artery disease
   D. all of the above

5. The differential diagnosis of a female student with chest pain and a cardiac exam with midsystolic click includes which of the following?

   A. mitral prolapse
   B. atrial septal defect
   C. ventricular septal defect
   D. aortic insufficiency

6. Psychostimulants are effective in the treatment of what percent of students with attention deficit hyperactivity disorder (ADHD)?

   A. 30%
   B. 50%
   C. 70%
   D. 90%

7. Side-effects of methylphenidate treatment for ADHD include:

   A. insomnia
   B. anorexia
   C. dry mouth
   D. all of the above

8. The optimal dose of psychostimulants is related to:

   A. age
   B. sex
   C. weight
   D. none of the above

9. The normal range for the menstrual cycle is:

    A. 21--28 days
    B. 21--25 days
    C. 21--42 days
    D. none of the above

10. Excessive menstrual bleeding can be described as all of the following EXCEPT:

    A. menses more frequently than every 21 days
    B. greater than 20 cc of blood loss per cycle
    C. lasting for more than 7 days
    D. greater than 80 cc of blood loss per cycle

11. Polycystic ovary syndrome (PCOS) is characterized by:

    A. anovulation
    B. androgen excess
    C. infertility
    D. all of the above

12. The long-term health risks of PCOS include all of the following EXCEPT:

    A. obesity
    B. type 1 diabetes
    C. dyslipidemia
    D. endometrial cancer

13. The most common cause of secondary amenorrhea in college-aged women is:

    A. hypothyroidism
    B. anorexia nervosa
    C. pregnancy
    D. sexually transmitted diseases

14. The most commonly abused substances in the college-aged student include:

    A. alcohol
    B. marijuana
    C. tobacco
    D. all of the above

15. Adverse effects of anabolic steroid use include:

    A. testicular atrophy
    B. hepatic carcinoma
    C. hypertension
    D. all of the above

16. What percentage of cervical cancers are associated with infection with human papilloma virus (HPV)?

    A. 55%
    B. 75%
    C. 90%
    D. 99.5%

17. All of the following are correct about HPV infection EXCEPT:

A. 90% of young women will acquire HPV infection within 5 years of becoming sexually active
B. incidence increases with increasing number of sexual partners
C. characteristics of cervical epithelium of younger women increase vulnerability of the young cervix to infection
D. HPV virus 16 is associated with invasive cervical cancer

18. A careful history will identify what percentage of medical conditions that require limitation of exercise?

A. 10%
B. 30%
C. 50%
D. 75%

19. The American Academy of Neurology Grade 1 concussion score includes:

A. no loss of consciousness
B. transient confusion
C. resolution of symptoms within 15 minutes
D. all of the above

20. The American Academy of Neurology recommendations for return to exercise for patients with concussion:

    A. first episode with loss of consciousness - hiatus for one week if asymptomatic
    B. second episode - return if asymptomatic for one month
    C. terminate season if MRI/CT scan is abnormal
    D. all of the above

21. Sports injuries requiring surgery are highest in which of the following sports?

    A. wrestling
    B. football
    C. hockey
    D. soccer

22. What percentage of patients with depressive disorder have a close family member with depression?

    A. 10%
    B. 30%
    C. 50%
    D. 70%

23. Cardiac side-effects of tricyclic antidepressants include:

    A. orthostatic hypotension
    B. conduction delay
    C. tachycardia
    D. all of the above

24. Which of the following is UNTRUE about immunization of the college student?

A. meningococcal vaccine is mandated for all college students F
B. meningococcal vaccine is recommended for students residing in dormitories T
C. hepatitis B vaccine is mandated for all students T
D. hepatitis A vaccine is not mandated for all students T

25. Newer vaccines currently in development or soon to be licensed or released include:

A. acellular pertussis vaccine
B. human papilloma virus vaccine
C. herpes simplex vaccine
D. all of the above

26. The classical triad of arthritis, dermatitis, and tenosynovitis is characteristic of which sexually transmitted disease?

A. gonorrhea
B. syphilis
C. chlamydia N
D. hepatitis C N

27. Constitutional symptoms occur in what percentage of patients with initial infection with genital herpes?

A. 10--25%
B. 40--60%
C. 70--80%
D. 100%

28. Sexual transmission of which of the following is more common?

    A. hepatitis A
    B. hepatitis B
    C. hepatitis C
    D. none of the above

29. What percentage of healthy patients previously infected with Ebstein Barr Virus may be shedding the virus at any time?

    A. 20%
    B. 40%
    C. 60%
    D. 80%

30. Complications of infectious mononucleosis that may be improved with corticosteroids include:

    A. massive tonsillar hypertrophy
    B. thrombocytopenia
    C. encephalopathy
    D. all of the above

PROGRAM EVALUATION

1. Rate this *Clinics* issue for its coverage of the topic (identifies major controversies, alternative approaches, etc.)
   - A. excellent
   - B. satisfactory
   - C. unsatisfactory

2. Rate this *Clinics* issue for its balance, scientific integrity, and freedom from commercial bias.
   - A. excellent
   - B. satisfactory
   - C. unsatisfactory

3. Rate the appropriateness of the level sophistication of this *Clinics* issue for the intended audience.
   - A. excellent
   - B. satisfactory
   - C. unsatisfactory

4. How relevant were the topics presented in this *Clinics* issue to the patients in your practice?
   - A. very relevant
   - B. slightly relevant
   - C. not at all relevant

5. Do you plan to make changes in your practice as a result of reading this issue?
   - A. yes, definitely
   - B. possibly
   - C. no

6. Rate the test for its coverage of the topics in this issue.
   A. excellent
   B. satisfactory
   C. unsatisfactory

7. Rate the appropriateness of the level of complexity of the test for the intended audience.
   A. excellent
   B. satisfactory
   C. unsatisfactory

8. Rate the format and functionality of the online test. Were the instructions clear and was the process intuitive?
   A. excellent
   B. satisfactory
   C. unsatisfactory

What did you like most about this *Clinics* issue?

What can we do to improve the *Clinics*?

Please list the topics that you would like presented in future issues.

Approximately how many hours did your spend reading this issue?